MIGRANTS, MINORITIES AND HEALTH

How has twentieth-century medicine dealt with immigrants and minorities? The contributors to *Migrants, Minorities and Health* have studied a number of different types of migrant and minority groups from different societies around the world in order to examine the complex relations between health issues and ideas of ethnicity and race.

The collection explores the historical origins and the contemporary power of stereotypical views – of immigrants as importers of disease, for instance, or of minorities as a source of infection in the host society. The authors show how ideas of ethnicity and race have shaped, and in turn have been influenced by, the construction of medical ideas.

Challenging our common assumptions about migrants, minorities and health, this collection brings together new perspectives from a variety of disciplines. It will make fascinating reading for social historians, medical historians and social policy makers.

Lara Marks is Lecturer in the History of Medicine at the Centre for the History of Science, Technology and Medicine at Imperial College, London. **Michael Worboys** is Head of Research at the School of Cultural Studies, Sheffield Hallam University.

STUDIES IN THE SOCIAL HISTORY OF MEDICINE

Edited by Jonathan Barry and Bernard Harris

In recent years, the social history of medicine has become recognised as a major field of historical enquiry. Aspects of health, disease and medical care now attract the attention not only of social historians but also of researchers in a broad spectrum of historical and social science disciplines. The Society for the Social History of Medicine, founded in 1969, is an interdisciplinary body, based in Great Britain but international in membership. It exists to forward a wide-ranging view of the history of medicine, concerned equally with biological aspects of normal life, experience of and attitudes to illness, medical thought and treatment, and systems of medical care. Although frequently bearing on current issues, this interpretation of the subject makes primary reference to historical context and contemporary priorities. The intention is not to promote a sub-specialism but to conduct research according to the standards and intelligibility required of history in general. The Society publishes a journal, *Social History of Medicine*, and holds at least three conferences a year. Its series, Studies in the Social History of Medicine, does not represent publication of its proceedings, but comprises volumes on selected themes, often arising out of conferences but subsequently developed by the editors.

Life, Death and the Elderly
Edited by Margaret Pelling and Richard M. Smith

Medicine and Charity Before the Welfare State
Edited by Jonathan Barry and Colin Jones

In the Name of the Child
Edited by Roger Cooter

Reassessing Foucault
Power, Medicine and the Body
Edited by Colin Jones and Roy Porter

Midwives, Society and Childbirth
Edited by Anne Marie Rafferty and Hilary Marland

MIGRANTS, MINORITIES AND HEALTH

Historical and contemporary studies

Edited by
Lara Marks and Michael Worboys

Routledge
Taylor & Francis Group
LONDON AND NEW YORK

First published 1997
by Routledge
2 Park Square, Milton Park,
Abingdon, Oxfordshire OX14 4RN

Simultaneously published in the USA and Canada
by Routledge
711 Third Avenue, New York, NY 10017

First issued in paperback 2014

Routledge is an imprint of the Taylor and Francis Group, an informa business

Typeset in Times by
J&L Composition Ltd, Filey, North Yorkshire

British Library Cataloguing in Publication Data
A catalogue record for this book is available from the British Library.

Library of Congress Cataloging in Publication Data
Migrants, minorities, and health: historical and contemporary studies/edited by Lara Marks and Michael Worboys.
(Studies in the social history of medicine)
1. Immigrants – Health and hygiene – Australia – History.
2. Minorities – Health and hygiene – Australia – History. I. Marks, Lara, 1963–. II. Worboys, Michael, 1948–. III. Series.
[DNLM: 1. Disease – ethnology. 2. Emigration and immigration – history. 3. Stereotyping. 4. Prejudice. 5. Minority groups. 6. Ethnic groups. WA 300 M636 1997]
RA553.M54 1997
306.4′61′08693 – dc20
DNLM/DLC
for Library of Congress 96–22911

ISBN 978-1-138-86818-2 (pbk)
ISBN 978-0-415-11213-0 (hbk)

Publisher's Note
The publisher has gone to great lengths to ensure the quality of this reprint but points out that some imperfections in the original may be apparent.

CONTENTS

ILLUSTRATIONS

FIGURES

TABLES

CONTRIBUTORS

Maggie Brady is a Research Fellow at the Australian Institute of Aboriginal and Torres Strait Islander Studies (AIATSIS) in Canberra. She is a social anthropologist who has worked on Aboriginal health and substance abuse over the last fifteen years. She has published several studies of alcohol use and a book on solvent abuse, *Heavy Metal: The Social Meaning of Petrol Sniffing in Australia*, 1992.

John Eade is a Principal Lecturer in Sociology and Social Policy at Roehampton Institute. He has written numerous articles and chapters on Bangladeshi settlers in Britain. He has published *The Politics of Community, The Bangladeshi Community in East London*, 1989, co-edited *Contesting the Sacred*, 1991, and edited *Living in a Global City*, 1997.

Liam Greenslade was Research Fellow at the Institute for Irish Studies, University of Liverpool. He has published on many aspects of the contemporary Irish experience of Britain.

Lindsey Harrison is a senior lecturer in the Department of Public Health and Nutrition at the University of Wollongong, New South Wales. She has published widely on the nutrition of the Aboriginal population of Australia.

Mark Harrison is Wellcome University Lecturer in the History of Medicine at Sheffield Hallam University, England. He is a historian of medicine who has published widely on medicine in British India, including a monograph, *Public Health in British India: Anglo-Indian Preventive Medicine, 1859–1914*, 1994. He is currently completing a monograph on the history of the Royal Army Medical Corps and editing collections on war and modern medicine.

Lisa Hilder has trained as an epidemiologist and an obstetrician. From 1991 to 1994 she was a lecturer in reproductive epidemiology at Queen Mary and Westfield College, London University. Since 1994 she has worked as a researcher for the Department of Health and the Office for Population Census Statistics, and as a clinician for Homerton Hospital and Whittington Hospital. Much of her research and publications have concentrated on infant mortality in East London and issues of ethnicity and health care. She has also worked on primary health care projects in South Asia.

Alan M. Kraut is Professor of History at The American University in Washington DC. He is a historian of immigration and the author of *The Huddled Masses: The Immigrant in American Society, 1880–1921*, 1982, co-author of *American Refugee Policy and European Jewry, 1933–1945*, 1987, and editor of *Crusaders and Compromisers*, 1983. His recent book, *Silent Travelers: Germs, Genes and the 'Immigrant Menace'* was published in 1994.

Stephen Kunitz is Professor in the Department of Community and Preventive Medicine at the University of Rochester School of Medicine, New York. He has published widely on historical and social epidemiology and in medical sociology, and has undertaken field research among Navajo Indians in the American Southwest. His recent books are *Disease and Social Diversity: The Impact of Europeans on the Health of Non-Europeans*, 1994, and with Jerrold E. Levy, *Drinking Careers: A Twenty-five Year Follow-up of Three Navajo Indian Populations*, 1994.

Moss Madden is Professor of Planning and Regional Science at the University of Liverpool. He graduated in engineering and planning and took his doctorate in regional science. His research interests include: extended input–output analysis, demographic economic modelling, migration analysis, issues of race and urban planning, and urban planning theory.

Desmond Manderson is Senior Lecturer in the Law School, Macquarie University, Sydney. He has published widely in the area of drug law and history, including *From Mr Sin to Mr Big: A History of Australian Drug Laws*, 1993. He is now working on the relationship of law, aesthetics and symbolism, and *Songs Without Music: Aesthetic Dimension of Law and Justice* is due to be published in 1997.

Lenore Manderson is a medical anthropologist and social historian, and is Professor of Tropical Health in the Australian Centre for International and Tropical Health and Nutrition at the University of Queensland. Her books include *Women, Politics and Change*, 1980, *New Motherhood*, 1993, with Mira Crouch, and *Sickness and the State: Health and Illness in Colonial Malaya, 1870–1940*, 1996. She has also edited *Australian Ways*, 1985, and *Shared Wealth and Symbols*, 1986. Her primary research and publications relate to the anthropology of infectious disease, and to gender, sexuality and women's health.

Lara Marks is a lecturer based in the Centre for the History of Science, Technology and Medicine, Imperial College, London. She has published numerous articles and two books on the history of ethnicity and health, and on maternal and child health. Her books include: *Model Mothers: Jewish Mothers and Maternity Provision in East London, 1870–1939*, 1994; and *Metropolitan Maternity: Maternal and Infant Welfare Services in Early Twentieth Century London*, 1996. Her current work concerns the international history of the oral contraceptive pill, 1950–80.

Richard Meckel is Associate Professor of American Civilization and History, Brown University, Providence, RI, USA. He is the author of *Save the Babies: American Public Health Reform and the Prevention of Infant Mortality, 1850–1929*, 1990, along with numerous articles on historical demography and the history of child welfare and health policies and programmes. Among his most recent publications are: 'Open-Air Schools and the Tuberculous Child in Early 20th-Century America', *Archives of Pediatrics and Adolescent Medicine*, 1996, and 'Health and Disease', *Encyclopedia of the United States in the Twentieth Century*, 1996.

David Nash is a Visiting Fellow at the Australian Institute of Aboriginal and Torres Strait Islander Studies (AIATSIS) in Canberra and in the Department of Linguistics, Australian National University, Canberra. He trained in linguistics and has studied Australian languages for the last fifteen years. His work has concentrated on the languages of central Northern Territory, where he has also studied Aboriginal relationships with the land.

Maggie Pearson is Regional Director of Research and Development, NHS Executive North West and was Professor of Health and Community Care at the University of Liverpool, and Director of the Health and Community Care Research Unit, funded by the North West Regional Health Authority. As a social scientist working in health and health service research, with a focus on service users' and carers' perspectives, her current research interests include: households' management of their health and the interfaces between local communities and different agencies in health and social care.

John Powles is Lecturer in Public Health Medicine at the University of Cambridge. Prior to this appointment he worked in Melbourne, Australia. He conducted an epidemiological study comparing siblings who stayed on the Greek island of Levkada with those who migrated to Melbourne and has published on ethnic differences in health in Australia. More recently he has been studying reasons for high mortality in East European countries, with specific studies in Bulgaria.

Michael Worboys is Head of Research in the School of Cultural Studies, Sheffield Hallam University, England. He is a historian of medicine who has published widely on the history of tropical medicine and colonial science. He is currently working on a monograph on the history of germ theories of disease in Britain in the period 1860–1900.

1

INTRODUCTION

Lara Marks and Michael Worboys

This volume brings together studies from a variety of disciplines on the changing historical and contemporary health status of migrant and minority groups in different societies across the world. The essays cover a wide geographical range, including Britain, the United States, Australia, India, Malaysia and Africa. The chapters present many different types of migrants and minorities, and explore how health issues around these groups have interacted with developing ideas of ethnicity and race. Contributors examine the historical origins and contemporary power of stereotypical views of immigrants as importers of disease, and of minorities as sources of infection to the host or majority society. Ideas of ethnicity and race are shown to have been shaped by, and to have themselves influenced, the construction of medical ideas and the development of health services.

Together, the chapters challenge many of our common assumptions about migrants, minorities and health and offer new perspectives and interpretations. A major theme of the book is the balance between immigrant and minority health disadvantage and advantage, as well as shifting relations between migrant and minority groups, and medical and health care institutions. In this context, many contributors demonstrate that migrants and minorities have not always adopted the dominant medical culture, rather they have been active in promoting their own views of healing and health. Overall the chapters in this volume explore the general question of health and migration, as well as the changing dynamics between, on the one hand, *health*, *disease* and *medicine* and, on the other, *immigrant*, *ethnic* and *racial* minority groups.

MIGRANTS AND MINORITIES

One of the problems in studying migrants and minorities is the multiple meanings attached to the terms 'migrant' and 'minority'. Much of the literature on migrants is about immigrants – people settling in a 'new' country – but as all immigrants begin as 'emigrants' – people who leave a country – so questions about why and how people leave, and the consequences for the 'old' society should not be lost sight of. There has also been discussion of 'internal immigration', with the movement of African Americans from the southern to northern states coterminous with European immigration in the same period. While many minority groups are of immigrant origin, there are many groups, for example American Indians, Aborigines and Maoris, who have become minorities in their own land. A volume just on minorities and health might have considered migrants as one type of minority.

Immigrants or minorities have often been assumed to constitute specific 'ethnic' or racial groupings, which are again terms frequently used without consistency or precise definition.[1] Ethnicity is usually defined in terms of particular historical and cultural traits common to a group, such as a 'homeland', a shared language, similar religious beliefs, and characteristic dietary and personal habits, as well as a shared heritage.[2] As an identity it is normally self-defined, though other social groups may or may not accept the designation.[3] Words such as 'immigrant' and 'ethnic minority' can convey the impression of a unified, homogeneous and distinct group; indeed, labelling someone, or a group of people, as black, African, Asian or Caucasian often implies shared racial characteristics. Yet, there has been and remain tremendous variations within such groups and it is worth remembering that, despite its seemingly great physical diversity, humankind is one species. Unable to find any genetic or other markers that consistently distinguished particular human 'types', biologists gave up the term 'race' in the 1930s. The term has none the less remained in popular use for defining the superficial physical differences between human populations, especially skin colour. It would be convenient if ethnicity was always used with regard to culture, and 'race' with regard to physical characteristics, but the changing historical meanings and uses of the words, together with their modern political sensitivity, make them some of the most problematic concepts in historical and sociological work.[4]

Issues of categorisation and identity are especially problematic for migrants. For instance, those migrating from the same place to another do not always maintain the same social and economic status or identity. Migrants are not always distinct from the host society into which they settle, either in class or in ethnic origin. How long after settlement do migrants remain immigrants, and when do immigrants become minorities? It would be logical if the term 'immigrant' was used only for those who actually migrated and settled, that is, first generation migrants. Their children, born in the 'new' society, are not strictly speaking immigrants and ought to be regarded as members of a minority or some other group. However, the passage of time does not seem to be an important factor in determining the designation and use of these terms. Many immigrant groups have kept strong links with their home country, often returning on a regular basis, so that they retain many of the attributes of a 'foreign' identity. Some groups have integrated quickly, not least because they may not have been that different from the majority population in the host society to begin with. Some of the consequences of these complexities are evident in epidemiological studies that try to link immigrant and health status, as Marmot has explained:

> Should immigrants to England from the Indian subcontinent be considered ethnically different from native-born English? What if they are born of English parents? Are migrants to England from South Africa ethnically different from the English? Only if non-white? What if their parents were Portuguese?[5]

Additional complexity comes from the fact that immigrants have other identities and social positions, based on social class, gender, age, occupation and other variables.[6]

Immigrant groups that possess, develop, or maintain a distinctive culture and identity in the 'new' society have usually been designated ethnic or racial minorities. How quickly or completely this occurs has been a contingent matter and has depended on a host of factors: the receptiveness of the society, the communal links within the particular group, and the ties they maintain with their place of origin.[7] However, the origins and early history of settlement are never the whole story, for migration changes circumstances not only for the immigrant, but also for the host society. In this context, immigrants and minorities should not be seen as passive victims of circumstances and the dominant culture. Their responses, individual and collective, need to be studied, not least to counter any tendency to see integration and assimilation as the inevitable long-term outcome of immigration. As the case of the Jews demonstrates, ethnic identity and institutions can be maintained over many centuries of migration across many continents. At the same time, many groups are minorities as a result of characteristics and shared experiences that have only the remotest link to immigration, for example religious minorities. Indeed, it is arguable that modern pluralist societies are essentially composed of a whole cluster of different minority groups: from the rich to the poor, different occupations, religious affiliations, sex and gender orientations, regional identities, health status, etc., etc. The important point is that minority–majority status has not been centrally about numbers, rather it has been about power.

The notion of an 'ethnic minority' is fraught with ambiguities and complexities. Historically and socially contingent forces shape the process of categorisation and the meanings attached to the term. For instance, ethnicity implies very different power dynamics when it is a self-asserted identity by the migrants or minorities themselves, rather than a label imposed by others. While migrants have used and still do use ethnicity as a positive means of survival and communal bonding in a strange and sometimes hostile environment, groups in the host society can use it to maintain distance and legitimate inequalities. Where imposed from outside, the labelling of a minority as 'ethnic' has often resulted in the formation of stereotypes that are an important factor in the creation and maintenance of ideas of difference and 'otherness'. Just as the meaning of ethnicity is dependent on those who are deploying the term, the context in which it is used changes over time. Moreover, where groups share certain qualities that are seen to be a hallmark of their group identity, the degree to which they adhere to these characteristics can vary. This can be seen, for instance, in the context of religious beliefs and practices. Many devout Hindus and Sikhs, for instance, might not eat meat, while others of their religion do. Some devout Muslim women might be secluded from the outside world, particularly from men, because of the tradition of purdah, yet other devout Muslim women experience no such restrictions and train to be doctors, teachers and politicians without compromising any religious observances.[8] The experienced and perceived differences of an ethnic group might actually increase over time, for history and contemporary experience show that minorities are not always assimilated into the majority society.

The difficulty of defining 'ethnicity' is made even more problematic where the concept is used to denote 'race'; indeed, the words are often used interchangeably. In such cases ethnicity is used to designate 'biological' aspects of a group's characteristics, most notably skin colour, without reference to their cultural traits. In the nineteenth century, theories of social evolution biology and culture developed in parallel, so that 'advanced civilisations' were peopled by the more highly evolved 'white' races.[9] The extent to which biological and cultural factors are now routinely understood as constitutive of each other has been noted in anthropological studies, as Chapman has observed:

> In many societies, social and linguistic recruitment are entirely congruent with biological recruitment. A child is born into the society of which it is to become a part, whose language and manners it will learn. In such a context, there is no pressing need to distinguish carefully between biological, social and linguistic classifications of people, since these disparate classifications will all yield the same results, and will indeed have a unitary appearance to those involved in them.[10]

The idea of some degree of common inheritance for groups was assumed even before modern genetics. The observation that 'like begets like', and that blood lines should run true, were commonplace in nineteenth-century medicine and popular culture. These ideas gained credence and new meanings in the context of eugenics in the early decades of this century, though biologists in Britain and North America abandoned race as a useful concept in the 1920s and 1930s. The impact of Nazi eugenic programmes and the Holocaust was to break the link between biology and race. Yet, the word 'race' still means something different to the term 'ethnic'. Ethnicity is regarded as a more acceptable, seemingly neutral term that does not usually come loaded with the baggage of past abuses and biological connotations.

The history of minorities is by association the history of the majority in any society, for those in power often define themselves and legitimate their position by designating the 'otherness' of subordinate groups.[11] For example, 'Englishness', the identity of the majority and more especially elite groups in England, has been defined by what it was not, as much as what it was or stood for. Its meaning and uses changed against the background of the developing social and ethnic structure of the English population.[12] This identity was also taken abroad, to the colonial Empire where it defined white superiority and legitimated imperial rule and the civilising mission. However, in settler colonies, such as Canada, South Africa and Australia, it has had to struggle against other identities and social groups for hegemony, including emergent nationalisms. In this century, changing political and social relations meant that Englishness became more about national destiny, as in the two World Wars, though since the 1950s issues of colour and ethnic origin have come more to the fore. The older idea of historical (European) races has all but disappeared, though a new English identity, defined against New Commonwealth immigrants and other ethnic minorities, has emerged implicitly through the immigration legislation of the 1960s and 1970s, and some of the ideas of the so-called 'New Right'.

The ascription of minority status and identity usually plays on one aspect of difference and subordinates others, and tends to define 'otherness' in terms of categorical differences. This can be seen in the importance of binary oppositions in this area: minority–majority, black–white, ethnic–mainstream, immigrant–resident. As Derrida has pointed out, these are never equivalent terms, they are created and sustained as hierarchies, where the devaluation of one term and group empowers the other.[13] Such oppositions, with their focus on primary differences, also tend to homogenise and play down variations within social groups, as well as alternative designations, as we have already noted with regard to ethnic identity being one among many that an individual or group may hold. Many of the categories used by colonialists were already current in indigenous societies, where notions of difference were equally important and powerful, as in the Indian caste system. Much of the inspiration for the modern discussion of difference has come from Said's writings on Orientialism, which has recently been extended to the history of colonial medicine.[14] Arnold has explored how 'doctors and surgeons helped to form and give seeming scientific precision to the abiding impression of India as a land of dirt and disease', with Indian people understood in the same terms.[15] In her work on disease in colonial Africa, Vaughan discussed how the basis of dominant ideas on the pathological character of Africans moved in the inter-war years from medicine and the physical body to anthropology and culture.[16]

Studies of difference, with respect to immigrants and minorities in Europe and North America, have yet to explore the diseased–healthy polarity, with the exception of Gilman.[17] This is surprising as there are, at least superficially, many parallels between the 'sick role' and minority status – marginality, otherness, subordination. Sociologists of health and illness have talked about the 'double jeopardy' of being both a minority and sick, and also about the identification of certain diseases with immigrants and minorities, to the extent that the 'other' becomes the disease.[18] Immigrants and minorities were identified with AIDS in the early 1980s, when it was often seen as the disease of the '4-Hs' – Haitians, homosexuals, haemophiliacs and heroine users.[19] However, the concept of the 'sick-role' has many problems, some of which parallel new ideas about the complexities and power of notions of difference. For example, the distinction between sickness and health has been blurred by the growth of medical surveillance and of chronic illness, whilst mental illness and conditions treated by long-term medical intervention (e.g. renal failure, deficiency diseases) point to the possible 'invisibility' and multiple identities of the sick.

MEDICINE AND HEALTH

Historians of medicine have had very little to say directly about migrants and minorities, hence we know very little about the changing health status of these groups, or about their attitudes to the dominant medical culture, or about how dominant medical practitioners viewed them.[20] Yet, migration was an important implicit theme in the Hippocratic tradition; see, for example, the importance of 'location' in 'Airs, Waters and Places', while the writings on 'Epidemics' stressed the need for a physician who was new to an area to understand the ways in which the local environment affected the health of the people and influenced the possibilities and outcome of intervention.[21] The assumption in this tradition was that individuals and communities normally 'suited' their locale, and that epidemics arose when this harmony was upset by environmental changes or human movements, such as through pilgrimages or forced migrations due to famine or other pestilence. The interactions between body and environment were understood to be quite precarious, so any move had to be carefully managed and a period of acclimatisation was seen as inevitable.[22] Those who migrated to foreign lands had to adjust, and the more foreign the new environment, the greater the adaptation required and the longer this might take. Settlers in North America spoke of a period of 'seasoning' on arrival, but expected an improvement as their bodies adjusted and New Lands were tamed. However, some environments were so hostile, for example the tropics, that European acclimatisation or environmental control seemed impossible.[23]

The impact of European settlement and imperialism on the host populations of the New World is now a topic of considerable historical interest and controversy. The work of McNeill and Crosby, and more recently Kiple, has concentrated on the consequences of the transfer of infectious diseases between the Old and New World.[24]

Most see the post-Columbian exchange as grossly unequal, as Europeans brought with them more virulent pathogens than those present in the Americas. The consequences were dramatic, as the new diseases are said to have been the primary cause of the collapse of the host populations. However, just how isolated New World populations had been before the arrival of Europeans is questionable, as is the extent to which depopulation can be explained simply by the importation of pathogens. Recent work has put more emphasis on the social, material and environmental changes wrought by European settlement and extension, not least in the ways these destroyed existing human ecologies, created the conditions for infectious diseases to flourish and directly destroyed indigenous peoples.[25]

The notion that the body was influenced by its environment was commonplace in medicine and wider Western culture in the eighteenth and nineteenth centuries. This was expressed in the dominant medical model, which Rosenberg has characterised as one where the body was seen to be in 'a system of dynamic interactions with its environment', and where 'Health and disease resulted from the cumulative interactions between constitutional endowment and environmental circumstances'.[26] It followed that a 'change of air' or travel to a different area were ways to improve health, and doctors tried to match a person's constitution and illness with potential healing environments.[27] As well as being used in clinical medicine, this model informed public health, as people in the same place would be expected to experience broadly similar 'influences' on their bodies – positive and negative. Indeed, in the middle quarters of the nineteenth century, public health reform concentrated on environmental improvements, following the sanitarian view that clean water, efficient waste removal, pure air, clean streets and better housing would improve the public's health. In many countries, quarantines, which had previously been used to try to keep out contaminated goods and people, and hence diseases, were abandoned. Thus, in the 1840s, the association of the Irish with typhus in Britain and cholera in the US was more concerned with the conditions in which they lived and their behaviour producing disease, than about immigrants importing or spreading infection.[28]

From the 1880s, and especially after 1900, however, the environmentalist approach in public health was overtaken by a new preventive medicine that focused on the control of specific diseases and directly improving the health of individuals.[29] Informed by bacteriology, eugenics and ideas about the residuum, a new emphasis was now placed upon individual bodies as the sources and spreaders of infection. Now oriented towards specific diseases, public health officials adopted different strategies for different infections; for example, preventive inoculation for smallpox, isolation for measles, public education for tuberculosis. Medical surveillance and public health propaganda focused on the isolation of those with acute infections and halting the transmission of germs, which led some countries to reintroduce quarantine measures. There was no longer discussion of acclimatisation as such; what mattered now was exposure to germs and the conditions in which people would become open to infection – bad housing, unhygienic behaviour and socio-economic status.[30]

A major consequence of this change was that medical and public anxieties became focused on 'risk populations', and migrants were construed as especially dangerous. Indeed, modern anxieties about immigrants and health in Europe and North America date from the end of the nineteenth century, and in the United States such fears influenced public health after 1880. Equally, the link between immigrants and disease helped shape more restrictive immigration legislation, and medical officials were on the front line of controls at Ellis Island and other stations. Markel's study of cholera in New York in 1892 shows the new concern with the immigrant as the carrier of the germ as against older beliefs of immigrants as producers of insanitary and disease-making conditions.[31] However, Rogers' work on the polio epidemic in Eastern states after 1916 has shown the persistence of older ideas of immigrant and minority communities as sources of infection to the majority community.[32] Kraut's book on immigration to the United States discusses the ways in which ethnic groups were blamed for epidemic and other diseases.[33] That perceptions of immigrants as 'diseased' and 'dirty' both created and confirmed the fears of the host population, and supported wider cultural stereotypes and stigmas, was evident during the plague outbreak in San Francisco in 1900.[34]

After 1900, the new preventive medicine extended to the promotion of health, with campaigns on personal hygiene, infant welfare and physical deterioration. These were justified, not only for their immediate impact on the public's health, but also in their contribution to the future of the race. Haller and Kevles have stressed the importance of eugenics, especially fears about the hereditary worth of immigrants from southern and eastern Europe in the Eastern states and the 'yellow peril' in California.[35] Eugenists worried not only about the social costs of supporting inferior immigrant 'stock', but also about the consequences of miscegenation and its impact on national and racial efficiency.

One area where 'migrant' health became a major problem was in the tropical colonies of the imperial powers. Curtin's study of European health in the tropics, gloomily titled *Death By Migration*, does in fact show how the health prospects of colonial adventurers, soldiers, administrators and traders, who could be regarded as both migrants and minority – had improved markedly during the nineteenth century.[36] None the less, imperial rivalries and ambitions after 1880 required that the image of the tropics as the White Man's Grave should be cleared, so major investments were made in new medical institutions, research and sanitary improvements.[37] The hope was that the transfer of medical technologies would first protect the agents of the Empire and then, albeit slowly, be diffused to the indigenous population as part of the civilising mission.[38] However, colonial trade and economic imperialism created health problems at the periphery, notably due to urbanisation, the use of migrant labour in mines and plantations, and changes in land use.[39] These problems were addressed by colonial medical services, especially where economic interests or expatriate health was threatened. Control programmes rarely matched the scale of the problem, while the sanitary and health care infrastructure created was minimal. By the 1930s, there was growing evidence that the health of colonial peoples was poor, and possibly deteriorating.[40] Ironically, some of the disease problems that developed in the tropical colonies at this time came back to haunt the former imperial powers, like Britain, in the post-independence period, when New Commonwealth immigrants reintroduced diseases into the country, like tuberculosis, and suffered from deficiency and other diseases associated with poverty.

Since the first wave of post-Second World War immigrants to Europe and North America, there has been a common assumption that immigrants are always at a health disadvantage.[41] There are clear reasons why this should be the case. Many immigrants are economic migrants or political refugees who were marginal and had compromised health in their 'home' country. Migrants are also said to experience physical and psychological dislocation, and have to integrate with a new, perhaps very different, host society. In new countries immigrants mostly start at the bottom, in badly paid and insecure jobs, in poor housing and, if not supported by their fellow immigrants, may suffer isolation and loneliness. Their lot is compounded by the problem of marginality arising from communication difficulties, clashes of values and the pains of discrimination. As well as having a direct impact on physical and mental health, their marginality and difference also put immigrants and minorities at a disadvantage when seeking access to the medical and health care systems of the new country. How many of these features are unique to immigrants and minorities is a moot point. Many would apply with equal force to the poor and socially marginal in general; but then immigrants and minorities tend to be found in those socio-economic groups anyway.

There are many studies that question the notion that immigrants and minorities were or are uniformly unhealthy and always experience health 'disadvantage'.[42] In many cases immigrants can be shown to have enjoyed better health than the average in the host population.[43] Such assertions need careful interpretation, for immigrant populations may have a different age structure, being skewed towards youth, and in addition their health status will be affected by their socio-economic positions. Also, immigrants tend to be a 'select' group, they may have been amongst the more socially mobile and healthier citizens of their home country. The obvious point is that it is impossible to generalise and it is in this context that historical and comparative studies are so useful.

The question of disadvantage and advantage is bound up with questions of difference. Difference is an ascribed category as well as an experienced reality. In the case of migrants and minorities a perennial question, more commonly asked than with other social groups, is about the role of heredity in health.[44] In this context, there is a growing body of work on specific diseases that can be linked to specific genetic traits, if not yet to genes. However, even where people have similar genetic dispositions, the occurrence of disease cannot be attributed merely to biological inheritance. Modern medical researchers, with views in many ways analogous to those current a century ago, increasingly acknowledge that biological factors cannot be disentangled from wider environmental influences such as diet, lifestyle, behaviour, living conditions and socio-economic status. In some cases these external factors might outweigh the inherited biological traits, while in others they might exaggerate them. Just as it is difficult to justify the existence of completely discrete races, so it is problematic to dichotomise disease in terms of environment versus heredity. Anthropologists have been particularly sensitive to the interplay of biological and cultural determinants of disease, as Macbeth has suggested:

> The aim of finding some way to disentangle the multifaceted causes adequately can probably never be achieved when 'culture' itself has so many facets that cannot be reduced to the numerical data needed for epidemiological analysis. Furthermore, when the geographic and ethnic origin of those lumped together by external observers is as diverse as in 'Asians' or 'Afro-Caribbeans', not only would daily activities be quite variable, but the gene frequencies would also be highly heterogeneous.[45]

This is not to deny the reality of genetic diseases, for example sickle cell anaemia can cause suffering and death, but in countries where malaria is endemic, 'sickle-shaped' red blood cells can actually protect against malaria.

Assumptions of difference between individuals and groups in medicine are shaped in large part by professional interests, the context in which knowledge has been framed and published and wider cultural influences. It might be easier to show the social construction of medical knowledge in historical studies, but there are examples where Eurocentrism has directly shaped contemporary medical knowledge. Recent medical debates over the cause of lactose intolerance were initially based on work with northern European adults whose normal level of lactose rose after childhood.[46] Subsequent studies showed much lower levels of lactose among healthy adults from certain ethnic groups, who were regarded as abnormal and suffering from 'lactase deficiency'. This was not just a matter of definition – a disease entity had been created and 'lactase deficiency' was treated as a manifestation of malnutrition and chronic gastrointestinal disease. However, further research, in other continents and with a greater range of population groups, showed that it was the northern Europeans who were if anything 'abnormal'. There was in fact a range of 'normal' lactose levels across the world, with Europeans at one end. It took over thirty years for medical practitioners, biochemists, nutritionists and geneticists to appreciate that high and low levels of lactose in adults represent a normal variability. Moreover, the extent to which this variability is attributable to heredity or environment may be unanswerable.

MIGRANTS, MINORITIES AND HEALTH

This volume could have been ordered in a number of different ways, for each chapter addresses the main themes of the book in a variety of ways: i.e. health and migration, minority status and difference, racial and cultural determinants of health, and the medical beliefs and practices of minority and majority cultures. We have chosen to group the chapters under the broad categories of: (1) stereotypes and disease, (2) race and health, (3) ethnic disadvantage, (4) ethnic advantage and (5) the cultural variability in meaning of health.

Chapters 2 and 3 by Desmond Manderson and Lenore Manderson respectively, illustrate the tendency to designate migrants and minorities as 'other', and show how health has been central to the creation of powerful stereotypes. Desmond Manderson's discussion of Chinese immigrants in Australia highlights the complex nature of the fear immigrants evoked. He shows how white Australians viewed Chinese immigrants as sickly and sickening and potential sources of disease, but goes on to argue that this stemmed as much from their aesthetic, almost visceral, feelings of revulsion to 'other' races, as from fears of contagion. Drawing on Mary Douglas's notion of pollution as 'matter out of place', he suggests that the Chinese in Australia, like most other ethnic minorities, were not simply 'people out of place', who violated and threatened dominant social and cultural norms; they were, he contends, experienced to be sensually different. Desmond Manderson highlights the continual references made by health officers to sickening odours and the different facial and bodily form of the Chinese. Their inferiority was also assessed against the dominant notions of beauty and health. Hence, Chinese immigrants represented a moral and physical threat to white Australia, allowing the language of health to give racist beliefs greater authority.

The idea that Chinese immigrants could be seen as something unclean and as potential carriers of disease is also pursued by Lenore Manderson in her chapter on prostitution and medical surveillance in colonial Malaya. Discussing the Chinese alongside other migrant prostitutes of different nationalities, Lenore Manderson highlights the importance of ethnicity and race in shaping medical and state policies towards prostitutes. She shows that prostitutes of different ethnic origins were treated differently by the colonial administration and medical services. Chinese prostitutes were seen to be the most difficult group to control and were considered to be the greatest threat to the public health of the colony. They were regarded as dangerous, not only because they avoided state and medical regulation, but because they served clients from a variety of races and classes. This contrasted with Japanese prostitutes who tended to serve an elite clientele and conformed with hygiene and colonial regulation. Also less threatening were Tamil, Malay and Thai prostitutes, who largely worked within their own community and whom, when they partnered with Europeans, complied with their hygienic practices. Prostitution, because of the sexual taboos it raises, is a particularly interesting area for understanding the categorisation of migrants and minorities. What was at stake in Malaya was the degree to which immigrant prostitutes, and by extension the communities from which they came, threatened European 'norms' and sensibilities as well as European health. On the other hand, Lenore Manderson's chapter highlights the importance of understanding the immigrant experience on a number of different levels. She contends that Chinese prostitutes experienced triple marginality and subordination: as colonial subjects they were a minority in terms of social, economic and political power; as women and Chinese they were numerically a minority in terms of their sex and race; and as prostitutes they were vulnerable and stigmatised as the active transmitters of dangerous diseases.

The changing nature of racial stereotypes is the central theme of Richard Meckel's chapter on the infant welfare movement in the United States. In the north-eastern states and urban areas, the campaigns to reduce infant mortality were similar to those in Europe, concentrating on environmental and behavioural factors. Both campaigns expressed concerns about race, but in the United States this was largely influenced by anxieties about the impact of immigrants from eastern and southern Europe as well as the eugenic deterioration of the health of the native population. In the southern states there were no similar concerns or campaigns to diminish infant mortality amongst Negroes. Instead, infant mortality was subsumed in larger concerns about the deteriorating health of Negroes as a racial group. Their declining health was explained by southern physicians largely in terms of degeneration, racial inferiority and the abolition of slavery, which they claimed had been a boon to Negro health. From the 1900s this view was challenged by black physicians and anthropologists like Franz Boas, who attributed high Negro morbidity and mortality (infants were still not separated for special attention) to environmental and social factors. When a special concern about Negro infant health eventually emerged in the 1920s, this was framed in the same terms as the earlier northern campaign. However, racial differences remained a key explanatory variable, though Meckel notes that in the interwar years race was increasingly associated with culture rather than with biology. None the less, even in this context

Negro inferiority continued to be seen as a cause rather than as a consequence of poor health.

The question of race is also discussed by Harrison and Worboys in Chapter 5 in relation to British medical debates on the reasons for the spread of tuberculosis in Africa and India. Historical epidemiology of the disease is not the focus of the chapter, rather they seek to explain the changing interpretations of the rising incidence and mortality from the disease. Their argument is that what was termed 'tropical' or 'primitive' tuberculosis was framed by metropolitan experts not colonial medical officers. These experts maintained that tuberculosis was a 'disease of civilisation', and that its spread and rise in any country was primarily due to the social and environmental changes, in this case how European imperialism had brought urbanisation and industrialisation to Africa and India. In Africa the disease was understood to constitute a 'virgin soil' epidemic, where African vulnerability was due to a lack of prior exposure to the disease and hence an absence of immunity. The extent to which African vulnerability was inherited and racial, as opposed to acquired and environmental, was hotly disputed throughout the period. The majority view of tuberculosis experts in Britain and in other imperial powers linked 'virgin soil' status to the absence of acquired immunity; India was seen as an important test case, for it was an area where the disease had been present for many decades and had spread only because of the migration of populations to towns, and to industrial employment. However, while tuberculosis experts stressed environmental factors, their references to 'primitive tuberculosis' and the analogies they drew between children and 'tribal Africans' seemed to confirm ideas of racial inferiority and backwardness.

Racial assumptions in health policy have both explained inequalities and often negated the possibility of even attempting to change the status quo. This is most clearly shown in Chapter 6 in Lindsey Harrison's examination of government policy on the health of Aborigines in the Northern Territory of Australia. Until the Second World War, Aborigines were assumed to be a group that would probably become extinct in the face of civilisation, either by assimilation or race mixing. Their geographical and social marginality meant that few health services were provided for this group. However, with the reversal of such assumptions and the increasing visibility of the Aboriginal population within Australian society, protective and preventive measures were introduced by the government. The ultimate aim of this policy was to promote the greater integration and assimilation of Aborigines. Nutritional programmes became an essential component in countering Aboriginal disadvantage, both as a means of improving physical health as well as inculcating the norms of the dominant society. Rather than promoting integration and self-sufficiency, such measures created dependence. Feeding programmes were based on racial stereotypes and assumed physiological differences that have since been shown to be inaccurate. The overall benefits of the scheme are now seen to be problematic, not least because the policy was formulated and executed without consultation with the Aboriginal communities.

The growing visibility of Aborigines and their health problems in Australia contrasts with the virtual invisibility of the health problems of second generation Irish immigrants in Britain. In Chapter 7, Greenslade, Madden and Pearson note the contrast between the neglect in health policy of first and second generation Irish in Britain, compared to the attention recently given to other immigrant groups in Britain, particularly those who came from the New Commonwealth in the 1950s. Recent research has shown the Irish to have some of the poorest indicators of health and mortality in England and Wales. The lack of attention paid by health professionals and others to the Irish is said by Greenslade *et al.* to be largely because they are white and therefore seen as no different from the majority population, though this does not mean they escape racist ridicule. Greenslade *et al.* also link the poor health of Irish immigrants to the contradictions they face in their daily life, of being seen as somehow different and yet not so different from the host society. They argue that this has directly influenced their physical and psychological health, as well as limiting the access they enjoy to health services.

While the Irish in Britain highlight features of migrant disadvantage, Marks and Hilder show in Chapter 8 some of the ways in which ethnic minorities can have health advantage, the fourth theme of the book. They compare the rates of infant mortality found in host populations with the remarkably low rates found in two ethnic minority groups at different moments in time. In looking at Jewish East European immigrants at the turn of the century and Bengali immigrants today, they are able to provide a novel historical comparison of 'then and now' in the same geographical area. They highlight the importance of selection and cultural factors, as well as ethnic behavioural patterns, in determining advantage in infant health. Marks and Hilder also show the role of specific ethnic values and practices, and the importance of communal and familial support in the survival of infants. Their exploration of the transition from immigrant to settled status also reveals how the interplay between ethnicity and patterns of health changes over time.

Chapter 9 by John Powles also shows how Greek immigrants in Australia can have a better health status than the host population and, indeed, the communities they left behind in Greece. In an argument reminiscent of Thomas McKeown's analysis of overall mortality decline since 1800, Powles discusses five factors that might explain Greek immigrant advantage: data bias, genetics, selection, low exposure to risk factors, and high exposure to beneficial factors. Finding the negative or inconclusive evidence for the first four, he then explores in detail what 'high exposure to beneficial factors' Greeks have enjoyed. He argues that cultural factors, especially dietary and social networks, best explain the advantage of Greek immigrants. However, he goes beyond this to speculate that ethnic behavioural and dietary patterns, which might be beneficial to health, could also influence the health of the majority population, through the pressures for multiculturalism and growing diversity they offer to Australian diets.

The final theme of the book, concerning cultural struggles over meanings of health, is explored in Kraut's chapter (Chapter 10) on Italian immigrants to the United States. The chapter details the negotiation over definitions of health and hygiene between the public health agencies and Italian immigrants. After 1900, native-born Americans regarded Italians, as they did other immigrant populations, as a source of disease. Hence, alongside calls for immigration control, public health officials sought the compliance of immigrants with their programmes and with this the beliefs and practices of modern medicine. This provoked conflicts between Italians, who had their own perceptions of the causes of disease, and those of the government and health officials. Much of this tension went beyond the familiar disparity between lay and expert opinion, as Italian beliefs and practices were bound up with ethnic identity and were reinforced by migration back and forth to southern Italy.

Chapter 11 by John Eade examines health beliefs among Bengali immigrants in Britain. He argues that despite the growing acceptance of multiculturalism and pluralism amongst health care planners and professionals, 'expert' perceptions remain dominant. Eade explores this both with regard to orthodox Western medicine as well as the health care offered by established Islamic figures. While he recognises that each system is diverse, he contends that both are authority systems and operate with little reference to lay beliefs. Eade suggests that the alienation that Bengali immigrants' experience from orthodox medicine and organised health care is but one cause of the gap that has developed between lay and expert ideas in modern societies.

Brady, Kunitz and Nash also illustrate, in Chapter 12, the ways in which the authority of Western models of medicine and health care can be resisted by minorities. Focusing on Western and Aboriginal conceptions of health in Australia, they challenge those who assume a division between Western and non-orthodox views of health, particularly between scientific reductionism and the holism of ethnic or alternative medicine. They are interested in how and why this model of polar opposite systems arose and they suggest the polarity was forged in political struggles over Aboriginal health care policy, being ideologically useful to all sides. However, it is argued that this has led to a one-dimensional characterisation of both systems that has obscured the diversity within both systems and impoverished debates on health care for minorities.

As a whole, the chapters collected in this volume show the variability of the experiences that migrants and minorities have had of medicine and of health across space and time. Yet they also show that much of that experience can be understood around common themes and point to the potential for comparative study, not least in how medical views of the body and disease have been used to create and sustain notions of ethnic and racial difference.

NOTES

We would like to thank David Cantor, Mark Harrison, Clare Harvey and David Mayall for their assistance with this introduction.

1 J.L. Donovan, 'Ethnicity and Health: A Research Review', *Social Science Medicine*, 1984, 19/7, pp. 663; J.K. Cruikshank and D.G. Beevers, eds, *Ethnic Factors in Health and Disease*, London, 1989, p. 5.

2 The word 'ethnicity' is a relatively modern one that became popular amongst social scientists in the early 1960s. First coined in its modern sense in 1950, the term can be traced back to Ancient Greece where the word 'ethnos' was used to denote a group of people with shared characteristics. M. Chapman, ed., *Social and Biological Aspects of Ethnicity*, Oxford, 1993, pp. 15–16. On nineteenth-century ethnology see: G. Stocking, *Race, Culture and Evolution*, Chicago, 1982.

3 B.B. Ringer and E.R. Lawless, *Race, Ethnicity and Society*, London, 1989. Ringer and Lawless use the terms 'we-ness' and 'they-ness' to develop the distinctions between a self-defined, experienced identity

and one that is ascribed or imposed. Also see: M. O'Donnell, *Race and Ethnicity*, London, 1991.
4 H. Macbeth, 'Ethnicity and Biology', in Chapman, *Aspects of Ethnicity*, pp. 62–3; N. Stepan, *The Idea of Race in History, 1800–1960*, London, 1984.
5 M.G. Marmot, 'General Approaches to Migrant Studies: The Relation between Disease and Social Class and Ethnic Origin', in Cruikshank, *Ethnic Factors*, pp. 12–13.
6 K. Blakemore and M. Boneham, *Age, Race and Ethnicity*, Buckingham, 1993.
7 Marmot, 'General Approaches', p. 13.
8 Cruickshank, *Ethnic Factors*, p. 5.
9 P.J. Bowler, *Theories of Human Evolution: A Century of Debate, 1844–1944*, London, 1987.
10 Chapman, *Aspects of Ethnicity*, p. 21.
11 L. Colley, 'Britishness and Otherness: An Argument', *Journal of British Studies*, 1992, 31/4, pp. 309–30.
12 R. Colls and P. Dodd, eds, *Englishness: Politics and Culture, 1880–1920*, London, 1986.
13 J. Derrida, 'Racism's Last Word', in H.L. Gates, ed., '*Race*': *Writing and Difference*, Oxford, 1988, pp. 328–38 and 354–69.
14 E. Said, *Orientalism*, London, 1985; idem, *Culture and Imperialism*, London, 1993.
15 D. Arnold, *Colonizing the Body: State Medicine and Epidemic Disease in Nineteenth Century India*, Berkeley, 1993.
16 M. Vaughan, *Curing their Ills: Colonial Power and African Illness*, Oxford, 1991.
17 S. Gilman, *Difference and Pathology: Stereotypes of Sexuality, Race and Madness*, Ithaca, NY, 1985; idem, *Health and Illness: Images of Difference*, London, 1995.
18 W.I.U. Ahmad, *Race and Health*, Buckingham, 1993.
19 A.M. Brandt, *No Magic Bullet: A Social History of Venereal Disease in the United States*, Oxford, 2nd edn, 1987; E. Fee and D. Fox, eds, *AIDS: the Burdens of History*, Berkeley, 1988; R. Shilts, *And the Band Played On*, New York, 1987.
20 W. Anderson, 'Disease, Race and Empire', *Bulletin of the History of Medicine*, 1996, 70/1, pp. 62–7.
21 G. Miller, '"Airs, Waters and Places" in History', *Journal of the History of Medicine*, 1962, 17, pp. 129–40.
22 D. Livingstone, 'Human Acclimatisation: Perspectives on a Contested Field of Inquiry in Science, Medicine and Geography', *History of Science*, 1987, 25, pp. 359–94.
23 M. Harrison, '"The Tender Frame of Man": Disease, Climate and Racial Difference in India and the West Indies, 1760–1890', *Bulletin of the History of Medicine*, 1996, 70, pp. 68–93.
24 A.W. Crosby, *Ecological Imperialism: The Biological Expansion of Europe, 900–1900*, Cambridge, 1986; idem, *The Columbian Exchange: Biological and Cultural Consequences of 1492*, Westport, Conn., 1972; K. Kiple, *The Cambridge History of Human Disease*, Cambridge, 1992.

25 S. Kunitz, *Disease and Social Diversity: The Impact of Europeans on the Health of Non-Europeans*, New York, 1994.

26 C.E. Rosenberg, *Explaining Epidemics and Other Essays in the History of Medicine*, Cambridge, 1992, p. 12.

27 J. Pemble, 'The Victorians Practised Alternative Medicine', *The Listener*, 22 March 1984, pp. 14–15, and 'When a Doctor was Identified with God', *The Listener*, 29 March 1984, pp. 10–11; J.M. Powell, 'Medical Promotion and the Consumptive Immigrant to Australia', *Geographical Review*, 1973, 63, p. 449; A.J. Proust, 'Tuberculosis in Australia: Part 1', in A.J. Proust, ed., *History of Tuberculosis in Australia, New Zealand and Papua New Guinea*, Canberra, 1991, pp. 5–17.

28 A. Kraut, *Silent Travelers: Germs, Genes and the 'Immigrant Menace'*, Baltimore, MD, 1994, pp. 31–49.

29 E. Fee and D. Porter, 'Public Health, Preventive Medicine and Professionalisation: England and America in the Nineteenth Century', in A. Wear, ed., *Medicine in Society*, Cambridge, 1992, pp. 249–76.

30 G. Rosen, *A History of Public Health*, New York, 1958.

31 H. Markel, ' "Knocking out the Cholera": Cholera, Class and Quarantines in New York City, 1892', *Bulletin of the History of Medicine*, 1995, 69, pp. 458–69.

32 N. Roger, *Dirt and Disease: Polio Before FDR*, New Brunswick, NJ, 1992.

33 Kraut, *Silent Travelers*, passim.

34 G.B. Risse, 'The Politics of Fear: Bubonic Plague in San Francisco, California, 1900', in L. Bryder and D. Dow, eds, *New Countries and Old Medicine*, Auckland, 1995, pp. 1–20.

35 J.S. Haller, *Outcasts From Evolution: Scientific Attitudes to Racial Inferiority, 1859–1900*, Urbana, 1975; D. Kevles, *In the Name of Eugenics: Genetics and the Uses of Human Heredity*, New York, 1985.

36 P.D. Curtin, *Death By Migration: Europe's Encounter with the Tropical World in the Nineteenth Century*, Cambridge, 1989.

37 R. MacLeod and M. Lewis, eds, *Disease, Medicine and Empire*, London, 1988; M. Harrison, *Public Health in British India: Anglo Indian Preventive Medicine, 1859–1914*, Cambridge, 1994.

38 Arnold, *Colonising the Body*.

39 R. Packard, *White Plague, Black Labor*, Los Angeles, 1989; S. Hewa, *Colonialism, Tropical Disease and Imperial Medicine: Rockefeller Philanthropy in Sri Lanka*, Lanham, MD, 1995.

40 M. Worboys, 'The Discovery of Colonial Malnutrition', in D. Arnold, ed., *Imperial Medicine and Indigenous Societies*, Manchester, 1988, pp. 208–25.

41 R. Balajaran and V. Soni, *Ethnicity and Health: A Guide for the NHS*, London, 1993.

42 R. Balajaran and V.S. Raleigh, 'A Health Profile of Britain's Ethnic Minorities', in A.H. Bittles and D.F. Roberts, eds, *Minority Populations: Genetics, Demography and Health*, London, 1992, pp. 119–42.

43 Kraut, *Silent Travelers*, pp. 105–35.

44 Roberts, *Minority Populations*, passim.
45 Macbeth, 'Ethnicity and Human Biology', p. 65.
46 R.C. Johnson, R.E. Cole and F.M. Ahern, 'Genetic Interpretation of Racial/Ethnic Differences in Lactose Absorption and Tolerance: A Review', *Human Biology*, 1981, 53/1, pp. 1–13.

2

'DISEASE, DEFILEMENT, DEPRAVITY': TOWARDS AN AESTHETIC ANALYSIS OF HEALTH

The case of the Chinese in nineteenth-century Australia

Desmond Manderson

HEALTH AND IMMIGRATION: TERMS OF ENDEARMENT, TERMS OF ESTRANGEMENT?

Keep young and beautiful, it's your dooty to be bootiful
Keep young and beautiful, if you want to be loved.

So crooned Eddie Cantor to a Roman bath-house full of women. Although we may be sceptical about whether the syllogism is or was as straightforward as Hollywood chose to present it in the 1930s, from the ancient world to the present, health has been a powerful rhetorical source in the battle to legitimate social values and beauty its primary aesthetic symbol.[1] Health, as René Descartes put it, is the 'chief among goods' and more, the *sine qua non* of effective individual action. But health is not simply a fact or an idea. It is also a compound of images, ranging from ideals of beauty about the human body, to the ugly and unsettling images that help construct our approach to sickness and death. We need look no further than the ways in which contemporary norms of female beauty encourage in women epidemics of sickness and debilitating unhealthiness to recognise that the connection of health to beauty and sickness to ugliness is neither unproblematic nor unrelated to broader social and political agendas.[2] When I write of 'beauty' then, as when I write of 'health', I mean a socially constructed and manipulable phenomenon and not a realist account that might claim objective truth for a particular 'natural' meaning.[3]

In the bath-house, the serried ranks of women to whom Cantor addressed his advice were all, of course, virtually identical – the ideal of beauty they represented allowed little margin for difference. Beauty, health and normality have always been closely connected in that way. Orthodox beauty often exhibits a certain sameness. Similarly health is defined as a question of normal functioning. Each idea demands conformity. The origins of this connection date back at least as far as ancient Greece, when the Platonic notion of 'ideal form' applied to physiology as much as to ethics, metaphysics and the natural sciences. From that time to this, our notion of beauty has been formed around a calculus of proportion and homogeneity. In the eighteenth century, the 'science' of physiognomy sought to categorise and define a vast array of deviations from a norm, and to give those deviations moral significance. Later still, phrenologists believed that the slightest 'imperfections' of the skull corresponded to imperfections of the mind. Both health and beauty, then, are here understood in terms of a single ideal of the appearance of the 'normal' human being.[4]

We do not have to travel back in time much further than the talkies to discover a great interest in eugenics and public health, in Australia and in Britain, that likewise presented an image of beauty and a promise of health based on conformity to a norm. The federation of the colonies in 1901 had raised for many people the question of what it meant to be 'Australian'; the health and virility of the Australian man formed an important part of that developing self-image. Australia was a bush nation, a land of pioneers, tanned and strong, relying on their physicality to tame the barren earth. Thus, Dr John Cumpston, the first Commonwealth Director-General of Health, described himself as one 'who dream[s] of leading this young nation of ours to a paradise of physical perfection'.[5]

This paradise of physical perfection was, for Dr Cumpston among many others, to be constructed using every means available, from legislation to genetic engineering. Another leading health bureaucrat of the day looked forward to the moment when 'serious acceptance of a doctrine of national physical morality will cause preventable disease to be regarded as somebody's crime'. The *Sydney Morning Herald* spoke of genetic selection and selective breeding as if Australians were like their sheep.[6] Whether it was to be accomplished through force of law or magic of science, we may note again the strength of an ideal of health and beauty understood in terms of conformity to a specific type.

The 'type' in question was, of course, racial. Eugenics, in Australia as elsewhere, expressed an ideal of beauty founded on racial purity. Consequently, the aesthetic of conformity was confronted at that time in history by the experience of immigration, and thus of visible difference. Racist attitudes to migrants stem from diverse cultural, emotional and economic sources – fear of change, employment insecurity and the disturbance of a community's complacent approach towards its own traditions. Such factors all play their part in generating an often intense and violent resentment. But whatever its causes, the feeling of hostility also involves an aesthetic element in which, especially in otherwise homogeneous societies, the different look and sound of newcomers seems to offend accepted parameters of beauty. Sometimes with a conscious eye towards the manipulation of our emotions, and sometimes as an instinctive and unquestioned reaction, xenophobia uses aesthetic arguments as well as economic and social ones: it appeals to a certain image of beauty and ugliness. Thus, New South Wales Premier Sir Henry Parkes, in his second reading speech on the Chinese Restriction Bill 1888, urged members:

> to preserve to ourselves and our children, unaltered and unspotted, the rights and privileges which we have received from our forefathers . . . to preserve the soil of Australia that we may plant upon it the nucleus of a future nation stamped with a pure British type . . . [7]

Like the *Bulletin* – whose masthead declared 'Australia for the White Man' – which expressed its horror at the danger of a 'piebald race', Parkes' language is not reasoned, and while his rhetoric is emotional, we are dealing with a specific use of emotion in which the image of purity bears the brunt of the rhetorical appeal. It is no coincidence that one says 'pure white' but never pure black or yellow. Beauty was a matter of remaining 'unspotted' and 'pure' – and therefore 'white' – and it was that beauty that was to be preserved.

There is nothing inevitable or natural about that understanding of beauty, predominant as it was and may still be. The point is not to approve a particular contingent norm of beauty, but rather to explore its explanatory force in the construction and legitimation of social values; to see how much a social conflict is, amongst other things, a conflict over aesthetic visions. How do the aesthetics of health – cleanliness and purity on the one hand – dirt, pollution and squalor on the other – interact with migrants, who are often already vulnerable to an aesthetic valuation based on their visible difference? How has 'health' been used as a weapon to generate hostility to migrant communities, and to what extent can this weapon be understood as aesthetic in character?

Using materials related to the experience of the Chinese in Australia in the late nineteenth century, I am proposing, therefore, an exploration of ways in which the rhetoric of health has been used in the treatment of migrant communities, the prism of aesthetics serving as an innovative explanatory tool. The inter-relationship of these variables is complex. For the purposes of this chapter, I use the metaphor of a triangle, a geometric figure with three sides and three angles. There are three separate axes operative here – aesthetics, health and immigration – each of which has a positive and a negative pole: for example, health can be understood as a discourse ranging between the poles of wellness at one end and illness at the other, and health as a discourse that ranges between the extremes of beauty and ugliness. These three planes, however, do not exist in isolation: on the contrary, each has a point of confluence with the other two, these points of intersection forming the angles of the triangle. The exact nature of this interactive dynamic will be refined and explored in the process of argument, in particular to explore how the immigration side of the triangle interacts with the others. At the moment, schematically, this is the point we have reached (see Figure 2.1).

To begin with, however, it is important to emphasise that the argument develops through two distinct phases. The first phase focuses on the axis of health, and the second is directed to defining the nature and role of the aesthetic axis. First, the rhetoric of health serves as a means of stigmatisation. The apparent scientific rationalism of a concern about health may be simply a device that legitimates oppression. By accusing the Chinese of being dirty or diseased, for example, hostility towards them was given a patina of scientific legitimacy. And, at the same time, the imagery of dirt and disease itself provokes an *aesthetic* reaction. The aesthetics of health gave xenophobia undoubted immediacy and legitimacy.

Second, however, aesthetics is more than a mere factotum of other concerns, marshalled with more or less conscious contrivance. It is, at times, a genuinely felt value in its own right. By aesthetics I mean in the first place a reaction to a sensory stimulus – a sight or a smell, for example – on the basis of its beauty or ugliness, and recognition must be given to the force of this feeling, or rather this mode of

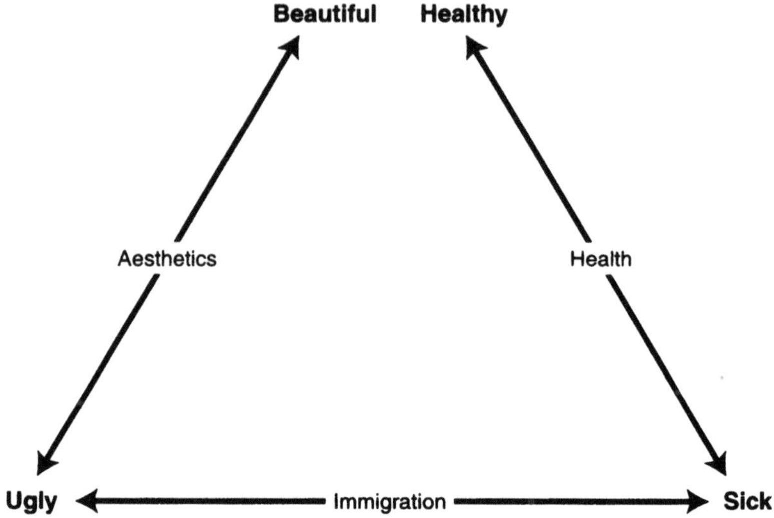

Figure 2.1 The triangle of aesthetics, health and immigration

apprehension. But where do these instinctively felt aesthetic valuations come from? What is their origin and purpose? To explore adequately the ways in which aesthetics governs perception, it is necessary to consider the images and icons that, representing cultural values in symbolic form, *ground* those judgements of beauty and ugliness. Aesthetics, then, is in part a felt judgement in reaction to an image. It is also about the other images – symbols – that generate that feeling. My argument at this point is that what might be labelled a 'health' issue is at times a misidentification or category mistake that conceals an aesthetic reaction stimulated by a complex of symbols. In particular, the passionate objection to Chinese opium use which radically changed drug legislation in Australia as around the world was, at heart, an aesthetic reaction to an alien habit perceived as disturbing because of the symbolic meaning attached to the drug.[8] In that case, an apparent concern about health masked a feeling of *revulsion* and a meaning that was not scientific or rational but symbolic.

THE CHINESE IN AUSTRALIA AND THE IDEA OF DIRT: FROM DEFILEMENT TO DISEASE

Of course, the effects of these associations operated both ways: the Chinese association led to the criminalisation of opium, certainly, but at the same time the opium association enhanced the image of evil attached to the Chinese community. Indeed, even the question of who belonged to that 'community' was by no means a pre-determined or neutral fact. Some 'respectable Chinese' were effectively excluded from being branded 'Chinese' in Australia, and their opposition to the opium trade, for example, was an important element in allowing them this status as honorary whites. The question of identity itself is not an unproblematic one, and being labelled 'Chinese' in Australia was in part about fitting into the stereotypes about the evil Chinese that were in the process of construction. I do not explore these issues here, but merely enter a caveat concerning the dangers of assuming the pre-givenness of the category 'Chinese'.

That said, however, in White Australia's long history of racism, the treatment of this community has a special place of ignominy.[9] Fear of being overrun by the yellow peril dated back to the early gold-rush years, when sizeable Chinese immigration to Australia began. The riot at Lambing Flat, which cost several lives, is notorious for its violence, but the attitudes and hostility it demonstrated were by no means atypical. From the 1860s through the 1880s, the colonial legislatures, sometimes over the objections of the British government, passed a variety of laws devised to limit or outlaw Chinese immigration, a legislative policy which, in one of the first Acts passed by the new Australian government in 1901, came to be known as the 'White Australia' policy. In practice, though not in form, that policy effectively prevented Asian immigration until the 1960s.[10] None the less, until the turn of the century, large Chinese communities were established, first on the goldfields and then in Australia's major cities. In 1877 the Palmer River goldfields in north Queensland, for example, had 17,000 Chinese and only 1,400 Europeans; 7,000 Chinese and only 1,000 Europeans lived in the Northern Territory in 1887, and Darwin has been a Eurasian city ever since.[11]

For some protagonists, the racism directed against the Chinese seemed an economic imperative. The Chinese, it was said, worked for long hours and seven days a week, when Australian unions had been fighting to reduce the hours of work. Further, most of the Chinese men who came to Australia did so to escape the poverty of China and to make some money for their families. They had no intention of staying permanently and often left their wives and children behind. In consequence, they were able to live on less than a labourer with a family to support. The *Bulletin* insisted that 'the badness of the Chinaman, socially and morally, is the outcome of his low wages'; they were, apparently, 'jaundice-coloured apostles of unlimited competition'.[12]

This was not just a debate, however, about economic protectionism. The Chinese, in language striking for its visceral hatred and excess, were portrayed as animals and as devils. A pamphlet written by the pseudonymous (and ironically named) 'Humanity' was by no means uncharacteristic in this regard:

> The Chinese amidst their evil surroundings, and their filthy and sinful abodes of sin and swinish devilry [will be] entered into by the servants of the Most High God! . . . It would never be believed that our Saxon and Norman girls could have sunk so low in crime as to consort with such a herd of Gorilla Devils.[13]

Already it will be apparent that the notion of filth was essential to this characterisation. The Chinese were not only portrayed as evil, but as 'filthy' and 'swinish'. Indeed, the imagery of the 'dirty Chinese' was a constant refrain in the hate literature that abounded. Here once more is the *Bulletin*, writing in typically purple prose for an infamous 1886 special edition entitled 'The Chinese in Australia':

> Disease, defilement, depravity, misery and crime – these are the indispensable adjuncts which make the Chinese camps and quarters loathsome to the senses and faculties of civilised nations. Whatever neighbourhood the Chinese choose for the curse of their presence forthwith begins to reek with the abominations which are forever associated with their vile habitations.[14]

There is no reason or argument here, only conclusory statements and an evocation to make our senses reel. The rhetoric of health – of 'disease and defilement' – validated the *Bulletin*'s invective, and that rhetoric was couched overwhelmingly in aesthetic terms – in expressions of disgust levelled at quarters that are not merely unsanitary, but 'reek' and are 'loathsome to the senses'. It is not *their* health about which the *Bulletin* is concerned, but its impact on *our* senses. The Chinese were said to be 'dirty' and this was at once an argument from the perspective of health and an image to revolt us. This is the essence of the aesthetics of health: what matters is not the well-being of the subject, but how they appear to the observer. 'Disease and defilement' sums up this dichotomy between health as a scientific and as an aesthetic value: you may be diseased, but *I* am defiled by it.

It would be a mistake to treat this use of language as purely calculated, a device to conceal other motives. The aesthetics of health expresses real sentiment and fear. Why is it that the Chinese were seen as 'dirty' – why did the ideas of 'disease' and 'defilement' congeal in this manner? It was surely the difference of the Chinese, in their appearance and manner, their customs, and their sequestration in separate communities, that provoked such a powerful need to label and condemn. Neither is it so surprising that the horror of difference should find typical expression in the language of health. Recall that, for Mary Douglas in *Purity and Danger*, dirt is properly understood as 'matter out of place'. It is culturally defined in terms of a breach of boundaries: dirt is the outside world brought inside (mud trampled on the carpet, for example, or dust on the mantelpiece), or our own insides made visible to the outside world (human waste not flushed away, or garbage loose on the streets); it represents a crucial breach in the ramparts we build between public and private spheres of life, both biologically and socially.[15] But immigration is itself, in a homogeneous and introverted society, a threat to the boundary between self and other. It exposes the rockpool of a culture to the oceans of humankind. That is why the use of terms like 'cultural pollution' or invasion is so endemic. The result is perhaps a feeling of being swamped, under the influence of which the migrant community *itself* is perceived as 'matter out of place'. Hence the suitability of the rhetoric of dirt and disease: the literal sense is substituted for the metaphorical one so that, from a feeling that the Chinese are a kind of 'pollution', we move quickly to a situation in which they are treated as if they really were polluted. To put it another way, the symbolic (in which A is taken to represent B) is treated as if it were a sign (in which the existence of A points to the presence of B).

Furthermore, it is with the image of dirt that beauty and health – or rather, ugliness and sickness – coalesce in a term through which the legitimacy of health and hygiene often mask an aesthetic reaction to violation. The result is a complex conjunction. 'Dirt' marks the point of collision between the three vectors: the experience of immigration, the language of health and the emotional power of aesthetics. It is for this reason that migrant communities such as the Chinese in Australia were readily characterised as diseased, and why this characterisation needs to be understood as stemming from an aesthetic and not a scientific concern. A metaphorical or symbolic disturbance understood aesthetically was translated into a rational and literal sign of ill-health. A twofold transformation therefore took place: 'dirt' was taken literally, and defilement was treated as if it were a synonym for disease.

THE IMAGE OF THE CHINESE: HEALTH AS A LEGITIMATING DEVICE

The prevalence of the use of the language of health in the manner described was itself an instrument of oppression, for it appeared to give legitimate reasons for anti-Chinese sentiment. There were, moreover, various commissions of inquiry that reinforced the idea that the Chinese were especially unhygienic. Preparing the 1876 Report of the Sydney City and Suburban Sewage and Health Board, for example, five members of the Board inspected the living conditions of some of the poorest parts of Sydney, including Chinatown, touring at all hours of the day and night for fifty-one consecutive days.[16] It was undoubtedly a difficult task, and their aesthetic reaction to the filth they encountered was both intense and unsurprising.

The inspectors did not particularly concentrate on the Chinese, and indeed quoted the New South Wales Chief Medical Officer, Dr Ashburton Thompson, who said of the Chinese that 'they are seldom quite so dirty, so indifferent to comfort and decency, or so squalid as some of our own poor often are'.[17] It is significant, however, that such a protestation had to be made. And it is also apparent that the Board, no less than their fellow citizens, were prepared to treat this squalor as a trait of the Chinese community in general, and not a function of poverty. 'If these people ever wash themselves, they do it by stealth,' commented Alderman Chapman and Dr Read.[18]

> For the next forty-eight hours, and that of the previous night, the horrible sickly smell of opium smoking which pervades all the Chinese quarters seemed to adhere to us, to say nothing of the fear of infection, which is not a pleasant sensation.[19]

About opium I shall have more to say presently. Let us note for the moment that the critique of 'the Chinese quarters' was of a 'horrible' 'smell'. It was the assault on the senses of the observers that was of prime concern here and not the health of the inhabitants: the smell, after all, adhered 'to us'. Furthermore, it was not the *experience* of infection that concerned the Board, nor was there any attempt to discern the extent to which infection constituted a real risk amongst residents. Rather it was the *fear* of infection about which they expressed anxiety. This fear affected them, and not the Chinese at all. At heart, the perception of the observer appears to be at stake – *their* fears and sensations – and not the well-being of the observed. This aesthetic of health, external in outlook and sensory in apprehension, could only serve as a weapon to be used against the Chinese and not in their interests.

At times, health arguments were used more specifically against the Chinese. The *Afghan* ship arrived in Australia in early 1888 along with three other ships containing a total of nearly 600 Chinese passengers. Those on board tried to disembark in Melbourne, and were refused permission to do so. They sailed on to Sydney, and again they were denied. There they waited, trapped in their floating world off Circular Quay for several weeks, hoping vainly for a change of heart, while angry crowds lined the shore and demonstrated against their presence, and the New South Wales parliament debated a new bill to ensure their exclusion.[20] Finally, defeated, the *Afghan* set sail, and eventually returned in failure to Hong Kong, its mast between its legs. The *Mayflower* was never so ill treated.[21]

The actions of the governments of Victoria and New South Wales were clearly illegal, since although the legislation in place at the time set a quota on the number of Chinese immigrants (calculated in proportion to the weight of the ship, no less) which the *Afghan* certainly exceeded, the Collector of Customs refused to land any Chinese, including those who were British subjects (such as passengers from Hong Kong).[22] But Sir Henry Parkes defended his actions with rhetorical flourish.

> I cast to the winds your permits of exemption; I care nothing about your cobwebs of technical law; I am obeying a law far superior to the law which issued these permits, namely, the law of the preservation of society in New South Wales.[23]

The question of smallpox was a crucial argument in defence of these actions. The *Afghan* was declared infected, and flew the flag of quarantine. The refusal to land its passengers seemed then the soundest of public health. But as it frequently was, the argument from health was sleight of hand. The *Afghan* had not been to an infected port and was not at risk. Furthermore, non-Chinese and, following an order of the Supreme Court of Victoria, fifty others, were finally allowed to land.[24] This was a strange virus then, discriminating in its contagion and apparently attuned to the finer points of the Influx of Chinese Restriction Act.

This was but one of many cases in which the fear of smallpox acted as a rationalisation and not a reason for action. It was a disease strongly associated with the Chinese. Phil May's famous illustration, 'The Mongolian Octopus-Grip on Australia', caricatured the Chinese

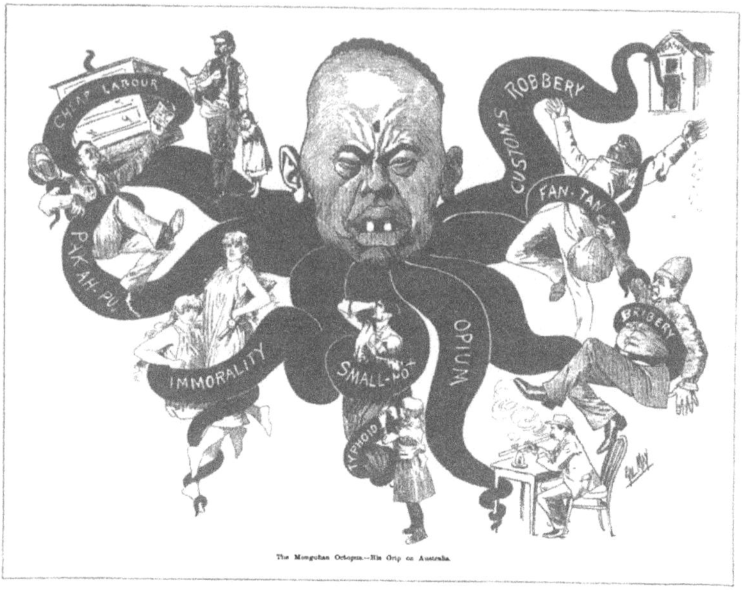

Figure 2.2 'The Mongolian Octopus-Grip on Australia' by Phil May

as a giant octopus, 'every one of [whose] arms, each of [whose] sensile suckers has its own class of victims or special mission of iniquity'. In this cartoon, alongside gambling, opium and 'immorality' among others, the arm of 'smallpox' and 'typhoid' can be seen squeezing the life out of two white children.[25] The fear was undoubtedly real, but it was a fear of Chinese immigration and not of disease.

At the same time, it is no coincidence that it should be a disease like smallpox that served the rhetorical and justificatory purposes it did. The effects of smallpox are immediate and visible: the pustules that form on the skin are disturbing and the scars they leave are permanent. Not all diseases are so unpleasant to behold, and the horror of smallpox is partly a consequence of its ugliness. We may contrast a sickness like consumption whose wounds are purely internal, whose pallor seemed to accord with a particular ideal of feminine fragility, and which even acquired a certain glamour in the nineteenth century.[26] Smallpox is exactly the opposite, and the revulsion associated with it and used to such effect against the Chinese was to some extent aesthetic. Moreover, smallpox is extremely contagious and was therefore a perfect metaphor for the pollution and violation that immigration itself represented. The ugliness, the virulence and the contagion of smallpox all made it a perfect symbol to affix to the Chinese. The question of health, then, was used in a powerful way: its aesthetic aspects, concealed beneath the rational, and its symbolic aspects, converted into the literal, intensified and justified the racism of white Australia.

Another dubious health argument cropped up frequently in the pages of the *Bulletin* and elsewhere. The Chinese were skilful and industrious market gardeners in and around Sydney. It was said of them, however, that they used nightsoil to fertilise their gardens and that this accounted for their success in growing vegetables. So horrifying was this allegation that it received considerable attention during the hearings of the 1892 New South Wales Royal Commission on Alleged Chinese Gambling and Immorality, and was there vociferously denied.[27] Again, the image of dirt which that attack employed suggested there was a genuine health risk at issue. A patina of scientific rationality surrounded the issue. But what is its basis? The practice of putting manure in and on the soil is and was standard and necessary. Even were the suggestions true, why should human waste be treated differently from that of a cow or pig? As far as the vegetables themselves are concerned, nightsoil is simply a nutrient like any other. Of course if vegetables have been doused with liquid manure, rather than it merely being mixed with the soil around them, then they must be well washed before use, but this is true whatever the species of waste used. It is only our discomfort with the processes of our own bodies, and our inability to abstract it into some neutral term such as 'manure'– a French word for dung and therefore tailor-made for euphemism, as we call a dead cow 'beef' and a dead sheep 'mutton' – that makes the difference; and it is then a difference of perception and not of reality.

The Report of the Royal Commission was clear in accepting the evidence of its medical witnesses that 'the objections often urged against the practice' had nothing but 'a sentimental basis'.[28] Yet for those who saw this as further proof of the dirtiness of the Chinese, no such reassurances sufficed. Some of the Commissioners, for example, stuck doggedly to a story about a cabbage they had seen, grown by 'a Chinaman at Forbes', in which the manure had somehow, miraculously, been absorbed in its raw form right up into the stem and head of the plant. No witnesses' insistence that such an event was botanically impossible would shake them from their belief.[29] In fact, much is made throughout the Commission of the question of smell: the smell of this mythical cabbage, the differing smells of different types of manure – even the smell of the water used to cook a 'Chinese-grown cabbage' was alleged to differ.[30] And clearly the Chinese themselves knew the indomitability of these myths and the power of disgust to affect their business. All of those interviewed by the Commission denied ever using human waste in their gardens.[31]

Once again, when the idea of dirt was used against the Chinese, an ostensible question of health turns out to be about the *imagery* of cleanliness and the stench of pollution. The disgust this imagery engendered became part of a whole folklore centred on an aesthetics of health – the Chinese as squalid, as faecal, as fetid, as infected – which, through the reactions of distaste it provoked, served to alienate the Chinese further and to entrench the hostility that their intrusion into white Australia had aroused.

THE HABITS OF THE CHINESE: OPIUM AS AN AESTHETIC OFFENCE

Taken at face value, as they often were (and still are), questions of health used against the Chinese rationalised fear. Understood as an aesthetic in which the look of something was of paramount importance, the image of health gave an emotional resonance and force to this fear. The aesthetic of health was therefore both a disguise and an intensifier. Further, as we have seen, it was the fact that immigration itself was often felt to be a confrontation, a violation of boundaries, that enabled those connections to be made so effectively. But the argument so far might suggest that the role of aesthetics in these episodes was as purely deceptive as the rational language of health: it concealed, it reconfigured, it emotionalised. It is time to render our appreciation of the aesthetic more sophisticated.

Let us start with the experience of feeling, as much a specialisation of human evolution as rational thought.[32] The experience of the aesthetic is keenly felt – as pleasure, awe, or disgust. But what causes these feelings and where do they come from? Aesthetic reactions undoubtedly gain force and meaning from their connotations and metaphors, as part of a semiotic system.[33] They are always built upon images or sensations that refer to other things. Nothing is inherently beautiful or ugly except in as much as it acts as a symbol. In this, the aesthetic realm is both quintessentially and invariably semiotic: it is the level on which cultural connections are felt and not thought. Symbols speak the language of aesthetics in a way that ideas and facts do not – they are the source material of the aesthetic as they are of the dreamworld.

A judgement of beauty or ugliness must therefore always be explained in terms of what it points to or symbolises.[34] The aesthetic reaction, say to an immigrant community, may therefore be a kind of displacement or transference – an economic or social fear *experienced as* a feeling of ugliness in much the same way as an illness in an organ may come to our attention as a shooting pain somewhere else on the body. But this is too reductionist an approach. If culture informs the aesthetic sense, so too does aesthetics inform culture; it is a *force* in the construction of values as well as a *mode* of their expression. Confronted with the intensity of an aesthetic reaction, unpacked from the casing of health rhetoric that rationalised it, we must also give it credit for its own sake. It is in this spirit, sensitive to both the persuasive force of aesthetics and the symbolic language that grounds it, that I wish to tackle the issue of opium.

Of all the indicators of difference that set the Chinese apart and served to label them as deviant, none was so powerful or so horrifying to the sensibilities of White Australia as their use of opium. From small beginnings on the Australian goldfields, opium imports increased dramatically. In 1857, when the governments of New South Wales and Victoria first imposed a duty upon the importation of opium, 328 pounds were imported into New South Wales, almost exclusively for the 9,000 Chinese.[35] By 1890, a Chinese population of about 21,500 in New South Wales and Victoria imported over 37,000 pounds of opium. In 1902, although the Chinese population Australia-wide had declined to 29,627, New South Wales still imported 14,000 pounds of opium, Victoria 10,000 and Queensland, with a large Chinese population working on the cane fields, 18,000 pounds. Almost all that imported stock was sold to the Chinese community.[36]

Yet White Australia was not a temperate society. Australians consumed, *per capita*, more patent medicines than any other country in the world. The active principle in these 'remedies' was more often than not alcohol, opium or a derivative thereof.[37] But the Chinese did not drink their opium, or take it in tablet form; it was their custom to smoke it, specially prepared in pipes and frequently in 'dens' fitted out for the purpose. Best evidence suggests that somewhere between 50 and 90 per cent of the Chinese population in Australia regularly smoked opium.[38] Smoking was at once a private reverie, and a convivial activity. Like any recreational drug, there were occasional users, regular users, abusers and addicts; there were houses in which the smoking of an opium pipe was regarded as a social courtesy, and others in which it was a serious business.

The smoking of opium was therefore the habit, at once ubiquitous and unique, of a minority. Many Chinese smoked opium: almost no Europeans did so. White Australians used different recreational drugs, while considerable opiate dependence was concealed as quasi-medicinal in nature. Opium smoking was in all these ways a 'Chinese vice', able to be set apart from other drug use in Australia.

Hostility to the Chinese use of opium masqueraded as a concern about the health risks of use. But we have learned enough about the role of health rhetoric in the construction of difference to be sceptical of such rhetoric. The addictive qualities of opium had been well established since the 1870s, but beyond the *fact* of addiction, evidence of the harm or ill-health consequent upon opium smoking was slight and anecdotal, then as now.[39] It was, rather, the *ugliness* of opium smoking that generated concern. When the *Bulletin* described the 'shambling gait, glistening eyes, and trembling muscles' of an opium smoker, its clear purpose was to provoke horror in the reader and not concern.[40] And what are we to make of this description of the dangers of opium uttered in 1893 by the Victorian Minister for Health, himself a medical doctor?:

> Who has not seen the slave of opium – a creature tottering down the street, with sunken yellow eyes, closely contracted pupils, and his skin hanging over his bones like dirty yellow paper.[41]

The offence given here was aesthetic; sympathy was not provoked, but rather pity (at best) or disgust (at worst). This slave of opium was not a man but a 'creature', and a creature moreover who was 'dirty' and 'yellow'. We have returned to the xenophobic image of the Chinese, dehumanised and polluted. And, once again, in a tell-tale aesthetic posture, we are *external* to the user: it is not what it feels like to be 'sick', but rather what it looks like.

The use of this kind of language suggests that the virulent hostility to Chinese opium use, while often couched in terms of disease, was aesthetic in nature and, moreover, intimately connected to racist attitudes to the Chinese in general. Opium smoking was perceived as a powerful symbol of difference, a violation of normality and conformity which the presence of the Chinese already challenged. But what generated this aesthetic interpretation? What was it about the smoking of opium in particular that made it such a powerful symbol to be marshalled against the Chinese? It was an image of such overwhelming negativity that between 1891 and 1908 every colony and state of Australia outlawed its use and possession in language of unique severity, while the Commonwealth government, for its part, declared it a prohibited import. It is not enough simply to emphasise the empirical connection of opium smoking with the Chinese community.[42] The particular aesthetics of the drug itself were vital in establishing that connection and entrenching that revulsion. Certain aspects of the aesthetics of opium made it especially well suited to take on the symbolic meanings it assumed.

In the first place, the very sensory novelty of opium smoking in the Australian context provoked an aesthetic reaction centred on the fear of difference. In the *Bulletin* article entitled 'Disease, Defilement, Depravity' there is a suggestive description of an opium den.

> Down from the fan-tan dens are stairs leading to lower and dirtier abodes: rooms darker and more greasy than anything on the ground floor: rooms where the legions of aggressive stinks peculiar to Chinamen seems ever to linger . . . Yet the rooms are not naturally repulsive, nor would they be so when occupied by other tenants; but the Chinaman has defiled their walls with his filthy touch; he has vitiated what was once a reasonably pure atmosphere with his presence, and he has polluted the premises with his disgusting habits . . . The very air of the alley is impregnated with the heavy odour of the drug.[43]

Although the *Bulletin* was ostensibly concerned about health and disease, it is immediately apparent that we are in the realm of aesthetic considerations. Strangeness was portrayed as ugliness, difference was aestheticised, and in the alien environment of the opium den, dark and close, everything impinged upon the senses at once, disordered and riotous, until only an all-encompassing sensation of dirtiness and a scent of strangeness remained. The pollution of being Chinese and the odour of opium smoking interacted and catalysed. What was wrong with both conditions was expressed and understood overwhelmingly in aesthetic terms.

I have so far argued that the reason for the symbolic importance of opium in epitomising hostility to the Chinese stemmed from the overpowering sensation of strangeness that opium presented to the uninitiated. It is not coincidental, however, that it was the *smoking* of opium that elicited this deeply hostile reaction. The imagery of the *Bulletin* was to some extent visual, using the familiar language of dirt and filth, of darkness and descent. But it was the peculiarity of the *smell* of opium to the European nose that in particular highlighted the difference of the Chinese, and stimulated revulsion. The 'pure' atmosphere of the room was polluted by the lingering 'aggressive stink' of opium; there was a sickly and overpowering odour that seemed to impregnate 'the very air'. We have noted much the same reaction to the 'horrible sickly smell of opium smoking' that clung to the inspectors of the Sydney City and Suburban Sewage and Health Board.[44]

Smoking is the one kind of drug consumption that most involves the observer. We experience others' smoke as we do not experience their taste or sight. Furthermore, in a more general sense, smells physically challenge our sense of boundary: they escape, they are shared, they envelop – they cling. The liminal and communal nature of the sense of smell is in itself a violation of autonomy. The olfactory system, moreover, is directly connected to our emotions and serves as a powerful trigger of feelings.[45]

Because of how the sense of smell operates, and because of what it signifies, it is unsurprising that drug smoking should in particular become characterised as pollution. An odour is already a boundary violation. An unfamiliar odour, even more so, violates the normal. A strange smell peculiarly associated with the Chinese was uniquely placed to become an important symbol of pollution and danger, and to be experienced as revulsion.

THE HABITS OF THE CHINESE: FROM DISEASE TO DEPRAVITY

Notice the equation of smell and infection at work here, the assumption of the dirtiness of the Chinese drawn from an aesthetic reaction to opium's unfamiliar odour. A further equation was made, too, namely that between dirtiness and immorality. The Sewage and Health Board wrote of 'the most revolting and immoral scenes' emanating from 'similar foul dens of Chinese depravity'. The transformation was thus completed. 'Defilement' was translated into 'disease', and 'disease' became 'depravity' – from ugliness to dirtiness, and from uncleanliness to ungodliness. That was the force opium exerted: an aesthetic difference rationalised using the language of health, and implicating moral values. Again, that transformation was accomplished by way of aesthetics: the ugliness of opium use came to *stand for* immorality, just as we saw the ugliness of dirt coming to stand for unhealthiness. In both cases, the metaphors prompted by an aesthetic reaction were literalised: ugliness, symbolising the unhealthy or the immoral, was treated as if it really were a sign of disease or depravity.

The power of aesthetics to accomplish this conflation – this boundary violation, one might almost say, between aesthetics, science and ethics – is apparent if we consider the image of the opium trader contained in the *Bulletin*'s fictional account of the life of 'Mr Sin Fat', which appeared at the time of the *Afghan* crisis.[46] In the story, Mr Sin grows wealthy by his ownership of dens 'reeking with the nauseating odour of opium and pollution and Chinamen, and always clouded with smoke'. Already the connections have been made: smell and the senses, invasion and pollution and the Chinese. Mr Sin Fat's particular pleasure is to entice innocent young girls into his lair, there turning them into hopeless addicts and sexual slaves. The story ends when one new victim turned out, unbeknownst to Sin Fat, to be the child of his wife. In a fit of fury, she stabs him to death with a pig-sticker.[47]

'Mr Sin Fat' is an image of evil, and his name says it all – 'Fat' implies bodily unhealthiness, and 'Sin', moral unhealthiness. The *Bulletin*'s main purpose was to link the two conditions. As Sin Fat prospers and becomes more and more sinful, so too he gets fatter, until at last:

> he was fatter than fat, his obesity was phenomenal – Layers of blubber bulged about his eyes – and his mighty neck rolled almost on to his shoulders, and vibrated like jelly with every movement.[48]

Fatness is ugly just as the scent of opium is ugly, and that ugliness was treated as if it were not merely a symbol of sin, but an unmistakable sign of it. Moreover, as fat suggests corporeal indulgence, sin suggests incorporeal indulgence. The parallel with opium as yet another kind of indulgence is obvious.

Together, obesity, sin and opium formed a triangle by which the drug was portrayed as creating a life at once both unhealthy and immoral: it was a connection accomplished above all through the power of images to generate revulsion and to make symbolic associations feel literally true. It was the ugliness of Mr Sin Fat that was relentlessly advanced, but that ugliness was taken to have genuine moral implications exactly as it was taken to have authentic health effects. The consequences of defilement were taken in fact to be disease and depravity, and so the ugly, the diseased and the immoral coalesced. Neither is this approach to ugliness unique. In the eighteenth and nineteenth centuries the sciences of physiognomy and phrenology were influential in likewise equating moral or intellectual capacity with a visual deviation from the norm. There too an imperfect body was read as a sign of deviance and imbecility.[49]

I am arguing that the smoking of opium, like the question of 'dirt', was never a question of health, no matter how much the rhetoric of health might have rationalised it. It was, instead, an aesthetic revulsion in response to images of metaphorical boundary violation. That revulsion was nowhere more apparent than in the kind of moral objection made to opium use. The central tenet of the demonisation of opium smoking, as tenacious as it was untrue, was that women who consumed it either lost all sexual control immediately or became so addicted that they were unable to resist seduction. The effect of opium was, it was said, to enable 'the criminal and sensual Chinese' to have their perverted way with white women.[50]

So it was that the *Bulletin* argued that there was 'only one possible result when a lustful and unscrupulous Chinaman is one of the parties and an unsuspecting, though perhaps instinctively cautious girl, the other':

> One of the girls now kept in a den on the Rocks, says . . . 'I went to the place when I was only about 16 because he used to give me presents. He then wanted me to smoke, but I never would, because the pipes looked so dirty. But one day he put a new pipe before me, and made it ready, and after the first whiff from it, he or any other man . . . I was completely at their mercy, but so help me God I was a good girl before that.'

'Shall the monsters of sensuality grapple the youth and innocence of Australia?' fulminated the *Bulletin*, warning that 'so long as the sensual Chinaman and innocent girls are permitted to come into contact, so long will the results be disastrous to the latter'.[51]

Despite the repeated denial of this mythology – not least by a dozen European women who lived with the Chinese in Sydney's Chinatown, and who gave the lie to it uncategorically in evidence presented before the New South Wales Royal Commission into Alleged Chinese Gambling and Immorality[52] – the fanciful attribution of near-magical powers to a drug found in no less potent form in any number of commonly available patent medicines continued to have a powerful hold over the minds and imagination of Australians. What fear did this express, after all, but miscegenation? And what greater violation of the community's boundaries could there be; what more disturbing affront to the sensibilities of a homogeneous and prudish society? The

Chinese and opium alike were constructed in terms of invasion, violation and pollution. Miscegenation was the apotheosis of those very fears that the Chinese represented to xenophobic Australia and that opium, on the other hand, had come to symbolise. It was a marriage of convenience, between fear and the symbolic forms in which it was expressed, that could not be set asunder merely by evidence or argument. Neither myths nor nightmares are vanquished by reason.

The aesthetics and imagery of opium, therefore, made it particularly appropriate as a vehicle in the hostility against the Chinese and particularly vulnerable to legislative and social attack. Those aesthetics were a powerful force in the construction of values, through the feelings they provoked and the symbols they entrenched. At the same time, the sensory and symbolic nature of the attitude towards opium was legitimated through health and moral concerns, both more apparent than real. What was ostensibly about science and morality was, beneath the surface, a question of vile smells and the horror of dirt – not health but aesthetics governed the social reaction to opium. The look and smell of opium dens provoked feelings that in turn can be explained in terms of the semiotic system attached to those images. Images connoted other images, of great strength and urgency. The treatment of Chinese opium use took place within that world of symbols. It is not by any means the old Chinese addict alone, somnolent in his hazy den, who has visions and thinks them real.

CONCLUSION: TRIANGULATING THE AESTHETIC

Using aesthetics as an analytic tool, I have explored some of the complex interactions between health and migration, focusing on the Chinese in nineteenth-century Australia. Certain themes have emerged. Beauty and health alike are constructed around an ideal of conformity to a type, and the strength of this ideal has frequently led to hostility directed against migrant communities. The 'dirtiness' of the migrant has been a significant rallying-cry of this hostility, as it frequently still is. It is a mistake to try to understand 'dirt' as a question of health, for beneath the health rhetoric lies strongly felt *aesthetic* reactions built on a semiotic system of 'boundary violation'.[53] The images of smallpox, or nightsoil, or opium provoke intense reaction in juxtaposition with the Chinese, in part because of their complex symbolic associations. As beauty and health share an ideal, so health and migration share a symbolism. The effect of the rational language of health, however, is to cloak these symbolic and aesthetic sources of ill-feeling, and to legitimate an aesthetic reaction by treating it as if it were rational and scientific.

The migrant experience of health, and I would suggest that it is an experience that can be extrapolated far beyond the Chinese, thus involves a twofold dislocation.[54] First, the aesthetics of health – a matter of images, of external perception, of looking at someone – is treated as if it were equivalent to health itself – a matter of science, of community welfare and of concern about someone. And second, the symbols that prompt that aesthetic reaction – the metaphors that fuel cultural connections and hidden meaning and that are the raw material or grammar on which the aesthetic language is built – are treated as if they were signs of an external reality: defilement is construed as if it were really the symptoms of disease, and disease as if it were really the stigmata of depravity. But the process of these dislocations remains unacknowledged. The symbolism in aesthetics and the aesthetics in health are alike erased.

Trying to map this inter-relationship is a difficult task. All I have suggested is that we cannot take what is said and done in the name of 'health' or about 'migrants' at face value; and that part of a more careful understanding requires an appreciation of the aesthetics of health and the aesthetics of immigration. Aesthetics is both an important influence on our judgements and values in its own right, and a lens through which we interpret both health and immigration. In this light, we can understand aesthetics as a mode of perception, and as the storehouse of symbols on the basis of which it judges what it perceives. The aesthetic is the agency through which the symbolic world finds expression. The ideas and experience of health is one of the many resources for that semiotic and interpretative system, while the Chinese, in this case, were merely the objects upon which symbolic meaning and aesthetic valuation were imposed. Figure 2.3, exploring the idea of a triangle in a presentational rather than a discursive manner, perhaps suggests some of these interwoven dynamics – here we find three distinct axes or planes, each of which includes a variety of attitudes ranging between positive and negative poles, and each of which connects with each of the other two axes to produce three distinct angles of intersection.

The danger of failing to distinguish between health rhetoric and the aesthetics of health continues, in relation, for example, to mental illness or AIDS, which we could substitute along the baseline of our pyramid to develop a parallel analysis. We might begin by con-

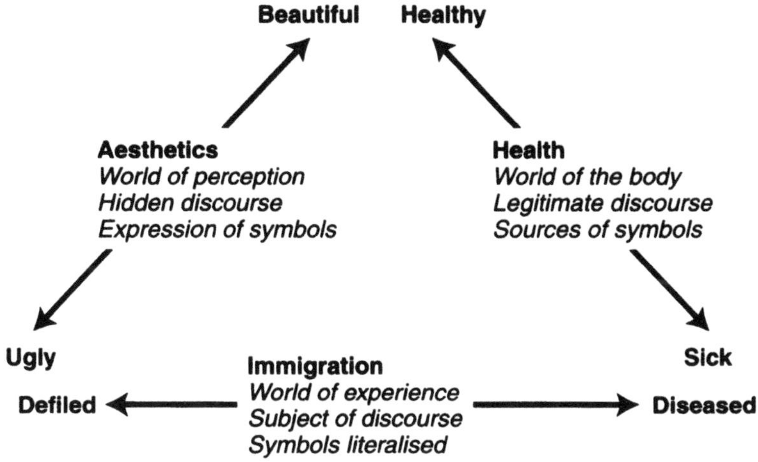

Figure 2.3 The interwoven dynamics of the triangle

sidering the extent to which imagery about the 'mentally ill', our disturbance at the way they look rather than how they feel, influences the social treatment they receive.[55] Similarly, as Susan Sontag has suggested, the *symbolic meaning* of AIDS, in relation to disease and sexuality, is a powerful determinant of the depth and nature of our concern.[56] More generally, how are we to explain our culture's obsession with youth, and ergo the popularity of cosmetic surgery, except as the socio-medical reflection of an ideal of beauty based upon an unattainable and homogeneous normality? – a reflection which, again, we find in, for example, legal cases of 'wrongful life' which have succeeded in arguing before the courts that it is better not to be born at all than to be born 'imperfect'.[57] The rhetoric of health is a powerful legitimator of alienation and discomfort, and an enforcer of a monolithic ideal of beauty. The conflation of difference and defilement with disease and depravity is of continuing significance.

To emphasise the importance of the aesthetic does not, however, imply that these judgements of beauty or symbolic associations are infrangible. Kant argued that an aesthetic judgement is accompanied by the feeling that it is universal, and used that conclusion to defend the absolute truth of beauty.[58] But this argument raises to a level of principle Kant's own desire for objectivity and universality. Aesthetics is cultural and temporal, as my emphasis on the symbols that drive it has made clear. At the same time, this relativism does not render it any less amenable to change or discourse than politics or ethics. There is beauty in difference, though some do not see it; there is delight in change, though some may fear it. Monism can be replaced by an aesthetic pluralism, in which variety is beauty and sameness a living death.[59] A greater awareness of the power of imagery and perception in the construction of social values does not imply that they have no legitimate role to play, only that, without that awareness, there can only be confusion.

NOTES

1 See M. Foucault, *The Care of the Self, The History of Sexuality*, Vol. 3, trans. R. Hurley, New York, 1988, for a detailed discussion of the construction of sexual relations in the Golden Age of Rome.

2 For recent discussion of these issues, see S. Faludi, *Backlash, The Undeclared War Against Women*, London, 1992; N. Wolf, *The Beauty Myth*, New York, 1991.

3 The notion of a scientific and objective state of 'mental health', in particular, has come in for considerable criticism in recent years: M. Foucault, *Madness and Civilisation, A History of Insanity in the Age of Reason*, trans. R. Howard, New York, 1988; T. Campbell and C. Heginbotham, *Mental Illness, Prejudice, Discrimination and the Law*, Aldershot, Dartmouth, 1991; T. Szasz, *The Manufacture of Madness*, New York, 1977; idem, *The Myth of Mental Illness, Foundations of a Theory of Personal Conduct*, New York, 1961. As for the question of beauty, the asserted objectivity of aesthetic value has an illustrious pedigree, see I. Kant, *Critique of Judgement*, trans. W. Pluhar, Indianapolis, 1987; Plato, *Gorgias*, trans. W. Helmbold, New York, 1952; Plato, *The Republic*, trans. D. Lee, London, 1974. It is unlikely that such a view would command general assent today – see in particular the discussion of the social construction of aesthetics in T. Eagleton, *The Ideology of the Aesthetic*, Oxford, 1990 – although in works such as L. Tiger, *The Pursuit of Pleasure*, Boston, 1992, there is an uncritical assumption of the universality of the author's own ideals of beauty which, were it in the least self-conscious, would owe a debt to Kant.

4 This is an argument developed further in B. Stafford, J. La Puma and D. Schiedermayer, 'One Face of Beauty, One Picture of Health, The Hidden Aesthetic of Medical Practice', *Journal of Medicine and Philosophy*, 1989, 14, pp. 213, 215–22.

5 Dr J. Cumpston discussed in M. Roe, 'The Establishment of the Australian Department of Health, its Background and Significance', *Historical Studies*, 1976–7, 17, pp. 176, 186.

6 N. Elkington discussed in ibid., p. 188; *Sydney Morning Herald*, 13 February 1914, p. 8.

7 George Dibbs paraphrasing Sir Henry Parkes, in *New South Wales*

Parliamentary Debates, Session 1887–8, 51 & 52 Vic. Vol. 33, pp. 4789, 4793.

8 See in particular D. Manderson, *From Mr Sin to Mr Big: a History of Australian Drug Laws*, Melbourne, 1993, pp. 17–58 and sources there cited.

9 See, for extensive material, A. Yarwood and M. Knowling, *Race Relations in Australia*, North Ryde, 1982; E. Rolls, *Sojourners, Flowers and the Wide Sea*, St Lucia, Queensland, 1992; I. McLaren, ed., *The Chinese in Victoria*, Melbourne, 1985.

10 See, for example, Chinese Restriction and Regulation Act, 1888, NSW, 52 Vic. No. 4, s.2; NSW Legislative Council, *Conference on the Chinese Question*, Sydney, 1888, pp. 5–6. See also, SA 51 and 52 Vic. No. 439; 52 Vic. No. 1005; WA 53 Vic. No. 3; Qld 53 Vic. No. 22; *Immigration Act*, 1901, Cth., No. 4 of 1901.

11 Yarwood and Knowling, *Race Relations in Australia*, pp. 176, 185.

12 *Bulletin*, Sydney, 12 January 1889, p. 6; 10 March 1888, p. 5.

13 'Humanity', *Sketches of Chinese Character*, Castlemaine, 1878, pp. 3–4.

14 *Bulletin*, Sydney, 21 August 1886, pp. 11–14. See also P. May, 'The Mongolian Octopus Grip on Australia', in ibid., pp. 12–13 and *Bulletin*, Sydney, Supplement, 14 April 1888.

15 See M. Douglas, *Purity and Danger*, London, 1966; and see also the discussion of the meaning of bodily waste in E. Becker, *The Denial of Death*, New York, 1973. For further discussion on the rhetoric of dirt and 'defilement' specifically in relation to racism, see K. Thomas, 'Strange Fruit', in T. Morrison, ed., *Race-ing Justice, En-gendering Power*, New York, 1992, pp. 364–89 and, more generally, J. Kovel, *White Racism*, New York, 1984.

16 Sydney City and Suburban Sewage and Health Board, *Eleventh Progress Report*, in NSW Legislative Assembly, *Votes and Proceedings 1875–6, Vol. V.*, pp. 535–661.

17 Dr J. Ashburton Thompson in ibid., p. 660.

18 Alderman Chapman and Dr Read in ibid., p. 569.

19 Ibid., pp. 568–9.

20 Archive Office of New South Wales, Colonial Secretary Special Bundle, *Chinese 1888, 4/884.1.*

21 See also the discussion in Rolls, *Sojourners*, pp. 464–504; Manderson, *From Mr Sin to Mr Big*, pp. 17–18.

22 Influx of Chinese Restriction Act, 1881, NSW, 45 Vic. No. 11, ss.4, 5 and 10. See also, for example, Vic. No. 45, Vic. No. 723; Qld 47, Vic. No. 13.

23 *New South Wales Parliamentary Debates, Session 1887–8, 51 & 52 Vic. Vol. 32*, p. 4787.

24 A.O.N.S.W., *Chinese 1888, 4/884.1.*

25 *Bulletin*, Sydney, 21 August 1886, p. 11; P. May, 'The Mongolian Octopus Grip on Australia' in ibid., pp. 12–13.

26 As to the social construction and imagery of consumption in this period, see S. Sontag, *Illness as Metaphor/AIDS and its Metaphors*, New York, 1990. The use of consumption as an artistic device in literature and opera is of course well known; although, given the average size of the diva who

sings Mimi in Puccini's *La Bohème*, 'conspicuous consumption' is a more accurate description.

27 New South Wales Legislative Assembly, Royal Commission on Alleged Chinese Gambling and Immorality (Mayor Manning, Chairman), *Report*, Sydney, 1892, p. 28 and various evidence given to the commission.

28 Ibid., p. 28; see also pp. 377–81.

29 Ibid., pp. 378, 421.

30 Ibid., p. 381.

31 Ibid., pp. 415 et seq.

32 See S.K. Langer, *Philosophy in a New Key*, Cambridge, Mass., 1942, 1978; idem, *Mind, An Essay on Human Feeling*, Baltimore, 1988.

33 I use the word semiotic in its broadest sense to refer to any system of signs. Far from the kind of structuralism and systemisation of writers such as C.S. Peirce or F. Saussure, I adopt the kind of flexible and broad approach to semiotic analysis represented by, for example, the variety of material presented in R. Kevelson, ed., *Law and Semiotics*, vols 1–3, New York, 1987–9.

34 See, in particular, for a more directly political analysis of the ways in which aesthetic values stand in for political ones, Eagleton, *The Ideology of the Aesthetic*.

35 NSW Legislative Council, *Votes and Proceedings 1858, Vol. 3*, pp. 305, 320; *Opium Duties Act* 1857, Vic. 21, No. 7; NSW Vic. 21, No. 1.

36 See Quong Tart, *A Plea for the Abolition of The Importation of Opium*, Sydney, 1887 (ML 178.82 B2), p. 11 and A. McCoy, *Drug Traffic*, Sydney, 1980, p. 72; NSW Census of 1891 and colonial censuses of 1891 and 1901; *Commonwealth Parliamentary Debates 1905, V Edw. VII Vol. 26*, pp. 1773, 1777.

37 Whisko, 'a non-intoxicating stimulant', was 28.2 per cent alcohol, Pe-runa 28.5 per cent, Warner's 35.7 per cent, and Hostetter's Stomach Bitters, 44.3 per cent. Mrs Winslow's Soothing Syrup, Bonnington's Irish Moss, Ayers' Sarsaparilla and Godfrey's Cordial all contained opium, while Ayers' Cherry Pectoral was morphine-based, and the quaintly named Cigars de Joy, 'perfectly harmless, pleasant to use, and contains no substance capable of deranging the system', were marijuana cigarettes, see Australian Archives, ACT, Prime Minister's Department CA 12; CRS A2 Correspondence files 1904–20, 1909/3562, Report on Secret Drugs by Mr O.C. Beale; *Royal Commission on Secret Drugs, Cures and Foods* (Octavius Beale, Commissioner), *Report, Vol. 1*, Melbourne, 1907. See also the discussion in Manderson, *From Mr Sin to Mr Big*, pp. 52–4; A. McCoy, *Drug Traffic*, pp. 52–70.

38 See NSW Legislative Assembly, *Votes and Proceedings 1878*; W. Young, 'Report on the Conditions of the Chinese Population in Victoria, Melbourne, 1868', in I. McLaren, *The Chinese in Victoria: Official Reports and Documents*, Ascot Vale: 1985, pp. 33–58.

39 T. Parsinnen and K. Kerner, 'Development of the Disease Model of Drug Addiction in Britain', *Medical History*, 1980, 24, pp. 283–4.

40 *Bulletin*, Sydney, 21 August 1886, p. 15.

41 Dr Scott in *Victorian Parliamentary Debates, Session 1893, Vol. 73*, p. 2640.

42 *Sale and Use of Poisons Act of 1891*, Qld, 55 Vic. No. 31, s. 13; The Opium Act, 1895, SA, 58 and 59 Vic. No. 644; *Opium Smoking Prohibition Act*, 1905, Vic. 5 Edw. VII, No. 2003; *Commonwealth of Australia Gazette No. 64*, Cth, 30, December 1905; Police Offences, Amendment Act, 1908, NSW, 8 Edw. VII, ch.12, ss.18–19. Despite a detailed analysis of the process of criminalisation in Manderson, *From Mr Sin to Mr Big*, pp. 20–58, it might yet be said that I have previously tended to base my argument mainly on the *association* of opium smoking with the Chinese, and inadequately on its particular symbolic significance.

43 'The Chinese in Australia' in *Bulletin*, Sydney, 21 August 1886, pp. 11–14.

44 Sydney City and Suburban Sewage and Health Board, *Eleventh Progress Report*, pp. 568–9.

45 See, in particular, D. Howes, 'Olfaction and Transition' in D. Howes, ed., *The Varieties of Sensory Experience, A Sourcebook in the Anthropology of the Senses*, Toronto, 1991, pp. 128–47; see also D. Howes, 'Odour in the Court', *Aroma, The Cultural History of Smell*, 1989–90, border/lines winter 28.

46 I am here sticking closely to my discussion in Manderson, *From Mr Sin to Mr Big*, pp. 26–7.

47 'Mr and Mrs Sin Fat', *Bulletin*, Sydney, 14 April 1888, pp. 8–9.

48 Ibid., p. 8.

49 See Stafford et al., 'One Face of Beauty, One Picture of Health', pp. 216–24.

50 'The Chinese invasion of Australia', in *Bulletin*, Sydney, 4 September 1886, p. 4. These attitudes and history are dealt with in much more detail in Manderson, *From Mr Sin to Mr Big*, pp. 24–30.

51 *Bulletin*, Sydney, 21 August 1886, pp. 11–14.

52 New South Wales Legislative Assembly, Royal Commission on Alleged Chinese Gambling and Immorality, *Report*, interviews recorded pp. 380–420.

53 For more on the rhetoric of dirt and 'defilement', specifically in relation to racism, see K. Thomas, 'Strange Fruit', in Morrison, *Race-ing Justice, En-gendering Power*, pp. 364–89; and, more generally, Kovel, *White Racism*.

54 There are obvious parallels here to the way the contemporary legal system translates questions of justice into points of law, and the content of law itself into issues of legal process, see R. Macdonald, 'Whose Access? Which Justice?, Review of Allan Hutchinson, ed., *Access to Civil Justice*, Toronto, 1990, *CJLS/RCDS*, 1992, vol. 1, p. 175; R. Macdonald, 'Theses on Access to Justice', *CJLS/RCDS*, 1992, vol. 2, p. 23; more generally, see R. Samek, *The Meta-Phenomenon*, New York, 1981.

55 The treatment of those we label mentally ill as somehow *sui generis*, as if their particular problems entitled us to dehumanise them, is considered at some length in Campbell and Heginbotham, *Mental Illness*.

56 See Sontag, *Illness as Metaphor*; see also R. Davenport-Hines, *Sex, Death and Punishment*, London, 1990.

57 See Stafford et al., 'One Face of Beauty, One Picture of Health', pp. 226–7; see also *Harbeson* v. *Parke Davis*, 1983, 656 P. 2d. 483; *Procanik* v. *Ciloo*, 1984, 478 A. 2d. 755.

58 See Kant, *Critique of Judgement*.

59 There are obvious parallels here with the recent development of legal pluralism; see, for example, M. Galanter, 'Justice in Many Rooms, Courts, Private Ordering, and Indigenous Law', *Journal of Legal Pluralism*, 1981, 19, p. 1; J. Griffiths, 'What is Legal Pluralism?', *Journal of Legal Pluralism*, 1986, 24, p. 1; S. Merry, 'Legal Pluralism', *Legal and Social Review*, 1987–8, p. 869. One might even propose an analogy between beauty and justice, although far removed from Plato's objectivist equation of the two; as there are different 'spheres of justice', there might also be different spheres of beauty, M. Walzer, *Spheres of Justice*, New York, 1983. Perhaps *meta*-aesthetic pluralism is more accurate since I am arguing not only for an appreciation of a variety of standards of beauty, but for an appreciation of the fact that different communities have varying standards of beauty.

So, too, from a medical perspective, Stafford et al., 'One Face of Beauty, One Picture of Health', pp. 228–9, condemns the 'mathematical model' of beauty and appeals instead for an alternative ideal based on diversity; difference then becomes not a flaw but a sign of humanity.

3

MIGRATION, PROSTITUTION AND MEDICAL SURVEILLANCE IN EARLY TWENTIETH-CENTURY MALAYA

Lenore Manderson

The concept of minority is an elastic one: it connotes both ideology and material difference; it captures and contains the notions of 'otherness' and subordination; it allows the exploration of the institutionalisation of difference, and the establishment and maintenance of control and dependency. In this chapter, it serves as a useful heuristic device to consider the prostitute, prostitution and sexually transmitted disease under colonialism.

In British Malaya, the minority status of Chinese women working as prostitutes occurred at multiple levels.[1] First, being a colonial subject created a minority status with respect to those in power, which was unrelated to population size. However, Chinese women were also a minority numerically, both in terms of race and sex. The powerlessness of prostitute workers within the brothel and their low status as prostitutes, together with their class and educational background – regardless of any cultural or political accommodation of prostitution – all positioned these women as marginal and vulnerable. As a result of recurrent infection and their perceived role in the transmission of venereal disease, these women were stripped further of personal and colonial subject status in clinical encounters and in discourses concerning public health, law and order. There were constant elisions in discourse between person and sex, and between sex and disease. The brutality, fear, violence and poverty that characterised the lives of most prostitutes was simply the most tangible dimension of their minority status.

In this chapter, I first discuss the historical position of prostitution in colonial Malaya, identifying the way in which labour migration strategies created the preconditions for immigrant prostitution. I then introduce colonial understandings of sexuality and prostitution, and examine the recruitment and employment patterns that affected most prostitutes during the period 1870–1920. Finally, I examine government strategies designed to limit or control venereal disease, and the role of doctors and other health professionals in providing medical services to brothel workers. The cavalier treatment that most women received and the profiteering of the doctors draws attention to the powerlessness of the affected women within the brothels, and to their vulnerability to state control.

MIGRATION, POPULATION AND THE DEVELOPMENT OF THE COLONY

A British military and commercial presence was established in Penang in the late eighteenth century, and in Singapore and Malacca from the early nineteenth century. Under East India Company governance, there was substantial voluntary migration of Chinese miners and merchants, with some 2,000–3,000 Chinese workers annually entering Penang and Province Wellesley to find employment on sugar and spice plantations and in tin-mines.[2] After the transfer of the Straits Settlements (hereafter Settlements) from East India to Colonial Office control (1867), and the extension of British political influence and administrative control over the Malay States from 1874, economic development and labour requirements expanded.

The nineteenth century saw the constant movement of peoples to colonial Malaya and between the colonies and adjacent areas. Labour demand was originally met by the spontaneous immigration of Chinese labourers, by way of Hong Kong. From around the turn of the twentieth century, however, with increased demand due to the rapid expansion of the rubber industry, the demand was met by the organised recruitment of Indian labourers, who were reputedly more compliant and cheaper than Chinese labourers.[3] Local migration also took place among the peoples of the peninsular Malay and Thai states and the Indonesian archipelago.

Most immigrants from Southern China and India travelled to Malaya on a temporary basis to seek their fortune or escape poverty, bondage or indebtedness. Over the 150 or so years of British colonialism, Ooi estimates that 14.5 million of around 17 million Chinese migrants were repatriated.[4] Even so, the population expanded rapidly, in Singapore almost doubling from 1881–1901 as the city established itself as the administrative, financial and commercial capital. In the Federated Malay States (hereafter FMS) of Pahang, Negri Sembilan, Perak and Selangor too, the population expanded rapidly as a result of migration.

Most of these migrants were men who had left their wives and children at home. In the Straits Settlement in 1871, the ratio of men to women was approximately 2:1; in Singapore in the Chinese community, the ratio was 6:1.[5] This imbalance continued, and where workers were concentrated there were approximately ten men to one woman. Intermarriage with local Malay women was relatively uncommon because of religious rules (i.e. men were expected to convert to Islam if they wished to marry Malay women), and there was no excess of local women in any case. The demography predetermined prostitution; under colonialism, prostitution flourished.

COLONIAL SEXUALITY

Colonial attitudes and policies towards prostitution were based on contemporary views of human sexuality and 'normal' masculinity, together with the pragmatic consequences of a colonial migration policy that recruited only men and the need to provide the workforce with recreational sex. Hyam has argued that for expatriates, sexual adventure was one of the few palliatives to the privations of foreign postings, and the distance between home and outpost, hence from social, moral and familial restrictions, gave British soldiers and administrators maximum opportunity for latitude and experiment.[6] This was so in the Settlements and the FMS, where British colonial staff, naval and ground troops, planters and company representatives took local women as mistresses, partnered their houseboys, and visited brothels as matters of routine. The health costs of this were no deterrent, and the venereal disease clinic in Kuala Lumpur was referred to as 'the other club'.

Hutchinson's description of prostitution in Kuala Lumpur in the 1920s captures something of the social and racial geography of the enterprise.[7] The Chinese brothels were located in High Street and Petaling Street, and had open fronts through which potential clients might view women 'painted thick with rouge and powder'.[8]

> Further down the Batu Road was 'the Malay kip-shop,' a huge ramshackle building presided over by 'moma,' a very fat jolly Malay woman – here you could get a cold beer or a Malay girl if you wanted one. Nearby was the 'Siamese house' with the Siamese girls . . . In the Batu Road and in Petaling St. and further on near the Princes Cinema were the more superior Japanese Hotels, wher(e) you could get Beer and almost any race of girl . . . [9]

Hutchinson's account notes that Chinese prostitutes were patronised by Chinese miners and planters, while women from other nationalities – Thai, Malay, European (often Jewish women from Eastern Europe) and Japanese women – provided entertainment and sex mainly for Europeans. There were also some Tamil women, who may have primarily worked with Indian plantation labourers or merchants; and some Japanese women who were patronised by Chinese men.[10]

The 'traffic' in women and venereal disease were always public issues and intermittently subjects of public debates from the 1870s to the 1940s.[11] Controversies concerned the legal status of prostitution and revealed its contradictions in colonial Malaya: the gross disparity of the sexes on the one hand, and moral issues on the other, in which questions of health and sickness tended to be embedded. Women in the brothels were routinely represented as vectors of venereal disease 'reeking with infection', but at the same time they were seen to provide an essential service within the colony to cater for men's natural sexual 'appetite'. According to Sir Frank Swettenham, writing to the Colonial Secretary of the Straits Settlements in 1891, '(n)ature endows men with desires and impulses without regard to their means of gratifying them', thus, without the possibility of marriage, these had to be met by prostitution or 'by unnatural and abominable vices'.[12] The Reverend W. G. Shellabear, giving evidence in 1894 to a Committee appointed by the Governor of the Straits Settlements to enquire into contagious diseases and brothels, held that 'unnatural vice' was the lesser sin: 'It seems to me more horrible for wicked men to ruin innocent young girls than that wicked men should ruin each other.'[13] This was a minority view in the 1890s; the dominant view was that male 'desires and impulses' needed to be 'gratified' and that, in the absence of sufficient women as wives, prostitutes supplied a 'public want' and were 'a necessary evil, to save us from something worse'.[14] Part of the argument for improving the physical conditions of the brothel buildings and ensuring the health of women working in the brothels was that 'intelligent Chinamen descend(ed) to forms of unnatural vice' rather than patronise the brothels which they regarded as 'centres of loathsome disease'.[15] The state regulations spoke of responsibilities in three areas: the protection of prostitutes 'irrespective of . . . the nature of their calling', the protections of those 'naturally driven to resort to the brothels', and the protection – by preventing congenital syphilis – of the unborn child.[16]

The alternative was to encourage greater numbers of women to immigrate, to encourage family formation, and so to provide for both sexual needs and other personal needs. Evidence before the Commission of Enquiry into the State of Labour in the Straits Settlements and Protected Native States in 1891 indicated that some estate employers limited the number of women, regarding them as both inferior labour and a diversion from work for male workers. However, this was not usual practice. Tamil men often migrated with their families, and the Commission felt that the presence of women, working also as tappers or labourers, 'rendered the (male) coolies more contented and willing to remain on the estates'.[17] The relatively larger proportion of women within the Indian community, plus the confinement of Indian men on often isolated rural estates, and their general penury compared with Chinese men, arguably contributed to a lower demand for prostitution. The sources are silent on the sexual behaviour of Tamil men. By contrast, Chinese men, who were not inclined to immigrate with their families, maintained a steady demand for brothels, and, Hyam suggests, 'famously knew how to take care of sexual needs without women anyway'.[18] The high incidence of anal syphilis reported among Hainanese houseboys would seem to support this, and official commentary is interesting in its silence on whether the infections were from other Chinese men or Europeans.[19]

Those who argued for legislation to control brothels maintained that (hetero)sexual desire was natural and that prostitution was an appropriate channelling of such desire, considering the demographic imbalance.[20] Those favouring regulation of brothels and prostitutes argued also that, among the Chinese, the institutionalisation of prostitution was 'cultural'; that is, they adopted a stance of cultural relativism that held that the practice of prostitution and the presence of brothel houses was a 'normal' aspect of Chinese society, a matter of 'Chinese character'.[21] This was not an argument extended to British colonial officials. Swettenham, however, opened up this possibility by arguing that morality was relative, 'dependent on influences of climate, religious belief, education and the feeling of society'.[22] Witnesses to the 1898 Committee of Enquiry held that most brothels were owned by 'well-to-do and respectable Chinese'. Racial character and cultural environment were understood to produce a range of behaviours: both Straits-born and immigrant Chinese accepted the brothel as a legitimate social institution, Indians allegedly did not value 'chastity as chastity', and even Europeans in Singapore, whilst they 'would not like their sisters or mothers to be engaged in prostitution', had few objections to it 'in the abstract'.[23]

These views were held relatively consistently to the 1920s, when it was still being argued that 'the Asiatic and Anglican points of view on questions of morality are wide as the poles apart'[24] and that 'the Asiatic does not recognise promiscuous intercourse as sin or vice . . . he sees no wrong of any kind in hiring casually as his inclinations dictate'.[25] Subsequently there was a change in opinion within government circles and, as reflected in the press in response to pressure from the League of Nations, from British reformers and others campaigning against venereal disease and the traffic in women.[26] However, the shift was not unilateral and the impact of the prohibition of brothels in 1930 in the Settlements, and 1931 in the FMS, was tempered by the growth of so-called 'sly' prostitution, casual soliciting and an increase of small boarding houses, coffee shops and other venues for commercial sex. There was also an apparent increase in venereal disease in the mid-1930s coincident with the upturn in the economic cycle; after all 'economic imposed abstinence and self-denial (were) potent deterrents for indulgence in vice'.[27]

PROSTITUTION IN THE COLONIES

The colonial government, I have suggested, was relatively casual about the practice of prostitution, but it did feel responsible for protecting young girls, providing women with ways to leave prostitution, and minimising the risk of venereal infection, particularly among British troops. In these objectives it appeared to have enjoyed the support of the wider community, and complaints about prostitution as such were relatively rare until the 1920s when external pressure led to its suppression.

We know most about the backgrounds of the Japanese and Chinese women who migrated to the colonies. The women from both these countries who ended up in the brothels came from families impoverished through recurrent floods, famines and poor harvests.[28] Cantonese and Teochiu families from Southeast China sold their daughters to brothel agents. Some women were tricked rather than sold into prostitution, with the promise of marriage or work as nurses, seamstresses, hairdressers or servants, and, with the promise of relatively good pay on arrival, would take on a loan of $50 to $100 to cover their passage. They were then forced into prostitution to repay their debts.[29] Other women were recruited openly as prostitutes. In most cases the women were auctioned to Southeast Asian traders in Hong Kong, who determined from which port they were sold on to local brothel owners, or secret societies from towns in the Straits Settlements and towns and mining camps in the FMS.[30] They were then held captive by the brothel keeper whilst they remained indebted for their 'original purchase price', the subsequent costs of their passage, food, lodging, loans for medicine and clothing, and 'everything else that the ingenuity of their masters could think of'.[31] Local women were sometimes also purchased by brothel owners to be trained as prostitutes, and others were born in the brothels or brought into them as the adopted infants, daughters or younger sisters of the brothel keepers in Malaya, or procurers in Hong Kong.

This account suggests that women had little control in decisions about entering into and remaining in prostitution. Whilst there is evidence that some Japanese women were willing agents in their migration, this does appear to be far less the case for Chinese women. Hershatter estimates that only 5 per cent of women in Shanghai brothels entered as 'free persons' able to control their own work, and most had been either mortgaged or sold outright to the brothel owner by their families or traffickers.[32] In colonial Malaya, Lai argues that the number of independent workers was also low and that these women still paid protection money to secret society members, and yielded half their earnings to brothel keepers for food, lodging, use of premises and the supply of clients.[33] Differences in recruitment to some extent shaped access to resources. Women reared as 'daughters' by the brothel keeper had no access to money earned. Those who had come on assisted passages, for whom freedom was technically a possibility, worked to discharge their debts; others paid room rent to the brothel keeper, but had control over at least some of their earnings. Other women worked privately with a degree of autonomy.[34] Women sold to brothel keepers were effectively enslaved and could be released only if bought.[35]

Large numbers of women were involved in prostitution as brothel keepers and brothel prostitutes, 'sly' prostitutes, taxi-girls, singers, dancers and waitresses, working especially in the three commercial and administrative centres of the Settlements, in Kuala Lumpur and

Ipoh in the tin-rich states of the FMS, and in smaller towns near mines. Women confined in brothels worked exclusively as prostitutes, but others supplemented low incomes with the occasional sale of sex. However, official accounts of prostitution, excepting when concerned with pimps and the clients, write always of women and always of full-time prostitutes in brothels. The discourses around prostitution, legislation, government policies and practices operate on this understanding, despite the well-known traffic in boys and the complex nature of the sex trade.[36]

Estimates of the numbers of women working as prostitutes are crude and based on registration figures, cases of STD, or both. Several thousand women, registered under the Contagious Disease Ordinance (1870–87), worked in brothels in Singapore in the later nineteenth century; large numbers continued to work in brothels until the 1920s, untouched by the legislation.[37] Several hundred women were registered with or known to authorities in the other settlements.[38] Until 1894 women were registered in the FMS with the Chinese Protector, and then registered under the provisions of the Women and Girls Protection Enactment.[39] Official figures, which may be unreliable, suggested around 5,500 women worked as prostitutes around the mid-1890s.[40] According to Warren these figures are probably an underestimation, and the real number was perhaps nearer 10,000. These figures are sustained in estimates for the early twentieth century, and whilst Hyam perhaps exaggerates when he writes that any town in the FMS large enough to have a post office had a brothel, prostitution was certainly common.[41]

Prostitution and the traffic in women and girls was subject, in varying ways, to legislative provisions and administrative procedures. A Contagious Diseases Ordinance operated in the Straits Settlements between 1872 and 1887. During this period brothels were registered and inspected periodically for conditions of hygiene and sanitation and to check on the presence of children (3–15 years). Brothel keepers were subject to fines for breaches of the regulations.

Women were subject to routine medical examinations for venereal disease, with the intention of protecting British soldiers and sailors from infection.[42] Japanese and other women were examined on a weekly basis, admitted to the Lock Hospital when indicated, and issued with health cards; they were said to be reasonably co-operative with the regulations relating to medical examinations. Chinese women and brothel owners were less compliant with examinations, and to some degree circumvented them by substituting brothel servants for prostitutes. Identity cards with photographs were introduced to identify women for examination, registration and surveillance. After a period of considerable antagonism between brothel owners and police, medical examinations commenced, though they were conducted in a perfunctory fashion and only once a month, therefore they had limited public health merit.[43] None the less, as can be seen below, the rise in the rates of venereal disease after the repeal of mandatory medical inspection in the late 1880s, suggests that even perfunctory examinations helped hold down infection rates in Singapore and the Straits Settlements.

From the time of the introduction of the Ordinance in the Straits Settlements, however, 'moral reformers, feminists, missionaries and civil libertarians' lobbied for the repeal of the Acts in Britain and succeeded in 1886.[44] The repeal was extended to the colonies at the close of the following year and the registration of prostitutes had been phased out by 1894. Thereafter, women were expected to present voluntarily for medical treatment. The impact was predictable and 'devastating': the incidence of syphilis, gonorrhoea and other venereal infections escalated rapidly.[45] Statistics are poor and the best figures are of hospital admissions of clinical cases, but they indicate a steady increase of cases among both Chinese and British troops. For example, the number of admissions for venereal disease among the Singapore Garrison increased from 123 per thousand admissions in 1884 to 567 in 1896.[46] Admissions to the Pauper Hospital, gaol, lunatic asylum and General Hospital showed similar rates of increase of infection for both secondary and tertiary syphilis.

Under pressure from the Straits Settlements Association, the colonial government found a technical means to reintroduce surveillance without reinstating the offending legislation. They gave the Chinese Protectorate discretionary powers to control brothels under provisions of the Women and Girls Protection Ordinance. At the same time, the medical profession introduced more medical clubs for routine examinations and treatment of infected women working in brothels. These clubs operated in both the Settlements and the FMS, and they were the primary and often sole source of medical care for brothel women.

The incidence of venereal diseases did not decline dramatically after these changes. Figures are disparate, incomplete, derived from clinical cases, and not aggregated except in the case of death, but they suggest that STD remained an important cause of morbidity (though not mortality) over the next several decades.[47] It is difficult, therefore, to gain an accurate picture of the epidemiological significance of

STD. However, annual medical reports indicate its general effect on community health. Among poor patients admitted to the Tan Tock Seng Hospital in Singapore in 1907, the primary causes of admission were, in order of importance, malaria, syphilis, beri-beri, dysentery, and tuberculosis; 21 per cent of all cases were of syphilis. In the General Hospital in Singapore, 5 per cent of admissions in 1907 were for venereal diseases, but these were wealthier patients than those at Tan Tock Seng Hospital, and others may have been treated privately. In the General Hospital in Malacca in 1907, syphilis and vulva ulcers combined exceeded all other causes of admission and represented 14 per cent of all admissions; at the District Hospital in Penang, 37 per cent of all admissions were for venereal disease.[48]

In the FMS, the number of cases admitted to hospitals with venereal diseases appears low compared with the Settlements, but was probably due less to a lower incidence of disease than to the reluctance of Chinese women and men to present for care.[49] Brothels were registered, and in Perak money generated from licence fees and prostitutes' registration fees were used to establish and maintain a home for 'indigent and decrepit Chinese', with a Lock Hospital attached to it to treat prostitutes.[50] However, compulsory medical examination of prostitutes and compulsory detention of patients with venereal disease was never enforced. The argument against regulation centred on the possibility that such surveillance would drive Chinese women from the state, 'seriously affect(ing) the Chinese male population'.[51]

In the 1890s, colonial officials were struck not only by the increased incidence and transmission of venereal disease, but by the difficulty of controlling it and with the general poor health of prostitutes. Swettenham, writing in 1898 of Perak, said that 'the condition of prostitutes in the Malay States now is probably worse than it has ever been', and that women were 'dealt with by their owners without the smallest reference to the health, comfort or wishes of the women whom they hold [in the] vilest form of slavery'.[52] Hare, then Secretary for Chinese Affairs in the FMS, associated this with the repeal of compulsory registration and argued that, in the FMS as well as the Settlements, the brothels had fallen into a 'disgraceful state' and 'their sanitary conditions (had) immensely deteriorated'. In addition, the women and girls in them were described as being 'absolute slaves' and grossly ill-treated.[53] It was also argued that legislation governing infectious disease was inadequate to control venereal disease, because of the propensity of brothel keepers not to provide treatment for infection and forcing infected women to continue to work.[54]

Until the abolition of brothels and the beginning of moves to suppress prostitution, the solution to the spread of venereal disease was diagnosis and treatment, and the primary means of reducing disease was to increase patient access to care. This was largely effected through medical clubs, established from the late nineteenth century to provide routine examinations for women working in brothels. The initiatives taken to ensure the health of the prostitutes also worked to the advantage of the doctors who established the clubs and enjoyed retainers to provide the inspections and treatment.

BROTHEL SUPERVISION AND VENEREAL DISEASE

I have suggested that there is fragmentary evidence of the health of prostitutes and the incidence and effects of STD amongst them. In contrast, there is plenty of detail on the incidence of STD amongst troops, telling us more about the sympathies and concerns of the colonial authorities than about the epidemiology of venereal disease. It was reported, for example, that 'thousands of young men are ruined through sheer innocence' and

> an immoral woman may be known to be reeking with infection, and almost every man who has anything to do with her may become a new centre of infection. The woman is a public danger but there is no power to isolate her and put an end to the mischief she is doing . . . *one impure woman infects scores of pure men.*[55]

Further, although prostitution was rationalised in terms of the demographic imbalance amongst the Chinese, the victims of venereal infection were predominantly characterised as European. Hence, it was argued that, 'It is an intolerable idea to permit our own flesh and blood to contract infection from the lowest scum of Asia (the Chinese consider many of these women fit for coolies and rickshaw pullers only).'[56] The incidence of venereal disease amongst ground troops in the Tanglin district of Singapore, for instance, escalated once the compulsory medical examination of prostitutes ceased with the repeal in 1887 of the Contagious Disease Ordinance. Yet even during the final five-year period of the operation of the Ordinance, 144 per thousand men admitted to hospital had venereal disease, primarily gonorrhoea. From 1892 to 1896, without legislation, the average rate of admissions rose nearly threefold to 434 per 1,000 men, of whom two-thirds now had syphilis.[57] Estimates for the Navy show rates increased by around 50 per cent per annum once compulsory examinations and treatment ceased; this was also the case for men in prison.[58] Figures of infection for other populations were said to be even higher; Hare – who as Protector of the Chinese was concerned with the non-European population – estimated in 1898 that the incidence of gonorrhoea and syphilis among Hainanese servants ('houseboys') was around 60 per cent.[59]

Doctors were better placed to speak of infections among men – prisoners, troops, coolies and Pauper Hospital inmates – than women, although they regarded the latter as the 'chief disseminators of disease'.[60] In 1898, the Colonial Surgeon, Dr Mugliston, estimated that all of the 3,000 prostitutes working in Singapore were or had been infected, and that the majority at any time were unfit to work but were coerced to continue by the brothel keeper. Others shared his view that all women were infected at one time or another, those worst affected were said to have been brought 'second-hand' from Singapore to the FMS to continue working there.[61] As a result, the incidence of venereal disease was also believed to have increased in the FMS.[62]

The brothels were regarded as reservoirs of reinfection, women prostitutes as vectors, men – and especially European men – as their victims. Brothel workers were not the only source of infection in the colony, transmission amongst men as well as between men and other women was not uncommon. The incidence of anal syphilis in domestic servants and urban labourers was never cited in calls for a new Contagious Disease Ordinance, no doubt because of the difficulties of introducing interventions, because of unease about the public acknowledgement of homosexual practice, and because of the assumption that a fellow worker was a poor alternative to a female sexual partner. Hence, government control of venereal infection focused on the inspection of women to assure clients that they had a 'clean' bill of health.

The argument for the reintroduction of an Ordinance to ensure the compulsory medical examination of women prostitutes was premised on the belief that any voluntary system would fail. It was said that women would neither use hospitals nor accept medical help, that they were afraid of medicine, had an 'innate aversion' to examination, resisted more than perfunctory examinations, and were reluctant to go to a hospital except to die. In addition, medical examinations tended to be perfunctory regardless of women's attitudes towards them. In the 1890s, Chinese prostitutes were examined about once a month. A doctor might examine between 110 to 120 women per hour, the examination would consist of a check on whether the glands in their groin were enlarged as an indication of venereal infection. The view of the state surgeon, Dr Travers, was that these inspections were a 'farce'.[63] However, the committee appointed by the Governor of the Straits Settlements in 1898 to consider measures to check the spread of venereal diseases questioned the validity of these arguments, suggesting instead that Chinese women were indifferent rather than opposed to examination. Their report supported a formal system of examination and care, not because of women's reluctance to receive attention, but because this would be the most effective way of working around the restraints placed upon them: 'the largest proportion of women (had) absolutely no voice in any matter in connection with their own lives and thus any attempt to reach them as individuals whilst they remain working in a brothel would be useless'.[64] Dr Rogers and Dr Mugliston, the Colonial Surgeon, also argued that the major reason for delayed treatment was constraints on women's mobility by brothel keepers.[65]

Moral objections to the reintroduction of regulation – both because of the implied condoning of prostitution and because it was 'an indecent outrage . . . to examine a person's private parts' – led to consideration of non-legislative means of surveillance and medical treatment for prostitutes.[66] None the less, the majority of doctors and colonial officers in the Settlements and FMS wanted a return to legislation, claiming that the Ordinance had been repealed on the basis of English moral objections that had failed to take account of the realities of social and sexual life in the colonies. There was in addition a growing feeling that only legislative measures would overcome the resistance of the brothel keepers, a belief shared among prominent Chinese members of the community as well as European officials.

The first step towards reintroduction came in 1896 when the Women and Girls Protection Ordinance was introduced. This aimed to prevent the procuring, receipt, harbouring or use for prostitution of women under the age of 16, and provided state protection of women held against their wishes in brothels or imported without their agreement or foreknowledge to work as prostitutes. The Ordinance was broadened in 1899 to make it illegal for a brothel keeper to employ a woman with venereal disease as a prostitute. Before its introduction, officers of the Chinese Protectorate met with brothel keepers to explain the implications of the legislation; since brothel keepers were to be held responsible for disease in their brothels, they were advised to retain the services of qualified medical men to visit the brothels, inspect the women and arrange for those with serious infection to be treated at a private hospital or the government Lock Hospital.[67] Most brothel keepers of large establishments responded by employing their own doctor, while others arranged for medical inspection by a government practitioner, who provided medical care to the brothels in addition to undertaking his official duties.[68] Outpatient attendance at government hospitals also increased.

THE BROTHEL CLUBS

It had been common for doctors to be summoned only when venereal disease was advanced and, in general, brothel keepers resisted house calls and the inspection of their 'girls'.[69] However, a limited number of Japanese and Chinese brothels in Singapore, Penang and the FMS had employed doctors in the nineteenth century, and from the turn of the century, following the amendments to the Women and Girls Protection Ordinance in the Settlements and the FMS, a number of private hospitals for prostitutes, run by government employed medical practitioners, proliferated. Brothel keepers often shared the costs of retaining a doctor, and rented a house in the neighbourhood to use as a hospital to examine and treat brothel workers. Severely sick women were sent to the Lock Hospitals.[70]

The success of the private medical clubs attracted government employed doctors, who took advantage of the right to private practice to establish contracts with brothels. In 1903, two private Lock Hospitals were operating in Kuala Lumpur, Selangor, one run by Dr Travers.[71] Medical fees varied: in Kuala Lumpur medical club membership was $1 per month for each woman (cf. a daily wage of a labourer of about 25c); in Perak it was $2, but this included two examinations, treatment for any medical condition and free medicine.

The examinations provided through these arrangements were hastily conducted and usually involved a visual check of genitalia or, more often, a cursory glance at the woman's general appearance and a quick feel of her groin through her clothes. Quality of care varied. Under the provisions of the brothel clubs operating in the Kinta district of Perak, for example, Japanese women were examined routinely, but Chinese women were neither visited at the brothels nor examined regularly, and their examinations were perfunctory. According to Dr Cooper, who ran a brothel practice:

> I never visited the brothels. Once a month I used to send round to a particular brothel and say I would like to see the inmates at the

> private hospital: they would come forward one by one, and I examined the skin of the legs, thighs, abdomen, hands and feet and inguinal glands through the clothes, and the throat if necessary . . . To examine a dozen women it would take, as I did it, more or less a half an hour.[72]

Dr Wright, State Surgeon of Perak, argued that a full medical examination had to be both internal and external to identify disease, while other doctors argued that this would discourage Chinese (although apparently not Japanese or Indian) women from voluntarily joining a medical club.[73] Gimlette, who ran a private hospital in Ipoh, Perak, argued against government officers taking a fee for service, since it was impossible for them to examine thoroughly 400 women twice a month without neglecting their government duties.[74]

Private brothel practice was highly lucrative, causing a 'scramble for a share of it' by medical doctors.[75] This led to a series of enquiries into the role of doctors in soliciting patients, profiteering and exploiting their position as state employees for pecuniary advantage. Within a few years there had been an enquiry into the activities of Dr Travers in Selangor, and several senior medical officers in Perak. These included the Kinta 'case', a series of related legal and ethical enquiries into the medical practices of Drs Fox, Cooper and Brown, and an enquiry into the 'Connolly Campaign', involving state employed doctors and the State Resident, which was aimed at establishing monopolies in brothel areas of the state. The findings of the enquiries led to a prohibition on medical officers participating in brothel practices from September 1907, and thereafter they could only attend women unable to present to hospital if no other private practitioner were available. In addition, government medical officers were no longer allowed to attend or inspect brothels regularly, and were to have no financial interest in private hospitals or practices.[76] Brothels were subsequently notified that it was not necessary to retain a medical attendant and that examinations, treatment and drugs were freely available at government hospitals.

CONCLUSION

The problems venereal disease posed to the British colonial authorities revealed one of the contradictions of colonialism in Malaya. While economic policy encouraged prostitution and the spread of sexually transmitted disease, military and moral fears demanded its regulation. In other respects, however, medicine served a role under imperialism as a cultural agent;[77] in this context, without either moral power or adequate technical (pharmaceutical) fixes, doctors were still able both to police and to legitimise the brothels, and, for a while, to profit personally from the practice of prostitution and the need for surveillance.

Smart has characterised the nineteenth century as a period of regulation influenced by medical understandings of venereal disease and the role of individuals in its transmission, which highlighted women's uncontrolled sexuality.[78] In colonial Malaya, women's sexuality was not at issue, and women were systematically represented as objects, there to meet men's 'needs'. This did not reduce the need for regulation, of course. Legislative control (therefore also acknowledgement of prostitution) extended into the 1920s, and it was only then, under pressure from the League of Nations and social hygienists within the United Kingdom, that moves were made to suppress prostitution by both closing brothels and changing immigration policy to encourage the immigration of women as wives.

In the late 1920s too, medical advances in the treatment of venereal disease, and particularly syphilis, allowed an energetic drive to reduce the incidence of disease. Until then, the Contagious Disease Ordinance and its later legislative analogues sought to regulate the body and construed certain bodies – those of women sex workers – as pathogenic. More precisely, women working as prostitutes were regarded as vectors of disease, and the controls that were set in place to diagnose and treat disease differed little in approach from the systems of surveillance that operated to maintain hygiene and sanitation and reduce the risk of other epidemic diseases.

Race and ethnicity entered into the equation partly because of the numbers – the majority of prostitutes were Chinese – and partly because the Chinese Protectorate, established to ensure the well-being of this community, was relatively vocal regarding the welfare of Chinese women. As a consequence, Tamil, Malay, Thai and European prostitutes were largely ignored in contemporary debates, and Japanese women were the subject of attention only in specific contexts and cases. If there was any broader stereotyping in official discourse, it was this: Japanese women served an elite (like wealthy Chinese and Europeans), they were 'clean', compliant with any regulations imposed, and took good care of their health; they therefore did not constitute a threat to public health. Tamil, Malay and Thai women worked as 'sly' prostitutes within their own communities, beyond possible state surveillance but also not requiring such surveillance, or they partnered with European men and were therefore subject to European 'norms' relating to infection control and hygiene. European (and Eurasian) women constituted an elite minority, working in the same environment and with the same clients as Japanese women, and their nationality ('European') encouraged official silence. Chinese women, in contrast, were problematic: they partnered with men from various races and classes, did not readily subject themselves to medical authority, and the brothel owners resisted colonial (police and medical) control. Implicitly rather than explicitly, colonial discourse about prostitution was also about Chinese women, and the status of Chinese women within Chinese and colonial society.

In colonial Malaya, men were represented as possessing 'natural' impulses and desires. Such urges were represented as 'naturally' heterosexual, but in the absence of women men might partner with other men. Prostitution provided an institutional answer to the absence of women, and a palliative for workers in a rapidly expanding economy. For political and economic reasons, prostitution needed to be controlled, although the threat, in the late nineteenth and early twentieth century, was not explained in terms of the impact of disease on men's productivity, but rather, that disease, the absence of women, or both, might affect men's willingness to come to and remain in the colonies. At the same time, the continued transmission of STD posed a threat to British rule, since troops, British settlers and colonial officers themselves were vulnerable. In this context, women's bodies were monitored and controlled, with ideas of race, sex and sexuality informing both the discourse and legislative apparatuses of the state.[79]

NOTES

1 British Malaya as a political domain included the Straits Settlements (Singapore, Penang, Malacca), the Federated and Unfederated Malay States and parts of Borneo, corresponding in the 1990s to Singapore, Peninsular Malaysia, Sabah and Sarawak. In this chapter, I discuss prostitution in the Straits Settlements and Peninsula Malay States only.

2 Straits Settlements, *Report of the Commissioners Appointed to Enquire into the State of Labour in the Straits Settlements and Protected Native States*, Singapore, 1891, p. 8.

3 M. Stenson, *Class, Race and Colonialism in West Malaysia*, St Lucia, 1980, pp. 15–18.

4 Ooi Jin Bee, *Land, People and Economy in Malaya*, London, 1963, p. 13. See also V.W.W.S. Purcell, *The Chinese in Malaya*, London, 1948. R.J. Pryor, *Migration and Development in South-East Asia: A Demographic*

Perspective, Kuala Lumpur, 1979, p. 79, similarly notes constant movement of people together with the swelling of absolute numbers: 4 million Indians entered Malaya between 1860 and 1957, nearly 3 million left the country in the same period, and of the 1.5 million Chinese entering between 1911 and 1921, almost two-thirds returned to China.

5 J.F.A. McNair, C.B. Waller and A. Knight, *Straits Settlements: Census Reports and Returns*, London, 1873.

6 R. Hyam, *Empire and Sexuality: The British Experience*, Manchester, 1990.

7 G. Hutchinson, 'Rubber Planting in Malaya, 1928–1932', n.d., Files of the British Association of Malaya, BAM III/15, Library of the Commonwealth Society, London.

8 S. Garon, 'The World's Oldest Debate? Prostitution and the State in Imperial Japan, 1900–1945', *American Historical Review*, 1993, 98/3, pp. 717–18.

9 Hutchinson, 'Rubber Planting in Malaya', pp. 41–3.

10 S. Sone, 'The Karayuki-san of Asia 1868–1938: The Role of Prostitutes Overseas in Japanese Economic and Social Development', *Review of Indonesian and Malayan Affairs*, 1992, 26/2, pp. 44–62; J.F. Warren, *At the Edge of Southeast Asian History: Essays*, Quezon City, 1987; idem, 'Prostitution and the Politics of Venereal Disease: Singapore, 1870–98', *Journal of Southeast Asian Studies*, 1990, 21/2, pp. 360–83.

11 Warren, 'Prostitution and the Politics of Venereal Disease'; J.F. Warren, 'Prostitution in Singapore Society and the *Karayuki-san*', in P.J. Rimmer and L.M. Allen, eds, *The Underside of Malaysian History: Pullers, Prostitutes, Plantation Workers . . .* , Singapore, 1990; idem, *Ah-Ku and Karayuki-san: Prostitution in Singapore, 1870–1940*, Singapore and New York, 1993.

12 Great Britain, *Contagious Diseases Regulations (Perak and Malay States), Copy of Correspondence Relative to Proposed Introduction of Contagious Diseases Regulations in Perak or other Protected Malay States, H. C. 146*, London, 1894, p. 10. Swettenham was appointed Assistant Colonial Secretary for Native States 1876–1882, and in 1882 was appointed as Resident of Selangor. In 1896 he became the first Resident-General of the FMS, and subsequently the High Commissioner for the Protected Malay States and Governor of the Straits Settlements. Like a number of other colonial officials, Swettenham's contribution was literary as well as administrative, see F. Swettenham, *Malay Sketches*, London, 1896; and idem, *The Real Malay: Pen Pictures*, London, 1900.

13 Great Britain, *Correspondence Regarding the Measures to be Adopted for Checking The Spread of Venereal Disease, Ceylon, Hong Kong and Straits Settlements, H. C. 147, June 1894, C. 9523*, London, 1899, p. 75.

14 A.H. Capper, Memorandum on Registration of Chinese Prostitutes in the Federated Malay States, 6 April 1900, Files of the Colonial Office (hereafter CO), C0273/261/1900, pp. 9, 21; Great Britain, *Contagious Diseases Regulations*, p. 7.

15 E.A.O. Travers, Memorandum by the State Surgeon, Selangor, May 1897, in Great Britain, *Correspondence*, London, 1899, p. 90.

16 Great Britain, *Contagious Diseases Regulations*, p. 10.

17 Straits Settlements, *Report of the Commissioners*, pp. 51, 66–7.
18 Hyam, *Empire and Sexuality*, p. 143.
19 For some comment on homosexuality in British Malaya, see J.G. Butcher, *The British in Malaya 1880–1941: The Social History of a European Community in Colonial South-East Asia*, Kuala Lumpur, 1979.
20 Proposed legislation was directed towards controlling hygiene and sanitation conditions in brothels, providing legal mechanisms to search brothels for under-age girls, and examining prostitutes for signs of infection.
21 CO273/261/1900, 324.
22 Great Britain, *Contagious Diseases Regulations*, p. 10.
23 Great Britain, *Correspondence*, p. 71.
24 *Straits Times*, Editorial, 25 May 1921; also *Straits Times*, Editorial, 19 January 1921.
25 *Straits Times*, Editorial, 13 January 1921.
26 L. Fishbein, 'Harlot or Heroine? Changing Views of Prostitution, 1870–1920', *The Historian*, 1980, 43/1, pp. 23–35; B.A. Towers, 'Health Education Policy 1916–1926: Venereal Disease and the Prophylaxis Dilemma', *Medical History*, 1980, 24/1, pp. 70–87; P. Weindling, 'The Politics of International Co-ordination to Combat Sexually Transmitted Diseases, 1900–1980s', in V. Berridge and P. Strong, eds, *Aids in Contemporary History*, Cambridge, 1993.
27 M. Chambers, 'The Social Hygiene Campaign in Singapore', *Health and Empire*, 1938, 13/3, pp. 220, 225.
28 Sone, 'The Karayuki-san of Asia 1868–1938'; Garon, 'The World's Oldest Debate', p. 714; B. Mihalopoulos, 'The Making of Prostitutes: The *Karayuki-san*', *Bulletin of Concerned Asian Scholars*, 1993, 25/1, pp. 41–56; J.M. Ramseyer, 'Indentured Prostitution in Imperial Japan: Credible Commitments in the Commercial Sex Industry', *The Journal of Law, Economics and Organization*, 1991, 7/1, pp. 89–116; Sone, 'The Karayuki-san of Asia 1868–1938'; Warren, 'Prostitution in Singapore Society'.
29 Great Britain, *Correspondence*, p. 79; Federated Malay States, *Memorandum on the Protection of Chinese and other Asiatic Women and Girls*, Selangor, 1900, p. 1. The daily wage paid to male Chinese labourers in 1900 was 15–40 cents; a 'houseboy' or cook earned *c.*\$10–\$15 per month. Women usually earned less than men.
30 Lai Ah Eng, *Peasants, Proletarians and Prostitutes. A Preliminary Investigation into The Work of Chinese Women in Colonial Malaya*, Singapore, 1986, p. 28.
31 Great Britain, *Correspondence*, p. 6.
32 S. Gronewold, *Beautiful Merchandise: Prostitution in China 1860–1926*, New York, 1982; G. Hershatter, 'The Hierarchy of Shanghai Prostitution, 1870–1949', *Modern China*, 1989, 15/4, p. 476.
33 Lai, *Peasants, Proletarians and Prostitutes*, p. 70; Purcell, *The Chinese in Malaya*.
34 Federated Malay States, *Memorandum*, pp. 3–4.
35 Lai, *Peasants, Proletarians and Prostitutes*, pp. 29–30; Hershatter, 'The Hierarchy of Shanghai Prostitution', p. 477.
36 S.E. Nicoll-Jones, 'Report on the Problem of Prostitution in Singapore',

Colonial Records Project, Mss Indian Ocean S27, 1940, p. 17, Rhodes House Library, Oxford.

37 Warren, 'Prostitution and the Politics of Venereal Disease'.

38 Sone, 'The Karayuki-san of Asia 1868–1938', pp. 47, n.4, 56; *Warren, Ah-Ku and Karayuki-san*; CO273/2258, f.41.

39 CO273/261/1900.

40 Great Britain, *Contagious Diseases Regulations*, p. 6; Great Britain, *Correspondence*, p. 68; Files of the Selangor Secretariat (hereafter Sel. Sec.) 375/1886, f.4., Sel. Sec. 4434/1893.

41 Hyam, *Empire and Sexuality*, p. 109.

42 Warren, 'Prostitution and the Politics of Venereal Disease', p. 363.

43 Warren, in 'Prostitution and the Politics of Venereal Disease', p. 365, writes that '(a)fter threatening the law, possible riots, boycotts, the closing of shops, and making extraordinary scenes throwing down their licence boards, dancing on the floor with wooden clogs, and shouting furiously, they ultimately gave in to the measure'.

44 Warren, 'Prostitution and the Politics of Venereal Disease', p. 367.

45 Ibid., pp. 372–5.

46 Ibid., p. 374.

47 Case fatality from syphilis was relatively low, around 1 per cent of clinical cases, compared with around 30 per cent from malaria in the early twentieth century, and up to 50 per cent from tuberculosis, depending on the hospital.

48 Straits Settlements, *Annual Departmental Reports for 1907*, Singapore, 1909.

49 Great Britain, *Contagious Diseases Regulations*, p. 9; Selangor, 'Annual Report of the Medical Department for the Year 1905', 1906, Sel. Sec. P/KES/B.1, f.6.

50 Great Britain, *Contagious Diseases Regulations*, p. 8.

51 Great Britain, *Contagious Diseases Regulations*, p. 9.

52 Great Britain, *Correspondence*, p. 81.

53 Ibid., p. 85.

54 Ibid., pp. 113–15.

55 *Straits Times*, Editorial, 24 January 1921; my emphasis.

56 *Straits Times*, Editorial, 25 May 1921, text in brackets in original.

57 Straits Settlements Association (SSA), Minute Book, 11 August 1887–21 February 1899, Adamson, Chairman of the SSA, to Chamberlain, Secretary of State for the Colonies, 8 November 1897, Table A.

58 This estimate of 50 per cent infection among prisoners was one sustained into the twentieth century, see e.g. CO273/270/34212/1901, f.245.

59 Great Britain, *Correspondence*, p. 87. This was largely said to be anal syphilis, the result, according to Adamson, Chair of the Straits Settlement Association, of a particularly skewed sex ratio (70 men : 1 woman) which led to 'a large recourse by these men to low brothels' and to 'the common practice of unnatural vice'.

60 Great Britain, *Correspondence*, p. 87, Memorandum by Dr J. Welch, District Surgeon, Selangor, 21 April 1897.

61 Great Britain, *Correspondence*, pp. 52–3, 87.

62 CO273/262/25598/1900, f.100, *Medical Report for Selangor, 1900*.

63 Sel. Sec. 1731/1903, E.A.O. Travers, State Surgeon, Selangor, Memorandum on private medical examination of inmates of brothels and establishment of private hospitals, 14 April 1903, p. 1.
64 Great Britain, *Correspondence*, pp. 55–6; also CO273/261, f.358, A.H. Capper, Acting Protector of Chinese, Memorandum, 6 April 1900.
65 Great Britain, *Correspondence*, p. 47.
66 Ibid., p. 73.
67 CO273/256/4829/1900.
68 CO273/256/4829/1900, ff.56–7.
69 Great Britain, *Correspondence*, p. 115.
70 CO273/339/G1121, FMS 9181/1908, f.230A, Evans, Chinese Protector in Singapore.
71 Sel. Sec. 1731/1903.
72 CO273/339/FMS 11053/1908, ff.270–1.
73 Sel. Sec. 1731/1903, f.4.
74 Ibid.
75 CO273/339/G1121/FMS 11053/1908, f.65, Brockman to High Commissioner, FMS, 6 January 1908, p. 4.
76 Sel. Sec. 5405/1907, Circular 20/1907 (Private Practice of Government Medical Officers), 27 September 1907.
77 R. MacLeod, 'Introduction', in R. MacLeod and M. Lewis, eds, *Disease, Medicine, and Empire. Perspectives on Western Medicine and the Experience of European Expansion*, London and New York, 1988, p. 1.
78 C. Smart, 'Disruptive Bodies and Unruly Sex: The Regulation of Reproduction and Sexuality in the Nineteenth Century', in C. Smart, ed., *Regulating Womanhood. Historical Essays on Marriage, Motherhood and Sexuality*, London and New York, 1992, p. 11.
79 Smart, 'Disruptive Bodies'.

4

RACIALISM AND INFANT DEATH

Late nineteenth- and early twentieth-century socio-medical discourses on African American infant mortality

Richard Meckel

During the latter half of the nineteenth and the initial third of the twentieth century, the United States (US) was the site of a socio-medical discourse on the prevailing rates of infant mortality, the causes of that mortality, and the various measures that could be adopted to reduce it. Beginning as part of urban sanitary reform (*c.*1850s–1870s), the discourse gradually grew in scope, culminating during the Progressive era (*c.*1900–20) in wide ranging public discussion and both philanthropic and government infant welfare activities aimed at saving the nation's babies.[1] Americans, of course, were not alone in discussing the rates and causes of infant mortality and in debating and implementing measures to reduce it. Almost every other industrialised nation saw similar infant welfare discussion and activity.[2] Yet US infant welfare was distinct in a number of ways. Among the most salient was the amount of attention given to race. Indeed, while in other nations the question of race was bound up with the debates over infant mortality, in the US it played a much more critical role as a descriptive and analytic category in the collection, organisation, and interpretation of data on the levels, trends and causes of infant death.[3]

THE TWO DISCOURSES

During the late nineteenth and early twentieth century, the US socio-medical discussion of race as a determinant of infant mortality was structured in two overlapping but essentially discrete discourses that, at least initially, were regionally distinct in evolution, foci and participants. One discourse, which was centred in the Northeast and industrialised Midwest of the US, was primarily concerned with infant mortality among foreign-born immigrants residing in cities and industrial towns. It was created and elaborated by a large and varied collection of nationally prominent urban public health officials, vital statisticians, philanthropists, child and social welfare workers and activists, and paediatricians and obstetricians. Extensively documented, this discourse and its related infant welfare activities has received wide attention from historians.[4] This is not surprising, for if measured in anything from the volume of rhetoric to the number of well baby stations, the northern, urban-centred baby-saving movement produced the vast majority of American efforts to improve infant welfare before the New Deal and the creation of a federal maternal and infant health programme under the Social Security Act of 1935.

Yet taking place at the same time was another socio-medical discourse on infant mortality which has largely remained invisible historically. Focusing on the causes and rates of death among African American infants, this discourse originated from racialist debates on the social, moral and health impact of emancipation and the consequent migration of blacks to southern cities. Much of it was dominated by the views of southern physicians and public health officials who, by virtue of the concentration of the African American population in the south, assumed a type of proprietary expertise in all matters relating to black morbidity and mortality. Frequently, and often somewhat condescendingly, they shared their assumed expertise with northern colleagues, publishing essays that promoted racialist sociology alongside clinical observation in the *Journal of the American Medical Association*, the *Journal of the American Public Health Association* and other national publications.

In addition to being much smaller in scope and initially dominated by socio-medical analysts from the south, the discourse on black infant mortality differed in other significant ways from the concurrent discourse on urban immigrant infant death. For instance, unlike urban immigrant infant mortality, which by the late nineteenth century had been singled out and given sharp definition as a specific public health problem in and of itself, black infant mortality continued to be discussed within the context of black health in general. Indeed, it was not until the late 1920s that socio-medical analyses of African American infant mortality, apart from overall African American mortality, began to appear in medical and public health publications as a separate issue. Similarly, the socio-medical discourse on black infant mortality was more heavily influenced by racial theories of social evolution. As a result, during the early decades of this century, discussion of black urban infant mortality centred on the disparity between white and black infant death rates and on whether or not that disparity was the consequence of heritable, race-specific traits. While scientific racism did penetrate the discourse on immigrant infant welfare, it dominated the discussion of urban black infant mortality. This lent the debate over the causes of black infant mortality a specific orientation. Whether environmentalist or racialist, all analysts of black infant mortality were compelled to confront the causal significance of racial inferiority.

NINETEENTH-CENTURY RACISM

That African Americans, and especially those migrating to cities, experienced extraordinarily high rates of mortality among their young, first elicited comment from socio-medical analysts during and immediately after the Civil War. In 1862, the year Abraham Lincoln issued a preliminary edict promising to free the slaves in the rebellious regions, Joseph Camp Kennedy, the Superintendent of the Census, predicted that emancipation would most likely bring about a dramatic increase in African American death rates resulting in the eventual extinction of the race. By the mid-1870s, reports published by the US Sanitary Commission and the US Surgeon General's Office, along with data presented in the 1870 census report on population, appeared to confirm the accuracy of Kennedy's prediction, showing a drop in the decennial rate of natural increase in the African American population.[5] A decade later, the 1880 census, although countering somewhat the impression that southern blacks were failing to reproduce their numbers, lent further support to the perception that migration from plantation to city was resulting in a dramatic increase in African American mortality and a widening gap between the death rates of southern whites and blacks. Moreover, it connected that widening gap to exceptionally high rates of infant mortality, especially among urban African Americans. Noting that cities seemed particularly deadly for black infants, John S. Billings, Surgeon of the Army and author of the 1880 Census 'Report on Mortality and Vital Statistics of the United States', flatly declared that 'this excess of infantile mortality in the colored race . . . is the main cause of the excess mortality of the colored race over the white'.[6] Billings was offering support for what was already suspected: that along with tuberculosis, the diseases and disorders of infancy were becoming epidemic among southern urban blacks. Two years before Billings' report was published, S. S. Herrick, a New Orleans physician and vital statistician, stood before the American Public Health Association and reported that it was well known among his southern colleagues that urban migration was resulting in sharp increases in death rates among blacks with the consequence that 'mortality among the African race in this country is much greater than among the European, especially in the periods of infancy and early childhood'.[7]

In offering an explanation for this apparent rise in mortality among the African American population, a few southern physicians and public health officials adopted a perspective consistent with the principles of sanitary reform increasingly being articulated by their colleagues in the urban north. Drawing on the vital records of the few southern cities with passable registration systems, they sought to demonstrate both the extent and causes of the excessive mortality among recent black urban migrants and to connect it to the insanitary conditions attending urban poverty. Pointing to the ill-ventilated dwellings and insanitary neighbourhoods into which the new migrants crowded, sanitarian-oriented analysts suggested that it was little wonder that African American mortality, and especially infant mortality, was on the rise.[8] For, as most medical opinion held, infants were particularly susceptible to the morbific influences of filth and impure air.[9] Indeed, one physician opined that if black urban migrants occupied sanitary dwellings and neighbourhoods and enjoyed the comforts of life their poverty denied them, their infants would face a risk of death not appreciably higher than that faced by urban white infants.[10]

This, however, was a minority view among southern physicians and health officials. More common, especially as the century came to an end, was the opinion that if mortality among black adults and infants was on the rise, it was so for reasons that had less to do with the environment and more to do with the physiological and behavioural traits inherent to the African race. Holding that biological deficiency was at the root of the increase in African American mortality, socio-medical racialists in the late nineteenth century constructed a narrative on black health organised around the theme that the major consequence of emancipation had been the physical and moral degeneration of the freed slaves and their descendants. In this narrative, they contended that the diseases that were killing urban blacks and their infants had not been present during slavery because of the relatively good health conditions maintained by plantation owners interested in protecting their workforce. It was only when blacks were removed from the enlightened oversight of their plantation masters and allowed to succumb to their base instincts that excessive adult and child mortality had developed.[11]

This narrative of post-emancipation physical degeneration among blacks was, of course, part of a larger historical revisionism propounded by racist ideologues to promote and justify the subjugation of African Americans within a racially defined caste system maintained by political disenfranchisement and Jim Crow laws. It also found crucial support in a long tradition of racist medical thinking about the biological inferiority and distinctiveness of African Americans which in the nineteenth century had been shaped and granted considerable legitimacy by the evolutionary theories that had increasingly dominated the social and natural sciences, and had as a major project detailing the differences between the races of humankind and explicating their origin and evolution.[12] Providing a central focus to physical anthropology and human biology, the subject of racial evolution elicited considerable debate in the nineteenth century, especially in regard to primordial origin, the mechanics of hereditary transmission and whether physical and temperamental traits acquired by parents during a lifetime could be passed on to offspring. Nevertheless, whether Lamarckian, Darwinian, or some variant, most nineteenth-century evolutionary theory held that the human races possessed distinct biological characteristics that were the result of evolutionary interaction with specific environments; that mental, moral and temperamental attributes were anatomically determined and thus phylogenetic; and that evolution was essentially linear and thus that the various races could be ranked hierarchically according to the social and biological distance each had travelled from its primordial condition.[13]

Drawing on evolutionary theory, particularly Spencerian Social Darwinism, promoters of the idea of post-emancipation African American degeneration characterised slavery as a form of artificial selection, protecting blacks from the natural selection that guaranteed the survival of a race or doomed it to perish. They argued that with the end of slavery, blacks were forced to exist without the protective assistance of their white masters; and ill-equipped to do so, necessarily now faced decline and perhaps extinction.[14] Indeed, many viewed the blacks like Indians, who were also seen to be a dying race.[15] Alongside this was the view that the African Americans were anatomically and physiologically distinct. Borrowing from the theories of ethnologists, southern socio-medical writers, for instance, contended that blacks were not only handicapped by underdeveloped moral and intellectual competencies – as evidenced by small craniums – but also by other racially distinct anatomical and physiological features, such as small lung size, greater susceptibility and different responses to certain diseases, and constitutions unsuited by evolution for survival in a non-tropical climate.[16] In accordance with these ideas, throughout the latter half of the nineteenth and into the early part of the twentieth century, southern physicians fostered the notion that African Americans, because of their anatomical and physiological difference from whites, required distinct medical measures.[17]

Although they dominated this discourse, southern physicians were not the only promoters of such views. Indeed, such beliefs were a central tenet of nineteenth-century American physical anthropology and were widely accepted in the north as well as in the south. Social Darwinists in the north, for example, accepted as a matter of principle that blacks were inferior to whites and that their inferiority, which was racially heritable, doomed them in the competition between races that was the social complement of natural selection.[18] Similarly, it was not just southern physicians and public health officials who, in examining the mortality records for blacks in their cities, concluded that urban migration was followed by a level of mortality that threatened the race with extinction. As early as 1862, Nicholas Appolino, Boston's long-time vital registrar, noted that black mortality exceeded nativity and suggested that 'the colored race seems, so far as this city is concerned, to be doomed to extinction'.[19]

Moreover, the most authoritative and influential person in the discourse was not a southern physician, but Frederick Hoffman, chief statistician for the Prudential Life Insurance Company and a prominent figure in the American Statistical Association. In 1896, under the auspices of the American Economic Association, Hoffman published an exhaustive study of the economic, anthropometric, social and demographic condition of African Americans. Marshalling a wealth of municipal, state and national statistical data and quoting a wide variety of US and international studies, Hoffman sought to demonstrate beyond a doubt that the physical and moral condition of blacks had degenerated sharply since emancipation, that the primary cause of this degeneration was racial rather than environmental, and that the end result would be extinction of the race. Reiterating again and again that 'race and heredity [are] the determining factors in the upward and downward course of mankind',[20] he concluded his final chapter with the following summation.

> Nothing is more clearly shown from this investigation than that the southern black man at the time of emancipation was healthy in body and cheerful in mind. He neither suffered inordinately from disease nor from impaired bodily vigor. His industrial capacity as a laborer was not of a low order, nor was the condition of servitude such as to produce in him morbid conditions favorable to mental disease, suicide or intemperance. What are the conditions thirty years after? The pages of this work give but one answer . . . In the plain language of facts brought together the colored race is shown to be on a downward grade, tending toward a condition in which matters will be worse than they are now, when diseases will be more destructive, vital resistance still lower, when the number of births will fall below deaths, and gradual extinction of the race will take place.[21]

While concerned with illustrating all the physical, mental and social pathologies causing post-emancipation degeneration, Hoffman paid considerable attention to infant and child mortality among urban migrants, lending support to the widely held opinion that such mortality was inordinately high. Specifically, he showed that, following their migration to cities, African Americans suffered rates of infant and child mortality almost double that of urban whites. But in contrast to sanitarian theories that stressed the influence of the environmental conditions attending urban poverty, Hoffman attributed little primary causal importance to either poverty or poor sanitation. Although conceding that diarrhoeal diseases were connected to filth, he argued that the primary cause of infant diarrhoea, as well as that of the other disorders that carried away so many black urban infants, was racial rather than environmental. Indeed, he ridiculed 'those who believe in the all powerful effect of the milieux', and dismissed as unfounded the contention that, 'given the same social, economic and sanitary conditions of life, the colored race would enjoy the same health and death rate as the white population'.[22] In a sentence that would often be repeated by turn-of-the-century medical racists, Hoffman asserted that, 'it is not in the *conditions of life* but in *the race traits and tendencies* that we find the causes of excessive mortality'[23] (italics in original).

By 'race traits' Hoffman meant features that were both biological and social, arguing that the former determined the latter and that both were the product of racial evolution. After statistically demonstrating a high rate of infant mortality among urban African Americans, he contended that inferior racial organic and social development explained this death rate. Deaths in early infancy, and especially those from congenital debility, prematurity, inanition and atrophy, he maintained, were due to the comparatively weak vital powers and substandard organic efficiency with which evolution had equipped blacks. Also critically important, according to Hoffman, were the intemperance and sexual licentiousness to which he believed blacks were racially prone. Intemperance destroyed the health of parents who then bequeathed their infants weakened constitutions, while sexual excess led to enervation of the reproductive organs and venereal disease. Both conditions caused excessive stillbirths and deaths in early infancy. Deaths in later infancy, particularly those from digestive and respiratory disorders, Hoffman attributed to certain physiological and anatomical characteristics specific to the African race combined with neglectful and ignorant child-rearing practices which he ascribed to moral and mental underdevelopment. Like most sociomedical researchers, he considered blacks particularly susceptible to pulmonary tuberculosis and other respiratory diseases. Moreover, while conceding that the gastro-enteric disorders that killed so many black urban infants were directly tied to exposure to filth, he contended that such exposure was the consequence of black racial inferiority in parenting.[24]

Published as the south was politically disenfranchising its African American citizens and constructing a system of legally sanctioned apartheid, Hoffman's work was well received and widely quoted within southern elite medical circles, and continued to be so through the early decades of the twentieth century. Moreover, its anti-environmentalist thesis and its stress on biological and racial factors continued to inform socio-medical discussion of the rates of death among black urban infants even as significant advances were being made in bacteriology, physiology and pathology. Indeed, new understandings of the causes and processes of the major infant diseases were incorporated into racialist explanations, lending authority and specificity to claims that race traits specific to blacks made them ignorant and neglectful parents, unwilling and unable to follow hygienic regimens that would protect their children from infectious disease. Writing in 1910, H. M. Folkes, a physician from Biloxi,

Mississippi, connected such ignorance and neglect to race-specific fatalism among blacks, and argued that this fatalism resulted in irresponsible parenting and was the major cause of the rise in infant and child mortality since emancipation.[25]

However, not all late nineteenth-century socio-medical investigators fully subscribed to such views. Indeed, it was less that the published socio-medical discourse on black infant mortality mirrored the beliefs of the entire American medical, public health, vital statistical and sociological communities, than that it mirrored the beliefs of the relatively small and distinct segment of those communities who were particularly vociferous. As McBride has shown, prior to the First World War, literally the only participants in the socio-medical discussion on black health in general and black infant mortality in particular were physicians and public health officials from the south, where over 90 per cent of the nation's African Americans resided, and *laissez faire* conservatives and Social Darwinists like Hoffman.[26] As a consequence, the major themes propounded in the discourse were anti-reformist, anti-environmentalist and, for the most part, virulently racist.

THE NARRATIVE CHALLENGED

The thematic uniformity of socio-medical discussion of African American infant mortality began disintegrating in the early twentieth century as the community of those involved in the debate expanded. One of the first attacks came in 1906, when Atlanta University, perhaps the leading black institution of higher education in the US at the time, devoted its annual Conference for the Study of Negro Problems to 'The Health and Physique of the Negro American'. It was intended to be a forum for exploring social scientific and medical opinions at odds with the reigning racialist doctrine that the disparity between black and white morbidity and mortality rates was chiefly the result of the racial biological inferiority of African Americans. The overall argument of its participants was that the differences in disease and mortality patterns between blacks and whites were rooted in historically shaped social conditions and tradition or culture, rather than in racial traits.[27]

Among those at the conference most clearly articulating this argument was the anthropologist Franz Boas, whose writings on race and culture were to have a profound effect on American social science during the first third of the century. Although Boas had yet to publish his most influential work, he had already established himself as a dedicated opponent of the idea that variations in social status and mental capabilities were the product of inherited, race-specific, physical differences.[28] Indeed, a year before the conference, he had published in *Charities* a summation of an argument he would make again and again in regard to the status of African Americans. While accepting that the current social organisation, health status and mental accomplishments of American blacks were, on average, inferior to whites, he contended that 'everything points out that these qualities are the result of social conditions rather than hereditary traits'.[29] For him, and the analysts of the African American social condition whom he influenced, the deterioration of black health was rooted not in biological and racially defined causes, but in the wretched social conditions – and their influence on behaviour and custom – that blacks had been forced to endure.

A similar view was also advanced by a number of southern black physicians who in the first two decades of the century opposed racist explanations of high black mortality in papers delivered at the annual meetings of the newly organised National Medical Association and in essays published in black periodicals and journals. While generally accepting that the health of southern blacks had declined since emancipation, these physicians advanced an environmentalist and economic explanation for this change. One of the clearest and most forceful articulations of this theory was presented by C. W. Birnie, an African American physician from Sumter, North Carolina, at the 1910 National Medical Association Conference. Birnie readily agreed that blacks had enjoyed better health under slavery than after, and suggested that 'the cause is not hard to find. The owners insisted on a hygienic manner of living as a purely business matter. The slave was so much property that had to be hedged by every possible protection.'[30] But Birnie emphatically disagreed with the contention that the removal of that protection inevitably led to increased mortality because blacks were physically, mentally and morally ill-equipped for freedom. While characterising the death rates of black urban migrants from tuberculosis, pneumonia and the various diseases of infancy as appalling, Birnie argued that the primary reason for these high rates was that it was now in the economic interest of whites to impair rather than protect the health of blacks. Referring to the racialist explanations of rising black death rates, he complained that 'while the former slave owner and his descendants are making all the charges, they are not willing to assume their responsibility'.[31] Such responsibility, according to Birnie, lay in keeping urban blacks impoverished, denying them access to education, refusing to extend to their neighbourhoods adequate sewerage and water supply systems, and collecting high rents for crowded and insanitary housing. Castigating white tenement owners and employers for profiting from the misery of urban blacks, Birnie argued that white economic exploitation and the resulting continued poverty of blacks were the major reasons for the difference in mortality rates between the two races. 'Poor houses; underfed people, inability to provide by reason of the smallest wages, comfortable clothing, etc.; these make the high mark of mortality.'[32]

That poverty and its attendant ills, rather than biologically determined race traits, were the causes of high urban mortality was, according to black physicians like Birnie, nowhere more apparent than in the high death rates of African American urban infants. Calling such mortality truly alarming, Birnie contested ideas of racial inferiority in stamina and vitality, arguing instead that high infant mortality was the consequence of privations 'that parents are generally powerless to prevent'.[33] Given the conditions under which the average black urban infant is born and reared, Birnie observed, 'the wonder is indeed that the death-rate is not much higher'.[34] He also challenged the racialist characterisation of black parents as incapable of providing intelligent and protective care. While admitting that large numbers of black parents were ignorant of the basic rules of modern infant hygiene, and that many black mothers worked and therefore could not breast-feed or care properly for their infants, Birnie attributed this to poverty and lack of access to hygienic instruction.

Birnie was preaching to the converted. For among the black physicians who attended the annual meetings of the National Medical Association and who read and contributed to periodicals with a large black readership like *Crisis* and *Opportunity*, there was little doubt that ignorance and poverty, rather than racial inferiority, were the chief causes of high infant mortality among urban blacks. There was also little doubt that while poverty might be intractable and beyond the influence of the medical community, ignorance was not. As a consequence, black physicians in the south promoted and contributed to various infant welfare activities that had as their principal aim the reduction of infant mortality through the instruction of parents in hygienic infant nurture. Completely ignored by northern infant welfare activists and largely voluntaristic, since they received little if any financial support from municipal governments, these activities, while limited, constituted virtually the entirety, before the First World War, of organised infant welfare aimed at urban African Americans.[35]

PROGRESSIVE INFANT WELFARE DISCOVERS BLACK INFANT MORTALITY

In November 1909 the American Academy of Medicine organised a conference in New Haven, Connecticut, devoted to the prevention of infant mortality. Attended by many of the industrialised north's most prominent paediatricians, social workers and public health officials, the conference led to the founding of the American Association for the Study and Prevention of Infant Mortality (AASPIM). The conference more generally marked the beginning of a multifaceted public health campaign that has since been labelled the Progressive-era infant welfare movement.[36] Among the papers presented at the conference was one by Richard Cabot and Edith Richie, two medical researchers from Boston. Titled 'The Influence of Race on Infant Mortality' and based on analysis of over 3,000 death certificates, the paper reported the cause-specific death rates among the infants of what the authors considered Boston's major races.[37] Perhaps the most interesting feature of the paper is that, while it included blacks as one of the important races constituting Boston's population, it largely ignored them in the analysis. While listing black infant death rates, the paper provided little comment on these figures, focusing instead on a comparison between the rates and causes of death among the infants of native-born whites and those of foreign immigrants, particularly the Irish, Italians and Jews.

Such inattention to black infant mortality was typical of northern socio-medical analysis of urban infant mortality up until the First World War.[38] Although race had been at the centre of such analysis of infant mortality since the mid-nineteenth century, it had largely been defined and discussed in terms of national origin rather than colour. Part of this stemmed from the fact that during the latter half of the nineteenth and first quarter of this century, northern urban public health analysis and activity were shaped primarily in response to the in-migration of millions of foreign immigrants who swelled city populations, overtaxed housing, water supplies and sanitary facilities, and constantly challenged the ability of state and municipal authorities to safeguard the public health. Hence, when late nineteenth- and early twentieth-century northern socio-medical analysts discussed the 'racial aspect' of infant mortality, they tended to conceptualise it, as did New York's S. Josephine Baker, as 'the influence of the influx of alien races'.[39]

Infant mortality among northern African American urbanites was not, however, entirely ignored. It could not be, for tradition and law mandated that population and vital data be differentiated by colour. Black infant death rates were thus aggregated and published by states and municipalities. None the less, because the northern urban black population remained relatively small and was not seen as significantly influencing overall rates of morbidity and mortality, black urban infant death rates generally received little commentary, beyond the brief notation that 'colored' babies seemed particularly prone to death from respiratory diseases.

The perfunctory attention given to black infant mortality in the urban north changed with the massive migration of southern blacks to northern cities in the 1910s and 1920s. During the First World War articles began appearing in northern periodicals and medical and public health journals querying the extent to which the new migrants – believed to be suffering disproportionately high rates of tuberculosis – represented a serious threat to the general public health.[40] Municipal and state health officials also expressed concern that high mortality among the new migrants – who seemed to crowd into the most unsanitary, dilapidated and overcrowded housing – would reverse hard-earned declines in general mortality rates. Such concern found support in a US Labor Department survey in 1919 on the effects of the black migration to northern cities. Using local social work records and health surveys, the Department's investigators concluded that malnutrition, insanitary housing and overcrowding were producing appallingly high rates of morbidity and mortality among the new migrants. In particular, although data was scanty, it appeared that the death rates of the infants and children of the southern black migrants were exceedingly high and perhaps rising. Indeed, by 1920, it had become accepted wisdom among northern socio-medical analysts that however bad the health of southern blacks, it was far worse among those who had migrated north.[41]

The approach adopted towards the high black infant mortality was largely an extension of the measures that workers involved in northern infant welfare had already developed to fight infant mortality among impoverished foreign-born migrants. Influenced by innovations within paediatrics and bacteriology and convinced that the two major causes of mortality in later infancy – digestive disorders and respiratory diseases – could be prevented through hygienic feeding and care, infant welfare advocates in the first two decades of the century promoted instructing mothers as the most effective means by which urban infant deaths could be reduced. Intelligent, hygienic care, and especially breast feeding, they reasoned, could provide a buffer between the infant and the harmful influences of poverty and unsanitary conditions.[42]

Confident of the effectiveness of hygienic infant care, early Progressive infant welfare advocates, while conceding that inherited vitality and resistance to certain diseases might play a role, tended to view racial differences in the rates of infant mortality primarily as the consequences of different customs of infant care and of the extent to which those customs were ill-suited to the urban environment. If certain immigrant groups suffered higher infant mortality than others, it was largely because their infant rearing customs were more dysfunctional in an urban setting. In explaining why Jews generally seemed to have lower infant mortality rates than other of the new immigrant groups, Hull House's Alice Hamilton articulated a widely held belief when she told those attending the 1909 AAM conference on the prevention of infant mortality: 'the Jews have the advantage over other nationalities in that they have been for over 2,000 years accustomed to the conditions of over-crowded city life'.[43]

For the most part, participants in the Progressive infant welfare discourse applied this perspective to the new black urban migrants, viewing the high infant mortality rates they suffered as the consequence of the unsuitability to the northern urban environment of infant rearing customs shaped in the rural south.[44] Accordingly, the infant welfare programmes developed for the expanding black urban population were similar to those that had been established to reduce infant mortality among poor urban immigrants. One of the first of these was initiated in 1916 by the New York Association for Improving the Condition of the Poor in conjunction with the Child Hygiene Bureau of the Department of Health. Modelled on a 1911 programme aimed at immigrants, this initiative involved sending visiting nurses into the largely black Columbus Hill area to register babies for infant welfare station visits and to instruct their mothers in hygienic care and feeding.[45] Although the New York programme was soon followed by others, the amount of infant welfare activity nationwide aimed specifically at African Americans remained relatively inconsequential before the mid-1920s when states began using funds provided under the Sheppard-Towner Act (1921) to hire and train black visiting nurses and to establish infant, child and maternal welfare programmes in cities with large black populations.[46]

In emphasising the importance of good mothering in reducing infant deaths from gastro-enteric and respiratory diseases, Progressive infant welfare workers challenged the racist assumption that black infant death rates were the consequence of immutable race traits. While expressing the conviction that the excessive risk of death black infants faced was the result of the ignorant and unhygienic care provided by their parents, infant welfare activists stressed that this was remedial with instruction. Thus, they switched the question of adaptability from the biological to the cultural. Admittedly, this shift did not rid racist explanations from the discourse on African American infant mortality. None the less, conscious of the long history of racist assertions that blacks were phylogenetically neglectful parents and incapable of grasping all but the simplest ideas, liberals in the infant welfare community took great pains to stress that African American mothers seemed highly solicitous of their children's welfare and that they responded extremely well to maternal reform.[47]

Biological racism, however, was less easily discarded as an explanation for racial differences in death rates during early infancy or the neonatal period, deaths which were regarded as connected to the health, behaviour and reproductive efficiency of the mother during pregnancy and parturition. Originally little understood and generally seen as unpreventable, neonatal mortality had inspired little research, discussion or reform activity during the initial part of the Progressive infant welfare movement. By 1914, however, published mortality reports showing that neonatal mortality was remaining high while post-neonatal mortality was dropping prompted infant welfare activists to turn their attention to deaths in early infancy.[48] One result was that studies started to appear comparing the causes and rates of neonatal mortality among the different races and calling for renewed consideration of the role that race played in determining infant mortality differentials.

Somewhat surprisingly, the first of these studies revealed that neonatal mortality was highest among native-born whites and lowest among recent immigrants, most notably Italians, Slavs and Russian Jews, whereas the pattern of post-neonatal mortality was the reverse. By contrast, but less surprising, African Americans, and especially urban African Americans, were shown not to fit the pattern of native or foreign-born whites, for not only did their infants suffer exceedingly high post-neonatal mortality rates but also had the highest death rate during the neonatal period.[49] In explaining the differences in post-neonatal mortality, the studies underlined the importance of sanitary surroundings and hygienic infant care, contending that the infants of native-born white women tended to live in better sanitary conditions and to have mothers who were superior in intelligence and more educated in infant care than did immigrant and black babies.[50] Moreover, reflecting the common wisdom of socio-medical thinking on infant mortality, the studies considered the disadvantage suffered by immigrant and black babies to be remedial through maternal instruction.

The initial studies were less certain about the reasons for the racial disparity in neonatal death rates. One explanation for the lower immigrant neonatal mortality rates was that immigrant infants, descended from sturdy peasant stock, enjoyed 'greater vitality and superior constitutions' than did those of native-born white and African American women.[51] Another was that overcivilisation, nervousness and enervation of the reproductive organs among the well off, and overwork, chronic alcoholism and venereal disease among the poor, and especially the black poor, made it more likely that native-born white and African American women would experience problematic pregnancies and that their infants would be born premature or with congenital malformations and disabilities.[52]

This uncertainty over the causes of neonatal mortality, especially in regard to African Americans, continued on into the 1920s, keeping alive debate over whether biological racial inferiority was a determinant in infant mortality. As a *Journal of the American Medical Association* commentary noted in 1926, several of the studies thus far had suggested that 'the differences between the various groups in these [neonatal mortality] rates very probably have a biologic basis, and in this sense, may be termed racial'.[53] Yet many socio-medical researchers studying neonatal mortality in the 1920s were uncomfortable with such nebulous and unscientifically precise concepts as racially determined natural vitality. This was especially true of obstetric researchers who were in the process of legitimating their speciality and were inclined to identify specific and treatable diseases, pathological conditions and antenatal behaviour as the chief causes of interracial differences in neonatal mortality. For such researchers, two diseases in particular explained why so many African American infants were either stillborn or died in early infancy. These diseases were syphilis and tetanus.

One of the arguments of the socio-medical analysts who had constructed the narrative of post-emancipation African American degeneration in the late nineteenth and early twentieth centuries had been that syphilis and other venereal diseases were more prevalent among blacks than whites, and that along with tuberculosis and the diseases of infancy, contributed significantly to the increasing disparity in mortality rates between the races. Hoffman and others had argued that blacks were racially prone to sexual licentiousness and that they had inferior biological capabilities for resisting and surviving syphilitic infection.[54]

However, not until the First World War, a time of rising concern over foetal and neonatal mortality and over increasing venereal disease among the troops, did clinical researchers look closely at the connection between syphilis and deaths due to prematurity, congenital disease and foetal complications. While confirming that syphilis did indeed seem more prevalent and cause more foetal and neonatal deaths among blacks than whites, these studies explicitly challenged the notion that both the incidence of the disease and the death rates were in any way connected to biological racial inferiority. This challenge was reinforced after 1920 by the work of the eminent obstetric clinician J. Whitridge Williams at Johns Hopkins, which showed that pre-natal screening and treatment were highly effective in preventing congenital complications from syphilitic infection.[55] Moreover, by the mid-1920s, many socio-medical researchers were suggesting that pre-natal screening and treatment held the potential for reducing the gulf between black and white foetal and neonatal deaths from not only syphilis but also other causes of congenital complications such as toxaemia and eclampsia.[56] In short, while conceding the influence of maternal behaviour and environment on the survivability of newborns, most clinical research suggested that access to good medical supervision and treatment could effectively offset much of that influence.

A similar argument for the effectiveness of skilled medical treatment was offered in regard to what was viewed as an excessive death rate of African American new-borns from tetanus. Attributing the disease to the unskilled and insanitary practices of black midwives, commentators argued either for the replacement of midwives with skilled physicians or for training them in hygienic birthing methods.[57] The contention that skilled medical pre-natal supervision and attendance at birth would do much to reduce the recorded high rates of neonatal mortality among blacks received strong support during the mid- and late-1920s from studies conducted by the US Children Bureau, by municipal and state health departments, and by insurance companies, most of which indicated that black infant mortality rates had dropped significantly during the previous decade, especially among those African American families in which the mother had enjoyed access to pre-natal care and post-natal instruction.[58] One of the most influential of these studies was conducted by Louis Dublin on data collected on the families of Metropolitan Life Insurance policy holders. Quick to see the significance of his findings, Dublin proclaimed that the declining rates of black infant mortality – and black mortality in general – offered the final disproof of the old view that African Americans were racially ill-adapted for survival on the American continent and that they were a race whose biological inferiority doomed them to extinction. Quite the contrary was true, Dublin declared. Given the same material conditions, education and access to medical care, blacks could expect the mortality of their infants to continue to decline and ultimately to reach parity with that of whites.[59]

CONCLUSION

As was true in infant welfare in general, demonstration of the effectiveness of pre-natal screening and treatment and of following medical advice on infant hygiene made access to medical care and supervision an increasingly central issue in the discourse on black infant mortality. In the 1930s, which have been characterised by one historian of African American health, as 'the first time a national effort to curtail the excess disease mortality among blacks emerged', the provision of maternal and infant health care services became a favoured stratagem of those concerned with reducing black infant mortality and closing the gap between black and white infant death rates.[60] As it did so, the question of African American biological racial inferiority was increasingly shunted to the side and seen as made irrelevant by the proven effectiveness of medical care. Indeed, while racial prejudice would continue to mark socio-medical discussion of black infant mortality, its focus was shifted from biology to the extent to which black parents utilised available medical care and followed medical advice on pre-natal behaviour and infant hygiene.

NOTES

1 For an in-depth history of that discourse and the infant welfare activity it inspired, see R.A. Meckel, *Save the Babies: American Public Health Reform and the Prevention of Infant Mortality, 1850–1929*, Baltimore, 1990.

2 D. Dwork, *War is Good for Babies and Other Children: A History of the Infant and Child Welfare Movement in England, 1898–1918*, London, 1987; C.R. Comacchio, *'Nations are Built of Babies': Saving Ontario's Mothers and Children, 1900–1940*, Montreal, 1993; A. Klaus, *Every Child a Lion: The Origins of Infant and Maternal Health Policy in the United States and France, 1890–1920*, Ithaca, NY, 1993.

3 As in the United States, the infant welfare discourse in Great Britain, Germany, France and other industrialised nations was suffused with contemporary eugenicist and hereditarian ideas that made racialist concerns central to any discussion of infant mortality. Yet, unlike in the United States, race, or national origin, was rarely used as a descriptive category when dealing with intra-national, as opposed to international, infant mortality differentials. For further discussion, see Meckel, *Save the Babies*, pp. 130–2.

4 Meckel, *Save the Babies*; Klaus, *Every Child a Lion*; M. Ladd-Taylor, *Raising a Baby the Government Way: Mothers' Letters to the Children's Bureau, 1915–1932*, New Brunswick, NJ, 1986; idem, *Mother-Work: Women, Child Welfare, and the State, 1890–1930*, Urbana, Ill., 1994; C.R. King, *Children's Health in America: A History*, New York, 1993, pp. 106–19.

5 J.C. Kennedy, *Preliminary Report of the Eighth Census*, Washington, D.C., 1862, p. 8; J.S. Haller, *Outcasts from Evolution: Scientific Attitudes of Racial Inferiority, 1859–1900*, Urbana, Ill., 1971, pp. 40–1. Department of the Interior, Census Office, *Ninth Census of the United States, 1880*, vol. 1: F. Walker, 'The Statistics of the Population of the United States', Washington, DC, 1872, p. xviii.

6 Department of the Interior, Census Office, *Tenth Census of the United States, 1880*, vol. 2, Part 1: J.S. Billings, 'Report on Mortality and Vital Statistics of the United States', Washington, DC, 1885, p. xxxiv.

7 S.S. Herrick, 'The Comparative Vital Movement of the White and Colored Races in the United States', *Public Health: Reports and Papers of the American Public Health Association*, 1883, 7, p. 267.

8 H.W. Conrad, 'The Health of Negroes in the South', *Sanitarian*, 1887, 18, pp. 502–18; G.B. Thornton, 'The Negro Mortality in Memphis', *Public Health: Reports and Papers of the American Public Health Association*, 1882, 8, pp. 177–86.

9 For a discussion of nineteenth-century medical opinion concerning the ill effects of impure air on infant survivability, see Meckel, *Save the Babies*, pp. 22–6, 43–4.

10 Herrick, 'The Comparative Vital Movement', p. 266.

11 T. Afflect, 'On the Hygiene of Cotton Plantations and the Management of Negro Slaves', *Southern Medical Reports*, 1890, 2, pp. 430–5; J.M. Barrier, 'Tuberculosis Among Our Negroes in Louisiana', *Transactions*

of the Louisiana State Medical Society, 1902, 23, pp. 130–8; Conrad, 'Health of Negroes', pp. 502–18; J.T. Walton, 'The Comparative Mortality of the White and Colored Races in the South', *Charlotte Medical Journal*, 1897, 10, pp. 291–4.

12 For a summary of antebellum southern medical views of African Americans, see J. S. Haller, 'The Negro and the Southern Physician: A Study of Racial Attitudes, 1800–1860', *Medical History*, 1972, 16, pp. 238–53.

13 Haller, *Outcasts from Evolution*, especially pp. 40–68; R.F. Berkhofer, Jr, *The White Man's Indian*, New York, 1979, pp. 55–61; G.W. Stocking, Jr, *Race, Culture, and Evolution: Essays in the History of Anthropology*, New York, 1968, pp. 110–32; T.F. Gosset, *Race: The History of an Idea in America*, Dallas, 1963; P.J. Bowler, *Evolution: The History of an Idea*, rev. ed., Berkeley, 1989, pp. 299–306.

14 E.T. Easley, 'The Sanitary Condition of the Negro', *American Medical Weekly*, 1875, 3, p. 49; E.R. Corson, 'The Future of the Colored Race in the United States', *New York Medical Times*, 1887, pp. 47–8.

15 See, for instance, S. Harris, 'The Future of the Negro from the Standpoint of the Southern Physician', *Alabama Medical Journal*, 1902, 14, p. 65.

16 S. Cartwright, 'The Diseases and Physical Peculiarities of the Negro Race', *New Orleans Surgical and Medical Journal*, 1871, 2, pp. 421–7; R. Reyburn, 'Types of Diseases Among the Freed People of the United States', *Medical News*, 1893, 5, pp. 623–7.

17 Among the most influential of these was R. Matas, 'The Surgical Peculiarities of the Negro', *Transactions of the American Surgical Association*, 1896, 14, pp. 483–606, which served as a standard medical reference through the First World War.

18 On the conflation of social Darwinism and racial evolutionism, see Gosset, *Race*, pp. 144–75.

19 Boston City Registrar, *Registration Report for 1862*, Boston, 1863, 8. See also Rhode Island Board Of Health, *Second Annual Report, 1880*, Providence, RI, 1881, p. 107.

20 F.L. Hoffman, 'Race Traits and Tendencies of the American Negro', *Publications of the American Economic Association*, 1896, 11, p. 310.

21 Ibid., pp. 311–12.

22 Ibid., pp. 49–50.

23 Ibid., p. 95.

24 Ibid., pp. 65–9.

25 H.M. Folkes, 'The Negro as a Health Problem', *Journal of the American Medical Association*, 1910, 15, p. 1246.

26 D. McBride, *From TB to AIDS: Epidemics Among Urban Blacks Since 1900*, Albany, NY, 1991, pp. 16–18.

27 W.E.B. Dubois, ed., *The Health and Physique of the American Negro: Report of a Social Study Made Under the Direction of Atlanta University; Together with the Proceedings of the Eleventh Conference for the Study of Negro Problems, Held at Atlanta University, on May 29th, 1906*, Atlanta, 1906.

28 For a recent brief but cogent analysis of Boas' ideas on race and culture, see C.N. Degler, *In Search of Human Nature: The Decline and Revival of Darwinism in American Social Thought*, New York, 1991, pp. 61–83.

29 F. Boas, 'The Negro and the Demands of Modern Life: Ethnic and Anatomical Considerations', *Charities*, 1905, 15, p. 87.
30 C.W. Birnie, 'The Influence of Environment and Race on Diseases', *Journal of the National Medical Association*, 1910, 2, p. 246.
31 Ibid.
32 Ibid.
33 Ibid., p. 247.
34 Ibid.
35 A brief review of those activities, which have largely been ignored by historians of Progressive infant welfare, can be found in J.A. Kenney, 'Health Problems of the Negroes', *Annals of the American Academy of Political and Social Science*, 1911, 37, pp. 354–64.
36 For a description of the American Academy of Medicine and its orientation, see Steven J. Peitzman, 'Forgotten Reformers: The American Academy of Medicine', *Bulletin of the History of Medicine*, 1984, 58, pp. 516–28. For a description of the conference and the founding and aims of the American Association for the Study and Prevention of Infant Mortality (AASPIM), see Meckel, *Save the Babies*, pp. 108–16.
37 R.C. Cabot and E.K. Richie, 'The Influence of Race on Infant Mortality', *Prevention of Infant Mortality: Being the Papers and Discussions of a Conference Held at New Haven, Connecticut, 11–12 November 1909*, Philadelphia, 1910, pp. 113–25. A condensed version of the paper was published in the *Boston Medical and Surgical Journal*, 1910, 162, pp. 199–202.
38 Similarly, a 1917 study of the racial dimension of infant mortality in Boston also ignored African Americans. See F.H. MacCarthy, 'A Study of Mortality and Vitality of Different Racial Groups', *New England Medical Gazette*, 1917, 52, pp. 366–71. And as late as 1919, an influential and often cited study of infant mortality among the major races of the state of New York barely mentioned black infant death rates. See P.R. Eastman, 'The Relation of Parental Nativity to the Infant Mortality of New York State', *American Journal of the Diseases of Children*, 1919, 17, pp. 195–211.
39 S.J. Baker, 'Child Hygiene', in W.H. Park, ed., *Public Health and Hygiene*, Philadelphia, 1920, p. 675.
40 See, for instance, 'The Negro Menace to the Public Health', *American Journal of Public Health*, 1916, 6, p. 607.
41 McBride, *From TB to AIDS*, pp. 36–9.
42 On the adoption of breast feeding and maternal instruction as a means by which poor urban infants could be protected from the influences of poverty and insanitation, see Meckel, *Save the Babies*, pp. 92–123.
43 A. Hamilton, 'Excessive Child-bearing as a Factor in Infant Mortality', *Prevention of Infant Mortality*, p. 78. See also D. Dwork, 'Health Conditions of Immigrant Jews on the Lower East Side of New York, 1880–1914', *Medical History*, 1981, 25, pp. 1–40.
44 See, for instance, J.A. Tobey, 'The Death Rate Among American Negroes', *Current History*, 1926, 25, pp. 217–20.
45 J.C. Gebhart, 'Filling the Gaps in Child Life', *Survey*, 1919, 43, p. 313. See also 'Health Campaign Among Negroes', *American Journal of Public*

Health, 1917, 7, p. 510; H.L. Harris, 'Health and the Negro Family in Chicago', *Opportunity*, 1927, 5, pp. 258–60; A.G. Smith, S.S. Hobday, and L.E. Reid, 'Health Service in a Negro District', *Journal of the American Medical Association*, 1930, 22, pp. 68–74.

46 The Sheppard-Towner Act was the first federal social welfare measure to provide some measure of state maternity care. For more information on the Act see M. Ladd Taylor, '"Why Does Congress Wish Women and Children to Die?": The Rise and Fall of Public Maternal and Infant Health Care in the United States, 1921–1929', in V. Fildes, L. Marks and H. Marland, eds, *Women and Children First: An International History of Maternal and Infant Welfare, 1870–1945*, London, 1992.

47 L. Wald, *The House on Henry Street*, New York, 1915, p. 162; G. Abbott, 'A Message to Colored Mothers', *Crisis*, 1932, 39, pp. 311–12; P. Van Ingen, 'Why Negro Babies Die' *Opportunity*, 1923, 1, p. 195.

48 Typical of the general consensus was the recommendation by William H. Welch that AASPIM focus its attention on post-neonatal deaths since the causes of neonatal death were ill understood and probably unpreventable. W.H. Welch, 'Address', *Transactions of the American Association for the Study and Prevention of Infant Mortality, 1910*, Baltimore, 1911, p. 52. On infant welfare's new focus on neonatal mortality, see Meckel, *Save the Babies*, pp. 159–77.

49 Eastman, 'Parental Nativity', pp. 199–200; H. Ford, 'Racial Factors in Relation to Neonatal Mortality', *The Nation's Health*, 1924, 6, p. 254.

50 Eastman, 'Parental Nativity', p. 207.

51 Ibid., p. 207.

52 MacCarthy, 'Mortality and Vitality', p. 369.

53 'Current Medical Literature', *Journal of the American Medical Association*, 1925, 85, p. 466.

54 Hoffman, 'Race Traits', p. 95; Folkes, 'The Negro as a Health Problem', p. 1246; T. Murrell, 'Syphilis and the American Negro', *Journal of the American Medical Association*, 1910, 54, pp. 847–8; Thornton, 'Negro Mortality', pp. 185–6.

55 J.B. Holmes, 'Recent Work in Anatomy, Physiology and Pathology of Infancy and Childhood', *American Journal of the Diseases of Children*, 1924, 27, p. 262. Williams' two most important publications on syphilis and neonatal and foetal deaths are: J.W. Williams, 'The Significance of Syphilis in Prenatal Care and in the Causation of Foetal Death', *Bulletin of the Johns Hopkins Hospital*, 1920, 31, pp. 141–5; idem, 'The Influence of the Treatment of Syphilitic Women Upon the Incidence of Congenital Syphilis', *Bulletin of the Johns Hopkins Hospital*, 1922, 33, pp. 383–6.

56 H.W. Ford, 'A Statistical Study of Neonatal Mortality with Special Relation to the Factor of Mother Nativity', *American Journal of Hygiene*, 1927, 7, p. 91; J. Gebhart, 'Syphilis as a Prenatal Problem', *Journal of Social Hygiene*, 1924, 10, pp. 214–17; J.H. Mason Knox, 'Morbidity and Mortality in the Negro Infant', *American Journal of the Diseases of Children*, 1924, 27, pp. 398–400; idem, 'The Health Problem of the Negro Child', *American Journal of Public Health*, 1926, 16, pp. 805–9.

57 For a description of the socio-medical discourse on black midwives and of efforts to educate and train them, see M. Ladd-Taylor, '"Grannies" and

"Spinsters": Midwife Education under the Sheppard-Towner Act', *Journal of Social History*, 1988, 22, pp. 255–75.

58 US Department of Labor, Children's Bureau, *Results of a Field Study in Baltimore, MD*, by A. Rochester, Washington, 1923. This was the first of the Children's Bureau's highly influential series of local infant mortality studies to include a significant population of blacks. See also L.I. Dublin, 'The Effect of Health Education on Negro Mortality', *Opportunity*, 1924, 2, pp. 232–4; idem, 'Health Gains Among Negroes', *American Journal of Public Health*, 1929, 19, pp. 211–12; Smith, Hobday and Reid, 'Health Service', pp. 68–74; F.B. Washington, 'Health Work for Negro Children', *Opportunity*, 1925, 3, pp. 264–5.

59 L.I. Dublin, 'The Health of the Negro: the Outlook for the Future', *Opportunity*, 1928, 6, pp. 198–200.

60 McBride, *From TB to AIDS*, p. 85.

5

A DISEASE OF CIVILISATION

Tuberculosis in Britain, Africa and India, 1900–39

Mark Harrison and Michael Worboys

INTRODUCTION

On World TB Day at the end of March 1996, a World Health Organisation (WHO) report showed that global tuberculosis mortality has been on a steep upward curve since the 1950s; indeed, in 1993 the Organisation had declared the disease a 'global emergency'. The report described two epidemic waves: the first, which was concentrated in northern, industrialised countries, peaked around 1900 and went into decline before a second wave, concentrated in southern, Third World countries, picked up in the 1950s. During the trough in the 1920s and 1930s, mortality in the north fell rapidly, but an increase in the south became ever more apparent. In this chapter we discuss the development of medical awareness and explanations of the second epidemic wave in the first four decades of this century. More precisely, our focus is the debates amongst tuberculosis experts on how and why a disease, previously confined to industrial countries and imperial metropolises, began to become a serious health problem in colonial territories and amongst 'primitive' peoples.

Before 1940, tropical medical specialists and the colonial medical services paid little attention to the disease, being preoccupied with parasitic, vector-borne diseases and their control. Indeed, it was largely military medical officers who first reported a growing incidence of the disease at the imperial periphery after 1900, and it was subsequently European-based tuberculosis experts who mainly concerned themselves with the problem. One consequence of this was that 'primitive', 'tropical' or 'colonial' tuberculosis, as it was variously styled, was used to inform the anti-tuberculosis crusade in Europe and North America, especially on questions of immunity, race and migration. Those who reflected on the global situation regarding tuberculosis after 1900 found no difficulty in dividing the world's cultures and peoples into three levels of civilisation and tuberculisation – i.e. the process of the establishment of tubercular infection, though not necessarily tubercular disease, in a population.[1] The peoples of Europe and North America, who had been in contact with the disease for longest, were said to be more or less fully tuberculised. Tropical Africa, the Pacific Islands and other areas were regarded as 'virgin soil' – i.e. populations and individuals previously unexposed to the disease, and hence vulnerable because of a lack of immunity. In between were countries like India and China, where the bacillus had long been present, but where social, cultural and environmental conditions had limited the spread and severity of the disease. However, as these latter countries now underwent rapid urbanisation and industrialisation, it seemed that epidemic tuberculosis would result, as it had in Europe two centuries earlier. Contrasts were mainly drawn between 'civilised' and 'primitive' societies – the latter, mostly in Africa, were seen as comparable to Britain in Roman times. After 1930, the situation in India, said to be at the level of eighteenth-century England, which had been outside earlier discourses, was turned to as a possible model for events about to unfold in Africa and elsewhere in the Empire.[2]

The central notion of 'virgin soil' was interpreted and used in many different ways, though usually it was expressed in immunological terms. The main question was whether populations and individuals were vulnerable because they had no *inherited* immunity, or because they had not had the opportunity to *acquire* immunity. In practice the answer mattered little as both implied that adaptation to the bacillus in Africa and Asia would take many, many generations, as it had in Europe. However, the question of heredity was sensitive as it had implications for questions of racial susceptibility and difference. The dominant version of 'virgin soil' theory stressed acquired immunity, so that the social history and contemporary conditions of a population were felt to be more important than their innate biology. That said, distinctions between acquired and inherited immunity were often blurred, not least when the evolution of immunity in populations was sometimes confused with the development of immunity in individuals, and when race was defined culturally, and confused with ethnicity.

In this chapter we begin by considering developing ideas and models of immunity to tuberculosis after 1900, especially the physiological and social conditions in which infection could be controlled and in which resistance evolved, including questions of acquired and inherited immunity. Next we discuss how the key notion of 'virgin soil' was elaborated in the context of debates about the epidemiology of the disease in Europe, North America and South Africa. The key figure in the elaboration of the theory was Lyle Cummins, whose work and ideas on tuberculosis in different countries are discussed in detail, especially how these changed over time and how they were used by others. Finally, we consider the policies developed to deal with the growing menace of tuberculosis in the 1920s and 1930s: first, by medical officers in colonial Africa and second, by government, voluntary and professional agencies in India. We make no attempt to analyse or explain the historical epidemiology of tuberculosis in Africa or India. Rather our concern is with how the rising incidence of the disease was understood, what control measures were proposed and tried, and what the notion of a 'disease of civilisation' tells us about race, health and Empire in the first four decades of this century.

TUBERCULOSIS AND IMMUNITY

Koch's bacillary theory is usually said to have precipitated a revolution in the medical and social understanding of tuberculosis, from a disease that had been regarded as a complex, constitutional and hereditary affliction, to one that was a simple infection. However, there was no immediate abandonment of constitutional ideas; indeed, the notion of an inherited or acquired 'diathesis' or propensity to develop the affliction was reconstituted as an inherited or acquired susceptibility. The bacillus was seen to be a necessary cause of tuberculosis but not a sufficient one. Many historians have argued that the identification of the tubercular germ facilitated the adoption of more specific approaches to the control of the disease, allowing the disease germ to be attacked directly (by antiseptics, immune products, sunlight, etc.) and its spread to be controlled by specially targeted programmes (anti-spitting measures, isolation of sufferers, improving ventilation).[3] While this was certainly the case, of greater immediate importance in the anti-tuberculosis campaigns of the 1890s and 1900s were the observations of many clinicians and public health doctors that, despite up to 90 per cent of the adult population having been infected with the bacillus at some time in their lives, only about 10 per cent of these ever developed the disease. The evidence for this came from two sources: first, from autopsy findings of healed tubercular lesions in people who had died of other causes, and second, from surveys with the tuberculin skin test. Tuberculin was a filtrate of the culture medium on which tubercle bacilli were grown in laboratories, which, when injected under the skin, produced an inflammation in those who had previously been infected by the bacillus. While there was consensus that a positive skin test showed prior infection, there was uncertainty over whether a positive reaction showed that effective immunity had developed, or, as immunologists eventually came to accept, was merely an allergic reaction that signalled prior infection and nothing more. Whatever the meaning of individual test results, there was no disputing that many more people were infected than ever developed active disease. The implication drawn by anti-tuberculosis campaigners was that in the great majority of cases tubercular infection was contained and defeated, or cured naturally. This gave them further confidence that improvements in health coming from the 'natural' process of tuberculisation could be augmented by the systematic application of medical and hygienic measures to control and treat the disease.

The problem for tuberculosis specialists and immunologists was to explain this differential susceptibility or resistance: why were some people able to combat and defeat infection and others not? Why were some bodies 'stony soil' and others 'fertile'?[4] More often than not doctors spoke simply of a person's 'strength', the 'toughness' of their lungs, and their 'general vitality'; indeed, the open air treatment at this time was often spoken of in horticultural terms as being designed to 'harden off' patients. However, immunological theories, for example variables such as the numbers and activity of leucocytes, the body's ability to generate antigens and antitoxins, and its capacity to localise infection, played an increasingly important part. Clinicians regarded tuberculosis as a very variable disease, between individuals and even in the same individual over time, though epidemiological studies showed clear mortality patterns according to sex, occupation, geography and income, which might correlate to infection or susceptibility. Of course, any individual susceptibility was not fixed, it could vary in different environmental conditions, in relation to general health and concomitant afflictions and to age.

In Europe and North America mortality from tuberculosis was low during childhood, rose in adolescence to peak in adulthood, before tailing off in old age. Levels of infection, as shown in tuberculin surveys, showed steady increases by age, especially after adolescence, so that by old age over 90 per cent of the population had 'experienced' the bacillus. There were two seeming paradoxes with these findings, one with the old and the other with children. Old people had high rates of infection but low mortality. The preferred explanation was that they had acquired immunity from possibly numerous small infections at earlier ages, each of which their body had contained. Children had low mortality rates, except from tubercular disease of the joints which was believed to come from bovine sources. Yet tuberculin tests showed that they had few prior infections and ought to have been 'open' to the pulmonary form of tuberculosis.[5] The pre-bacillary explanation of their non-vulnerability had been that their general 'vitality' and rapid growth countered the wasting and degenerative effects of the disease. After 1900 the explanation given was that playing in the open air helped 'harden' their lungs, while their limited mixing with infected adults and exclusion from the kind of places where the disease spread (workshops, public houses, lodging houses), meant they received relatively low doses of the bacillus at any one time. In one sense, sanatoria tried to recreate idealised conditions of childhood: increasing weight and open-air living, plus close supervision, education in hygiene, freedom from worries and responsibilities and no sex.[6] Indeed, some sanatoria were called 'schools for consumptives', and the open-air school movement that developed in the Edwardian era worked with similar assumptions. However, in a tuberculised society children would not be expected to remain uninfected for very long, especially as they grew up and entered the world of work, frequented high risk environments, and adopted adult lifestyles. Adults who developed tubercular disease did so because either: (1) they had never acquired immunity in childhood or after; (2) they suffered such high doses of bacilli that any immunity was overcome; or (3) they had compromised any immunity they had through poor general health, 'irregular living', poverty or bad housing.

LYLE CUMMINS, TUBERCULISATION AND CIVILISATION

Lyle Cummins was born in Ireland in 1873 and graduated from Queen's College, Cork, in 1896. He began a career in the Royal Army Medical Corps (RAMC) in 1897, serving in Egypt from 1899 to 1909, and it was from this experience that he developed his interest in tuberculosis in Africa.[7] He then moved to the post of pathologist in charge of the Vaccine Department at the Royal Army Medical College, London, under Professor William Leishman. On

Leishman's retirement in 1914, Cummins took the Chair of Pathology and served concurrently with the British Army in France as head of pathology. He returned to the College full-time in 1918 and stayed until 1921 when he was appointed to the Chair of Tuberculosis at the Welsh National School of Medicine, Cardiff.[8] In the 1920s and 1930s, he was active in the National Association for the Prevention of Tuberculosis and the Welsh National Memorial Association, working on tuberculosis, mining diseases and the link between the two. From the late 1920s he was a consultant to the South African government and the country's mining industry, advising principally on tuberculosis in migrant workers. However, his experiences in the Rand led him to make significant changes to his ideas on the relative contributions that culture, environment and race made to the susceptibility of 'primitive' and 'civilised' peoples to tuberculosis.

In 1908, Cummins speculated on why troops drawn from the Sudanese interior were so much more vulnerable to tuberculosis than those recruited from Felaheen areas of Egypt on the Nile Delta.[9] Moreover, the pathology of the disease in the Sudanese was different: they suffered from an acute, disseminated type of the disease, whereas Egyptians showed the more familiar European chronic, localised, fibrous, pulmonary disease. Citing Pearson's work on tuberculosis and heredity, Cummins argued that the Sudanese were a 'virgin soil' population that had no inherited racial immunity because the prior absence of the bacillus meant that there had been no selection pressure for resistance, or insufficient time for the *survival of the immunest* to occur. In 1912, Cummins published again on the question but now stood out against any major role for heredity or race.[10] Instead, he now expressed 'virgin soil' ideas in terms of the absence of acquired immunity.

Cummins seems to have changed his mind, not due to any new evidence from Africa but rather to the new immunological theories he had adopted. By 1912 he was settled in London and in charge of the production of anti-typhoid vaccine for the RAMC, a procedure that gave the body artificial but none the less acquired immunity. He was clearly influenced by the ideas of Almroth Wright, who had been his teacher and mentor at Netley and who had developed the theory and practice of the protective inoculation Cummins now applied daily. Cummins' research and writing was cast squarely in Wright's terms and language.[11] Practically, Wright's ideas suggested new possibilities for both preventive and curative vaccines, as he stressed the importance of *active* immunity, based on the struggle in the body between 'infection and resistance'. Cummins also drew upon the work of other immunologists, notably those from the Pasteur Institute in Paris, such as Metchnikoff, Burnet and Calmette, who were also sanguine about the potential of antisera and vaccines to the control of infectious diseases by boosting natural immunity.

In the 1912 paper on tuberculosis and primitives, Cummins drew upon studies from Paris, Russia, Annan, German East Africa and French Guinea to construct a bar chart of percentage tuberculin positives amongst adult populations at different levels of civilisation (Figure 5.1). The important point for Cummins was the similar shape to that of the percentage of tuberculin-positives against age in industrialised countries. His conclusion was that the progressive tuberculisation of the population by age in a country like Britain was analogous to the same process in the history of civilisations. The two main tenets of 'virgin soil' theory were then spelt out:

1 That primitive tribes are highly susceptible to tuberculosis because in the absence of the tubercle bacillus they have never been obliged to protect themselves against the organism.
2 That civilised peoples are highly protected against tuberculosis because they have, in contact with the tubercle bacillus, elaborated protective substances against the organism.[12]

It is worth noting how the first tenet implies an active, perhaps Lamarckian, process in which 'tribes . . . have never been *obliged* to protect themselves' (emphasis added) not a blind Darwinian one. Cummins went on to argue that, 'The first proposition lays upon us a duty and the second opens to us the hope of fulfilling it with success', namely, to control the rate of tuberculisation of primitive tribes. Three possibilities were suggested: reducing the numbers of infected Europeans in Africa and other backward areas, slowing down the civilising mission, or ensuring that the mission always occurred in hygienic conditions. Cummins also speculated, as did French writers, on the possibilities of the accelerated tuberculisation of the world by vaccination. A key move for Cummins was the extension of the metaphor of 'virgin soil' from 'primitives' to British children, who likewise could be said not to have had the chance to acquire and develop immunity.[13] This notion, both played upon and reinforced wider ideas about the immaturity and naiveté of Africans and other non-white 'races', but at the same time it pointed to their vulnerability and the responsibilities that Empire brought.

Recognition of the growing incidence of tuberculosis in tropical

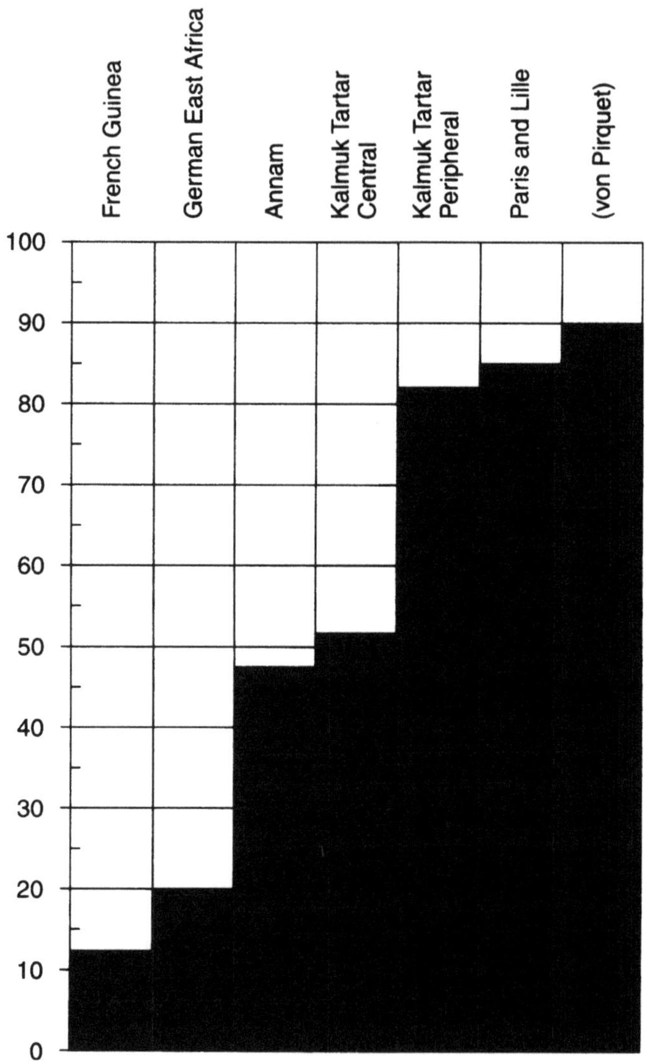

Figure 5.1 Comparative percentages of positive cutaneous tuberculin reactions in primitive and civilised peoples

Source: S.L. Cummins, 'Tuberculosis in Primitive Tribes and its Bearing on the Tuberculosis of Civilized Communities', in *International Journal of Public Health*, 1920, 1, p. 141

colonies was linked to wider concerns about the extent to which colonial rule had been a mixed blessing. In this case, the white man's civilisation had created the conditions for the white man's plague to flourish. However, the German pathologist Krause described tuberculosis as 'the price paid for civilisation', and many considered it worth paying. But against the background of influential metropolitan anti-tuberculosis movements, the question was, did it have to be paid?[14] In Europe and North America these movements were not proposing to turn back the clock and create rural, non-industrialised communities, though sanatoria were often seen in this light. None the less there was an ambivalence about the powers of modern civilisation as both the source and solution to the problem. This was illustrated by William Calwell's description of sanatorium treatment as 'the open air life of the savage, combined with the hygienic comforts of our own age, and systematised by military precision'.[15] In the anti-tuberculosis movement the modernisers triumphed and their programmes aimed to reform civilisation not abandon it; indeed, they trusted that more and higher civilisation, especially advances in medical and sanitary science, would provide the means to control, prevent and eventually eradicate the disease. Many on the Left understood the term 'social disease' rather differently and saw it in terms of inequality and marginality.

For most of those working on the epidemiology of tuberculosis, civilisation was constructed in terms of social and economic development, though cultural, ethnic and human factors were also considered, especially in the United States where there were fears about the importation of the disease by immigrants. Indeed, it was in relation to these groups, rather than to native Americans or African Americans, that the question of race and racial susceptibility was raised after 1900. However, leading American tuberculosis experts, like the Jewish physician Maurice Fishberg and the Army Surgeon George E. Bushnell, maintained confidently that the disease was not an ethnic or racial problem.[16] Both Bushnell and Fishberg disputed whether Jews, Negroes or any other such groups were 'races' in the sense of being distinct biological (genotype) groups. Fishberg, for example, suggested that any advantage enjoyed by Jews was cultural and derived from their social history and hygienic practices, while the experience of Irish and Italian immigrants pointed to economic factors being primary.[17]

After the First World War there was more interest in the causes of the high tuberculosis mortality rates amongst African Americans, if not native Americans. The health of African American soldiers had thrown up interesting questions, while domestically the consequences of the migration of blacks to northern cities was becoming an important public health issue. With regard to tuberculosis, the question was – why, after many centuries of contact with Europeans and the tubercle bacillus, had the morbidity and mortality rates of African Americans not approximated to that of Americans of European descent? A distinct racial susceptibility was an obvious explanation and was seemingly backed up by the pathological evidence that the disease took a different, more virulent and disseminated course in African Americans. Yet, more common than pathological studies were speculative historical epidemiologies that, while still giving a primary role to social factors, none the less mixed these with racial assumptions. For example, with regard to slavery it was suggested that plantation life had been open-air and healthy, and prevented exposure to the disease and hence the effective tuberculisation of African Americans. Thus, after the abolition of slavery, African Americans remained as vulnerable as their ancestors. However, mere exposure to a new pathogen did not seem to be the problem; instead the social conditions in which African Americans now found themselves and the lifestyles they 'chose' were seen as the main causes. The former senior Indian Medical Service (IMS) official, Sir Havelock Charles, explained with revealing stereotypes what the healthy, sanitary features of slavery had been and the 'suffering' caused by its abolition.

> Before the war [the African American] was a valuable chattel, under the care of his master, with good food, living in the open air, under the discipline of healthy labour and suitably clad. After the war, we have this race, immature mentally and morally, given its freedom. What followed? Released from the country, they herded into large cities, leading lives of comparative idleness, victims to intemperance and excessive venery, with bad food, bad air and weakened by the ravages of syphilis.[18]

Charles, in typical IMS fashion, suggested that the best hope lay with improved sanitation, which would, of course, encompass discipline and moral reform. Cummins agreed, though he placed more emphasis on ensuring that such vulnerable groups received small immunising doses of bacilli, not large and potentially lethal ones. Yet, the idea of distinct racial susceptibilities and pathologies had been undermined by the experience of the First World War, where under the same conditions the health status of African Americans rapidly began to converge with that of white Americans.

Bushnell's original intention, based on his military experience, had been to write a monograph on tuberculosis in the tropics and amongst the non-white races now under American rule, but, like Cummins, he was struck by the wider significance of his ideas for industrialised countries and for all races. He went furthest in suggesting that the tuberculisation of the population was both an inevitable and desirable consequence of modern civilisation.[19] But if tuberculisation was a marker of civilisation, where did that leave the anti-tuberculosis campaign and its aim of eradicating the disease? One answer was to argue that the type of epidemic that had accompanied urbanisation and industrialisation in Europe and North America could, with modern knowledge and technologies, be avoided. Latecomers to urbanisation and industrialisation ought, with modern knowledge and technologies, to be able to avoid the kind of epidemic seen in modern Europe. Thus, tuberculisation was not the result of civilisation as such, but was a feature of 'faulty' civilisations that ignored the 'laws of health' and had not balanced social and economic changes with 'necessary safeguards'.[20] Also, while it was acknowledged that 'Nature is carrying on in her own slow way her great anti-tuberculosis campaign' by the tuberculisation of the population, this was occurring too slowly, even in European countries.[21] None the less, there remained the problem that if the disease and the bacillus were to be eradicated, say, from the shores of the United States, then American citizens might again become 'virgin soil' and be vulnerable to immigrants carrying the disease or when they themselves travelled abroad.

The population movements of the First World War offered many new opportunities to explore the epidemiology of tuberculosis at home and abroad, including questions of immunity and tuberculisation.[22] Significant in confirming the label of 'social disease' were the correlations observed between increased mortality and morbidity rates and two 'environmental' factors: malnutrition and overcrowding.[23] Against this background Cummins published a seminal but controversial article on 'Tuberculosis in Primitive Tribes and its Bearing on the Tuberculosis of Civilised Communities', in the new *International Journal of Public Health* in 1920. In this he synthesised his earlier work, with new data from the war and studies of age-related mortality, into a fully developed model of 'active immunity acquired by contact with the bacillus', in which heredity played little or no part.[24] Cummins' article caused controversy in Britain for several reasons. First,

Karl Pearson objected that his views on heredity had been misrepresented and that Cummins was wrong in claiming no part for heredity in resistance to tuberculosis.[25] Second, Cummins was taken to task by Major Greenwood over his use of statistics and for confusing the acquired resistance of individuals with that of populations.[26] It seemed that Cummins was assuming the Lamarckian inheritance of acquired immunity between generations, or a version of recapitulation theory where the development of the individual repeated the evolution of the species. In fact, Cummins' theory of 'virgin soil' at this time did not depend upon evolution or heredity.[27] His point was that immunity was acquired by populations from progressive exposure to sub-clinical doses of bacilli, which allowed the build up of immunity in the individual. Over time such immunity would produce the tuberculisation of the population, as a higher proportion of chronic cases ensured a preponderance of sub-clinical infections that allowed the progressive establishment of immunity. Cummins anticipated an equilibrium between the germ and its human host in a few generations not on an evolutionary time scale. Put another way, he was suggesting that an infected population, with immunity, was potentially healthier than an uninfected, 'virgin soil' one, and that a tuberculised individual with 'arrested' or 'cured' infection was better off than someone who remained uninfected and hence vulnerable.

Anti-tuberculosis campaigners worried that their efforts would be undermined by any suggestion that low-level infections in childhood were beneficial, and an Editorial in the *Lancet* criticised Cummins, saying his whole argument was 'Barmecidal'.[28] Cummins denied that this was his message, but would only say that everything should be done to reduce the risk of lethal doses of bacilli reaching children. Two years later, in his Inaugural Lecture in Cardiff, he reiterated the point.

> [If] Nature is gradually getting rid of tuberculosis by a process of unconscious vaccination, then we should, in our efforts at prevention, give a great deal of attention to defending children and susceptible persons from massive doses, and we should concentrate research on efforts to discover a safe and efficient vaccine.[29]

In this lecture Cummins' once again expounded his ideas on acquired immunity and it is intriguing how he viewed Britain through the prism of tuberculosis as an imperial problem, especially in a suggestion that parts of North Wales resembled tribal Africa in being 'virgin soil'.[30] In passing, it is worth noting that there was no racial connotation here about vulnerable Celts, rather the parallel was in population density, levels of urbanisation and industrialisation, and migration patterns.

'VIRGIN SOIL' AND AFTER

In Cardiff, Cummins quickly developed research and practical interests in the lung diseases of South Wales coal miners and North Wales slate miners. This expertise, together with his earlier work in Africa, led to an invitation from South Africa in 1927 to be expert adviser to a Tuberculosis Research Committee (TRC) set up to advise on the control of tuberculosis amongst workers in the Rand's gold mines.[31] The work of the Committee and the impact of its report in South Africa have been discussed in detail by Randall Packard, who places it in the context of long-term concerns about mining and health in Southern Africa and, going forward, with the development of apartheid.[32] Tuberculosis was one of many disease problems amongst miners and in the 1920s there was some success in controlling its incidence by screening recruits and improving conditions, though mortality rates outside of the mines, in towns and in rural areas continued to rise. Packard shows that Cummins' ideas, fully elaborated in a final report of the TRC in 1932, helped foster a fatalistic attitude towards improving the health of miners because any major improvement would take several generations, if not centuries. More important for our argument is the revision of the 'virgin soil' theory that was prompted by his experiences in South Africa. First, he added an intermediate stage of immunity between 'virgin soil' status and fully tuberculised bodies and, second, he spoke again of racial differences with Africans having 'a real inborn lack of power to develop . . . resistance' and of 'a biological dissimilarity in the average response to tuberculous infection as between the black and the white races'.[33]

In the 1900s, the French immunologist Albert Calmette had elaborated a 'Law' which stated that, 'Peoples are more resistant to the attacks of the infectious diseases of their own countries and districts than to those of foreign diseases with which neither they nor their ancestors have been accustomed to come into contact'.[34] This had implications for all migrants as it suggests that first generation immigrants would always be subject to a health 'disadvantage'. In many ways the Law was simply a restatement of older ideas on 'seasoning'; however, it took a new significance in South Africa because of the importance of migrant workers in the economy. Would the health of these workers deteriorate when they left their 'homelands' whether or not they worked in the mines? Would improved diets, housing and health care for miners give significant benefits? If migrants' health deteriorated in the mines, would it improve again when they returned home? What prompted such speculation was the finding of the TRC that, amongst migrant miners, those who tested tuberculin positive on arrival were more likely to develop serious tubercular disease than those who reacted negative on arrival – i.e. those who were 'virgin soil'. F. J. Allen, from a study of native colliery workers in Witbank, had asked as early as 1927 about the balance of 'virgin soil' versus 'reawakened infection in previously contaminated soil'. This questioned the idea that tribal Africa was indeed 'virgin soil' and suggested that the high rates of the disease were due not to infection, but to the ways mine work weakened the bodies of Africans.[35] Allen was uncertain whether African vulnerability was due to a 'racial idiosyncrasy' or unfamiliarity with industrial work, but Cummins was clear that any difference was due to their 'imperfect individual and racial adaptation to the tubercle bacillus'.[36] Such speculations led Cummins to elaborate his 'virgin soil' theory in new ways.

In an article published in 1929, before the TRC report but after his visit to South Africa, Cummins complicated the parallel between British children and primitives by introducing 'adolescents' and equating them with migrant African miners. His argument was that such miners did not produce a mature immune response, rather their reaction was merely allergic or 'hypersensitive'.[37] This, he said, was similar to the 'latent' or 'larval' disease found in British adolescents where the disease had been localised but not successfully arrested. The fate of these individuals, between infection and resistance, was said to be finely balanced so that any emotional, physical or environmental stresses would lead to the development of active tuberculosis. A similar precariousness was often ascribed to adult sanatorium patients and was one factor in the revival of rest therapy in the 1930s.[38] According to Cummins, what was happening was that 'African natives' were not becoming fully tuberculised because the system of migrant labour meant that they enjoyed 'alternate periods of industrial stress and pastoral leisure'; indeed, in some accounts the picture he painted of 'tribal Africa' was of one large sanatorium.

There were said to be advantages in the system of migrant labour for the individual who benefited from 'the muscular work and good food' of the mines, followed by the leisured, outdoor life in his home village. The alternate periods of physiological stress and healing allowed them to maintain any infection in the hypersensitive or 'larval' stage. However, there were disadvantages for their communities and the nation, for as their tuberculisation was incomplete, hypersensitive individuals continued to be carriers and spreaders of infection. The two-way traffic in ideas between Africa and Britain was again evident in Cummins' summation of the problem.

> What has occurred has been, not a rapidly spreading epidemic . . . but the gradual establishment of endemic tuberculosis, leading, in the sunny open-air life of a native population, to a high average of positive tuberculin reactions in 'healthy' persons as well as to a fairly large number of chronic cases such as might be found in a country town in Ireland, Scotland and Wales.[39]

His conclusion was that Africans could safely remain hypersensitive in their home communities, but would continue to be vulnerable every time they returned to mine work. One hope for improvements was to create a permanent workforce by establishing townships, for he noted that already a few 'long service' Africans had been able to survive without returning to their homelands.

In the 1930s, Cummins returned to his earlier notion that the African response to the tubercle bacillus was different, in a way a 'hypersensitive' response was a 'primitive' one. He also talked again of there being distinct racial pathologies, with Africans suffering acute, disseminated disease. Hereditary ideas with respect to tuberculosis had never disappeared and there had been a reluctance amongst clinicians in Britain to attribute everything to infection and social conditions, given that they saw so much individual variation. This was also true of senior British tuberculosis experts; for example, in 1925 Louis Cobbett wrote of a transmitted factor 'deeply fixed in the blood of each race'. A decade later, Harold H. Scott argued that 'African racial peculiarities' explained much more than 'virgin soil' ideas, citing continuing high levels of the disease amongst African Americans, 'even after some hundreds of years of racial life on another continent'.[40] Similarly, American authorities, like E. R. Long, asked in the mid-1930s that attention should be given once again to ideas that had not been stressed recently, like the 'constitution'.[41] The combination of 'racial peculiarities' and hypersensitivity suggested to Cummins that African adaptation to urban, industrial lifestyles could not be rushed; a period of 200 years was expected to be necessary for adaptation to the disease, which in terms of practical policy was an eternity.[42]

From the first recognition of the problem in Africa and India, as in Europe, responsibility for the rise of the disease had been passed to some degree to the indigenous population. Amongst colonial peoples the highest rates of the infection were amongst internal migrants, that is, those who had 'chosen' to move to towns, to join the army, to end up in jail, or to work in mining and other industrial employment. Migration as such was exacerbated by ignorance, immaturity, overcrowding and insanitary conditions. While it was accepted that these were tolerable in remote, sparsely populated villages, when introduced into burgeoning towns and other settlements the consequences were inevitable.[43] However, like Cummins, there were many colonialists and medical experts who felt a sense of responsibility for the fact that 'primitive' peoples had been exposed too rapidly to the rigours of higher levels of 'civilisation'. With this went fears about the disintegration of 'tribal' societies and the possible physical degeneration of Africans. In the African context, it was social diseases like tuberculosis, syphilis and leprosy that were the diseases of civilisation in the first half of this century, not those we now place in this category – cancer, heart disease and diabetes.

TUBERCULOSIS IN COLONIAL AFRICA IN THE 1930s

In the 1930s the main constituency discussing tuberculosis in Africa shifted from experts based in Britain to medical officers working in Africa and elsewhere. Their view was not so much that the theory of 'virgin soil' needed revision, but that its historical moment had passed. They contended that the colonial state, together with the army, traders, missions, mines and other commercial ventures, had permeated Africa so deeply that few places remained uncontaminated by the bacillus, or affected by 'civilisation'. Charles Willcocks, in several studies of tuberculosis in Tanganyika (now Tanzania), concluded in 1938 that 'In no part of the territory I visited could the Natives be regarded as virgin soil.'[44] A review of the literature on tuberculosis in the tropics in 1937 said that the evidence showed that 'even in the more remote portions of Africa tuberculous infection is widespread'.[45] Bezançon and Arnould, from evidence of French African colonies, now argued that Africa had never been 'virgin soil' and that it was the recently deteriorating social and economic conditions that had allowed the disease to spread from indigenous foci as well as from migrants.[46] Whatever the history of the tubercle bacillus in Africa, with the end of 'virgin soil' status and the spread of the disease, the prospects of Africans were expected to improve.[47] Tuberculisation was now likely to be more rapid and effective, and the disease easier to control and treat.[48]

The reframing of tuberculosis in Africa as an endemic disease, made worse by the social and economic dislocation of imperialism, resonated with the wider picture of colonial health and welfare that developed in the 1930s. Economic recession, colonial indebtedness, emergent nationalism, a loss of self-confidence in the 'civilising mission' and the ideal of the 'dual mandate' combined to create what contemporaries called the 'colonial problem'.[49] In health, there was evidence of deteriorating mortality levels in many colonies, compounded by malnutrition and uncontrolled urban growth. As early as the 1920s, colonial medical officers had expressed a sense of foreboding about the spread of tuberculosis in Africa and of 'the duty of bearing the white man's burden to relieve some of that which we ourselves have imposed'.[50] Africa had long been seen as the dark, diseased continent, but the hope of tropical medicine was that the control of disease would be the first step to development. Now it was evident that economic, social and cultural development had made some disease problems, like tuberculosis, much worse.

By the end of the 1930s, however, little or nothing had been done in most colonies with regard to tuberculosis and other non-tropical diseases. At the Empire Conference on the Care and After-Care of the Tuberculous in 1937 many speakers from African colonies admitted frankly that they had no idea of the extent of the disease in their territory.[51] Only in East Africa, where officers like Willcocks and H. N. Davies had made special studies, was there any detailed picture of the problem, or any developed ideas on the control of the disease.[52] At the NAPT Conference in July 1938, the close links between the problem in Africa and Britain were again evident when Willcocks, who was by this time Tuberculosis Research Officer for British Africa, recommended a control programme based on the one recently introduced in Lancashire.[53] Davies, who worked in Kenya, had tried to adapt the up-to-date treatment of collapse therapy to African hospital conditions, feeling that technical interventions could achieve more in the short term, for effective social interventions were a distant prospect.[54] Cummins now looked to the adaptation of control measures to 'native customs and preferences' and suggested following the lead of missionaries to concentrate on the medical treatment of individuals rather than administrative measures with communities.[55] His idea was for a modified dispensary system, including educational measures and tuberculin testing, backed up by the segregation of sufferers in village settlements rather than sanatoria.[56] A more radical view was that Africans be offered intermediate forms of urbanisation and industrialisation that would slow down the rate of tuberculisation. In 1934, J. A. Young, a colonial medical officer in Nigeria, called for the establishment of special settlements on the outskirts of existing towns and cities, where population densities would be low and where healthier industrial environments could be maintained.

> If groups of industries were established along these lines small townships, limited in size could be set up which would be sufficiently near to agricultural areas to enable workers to obtain their natural foodstuffs cheaply and further would not estrange them entirely from their old methods of living.[57]

The sense that Africa had moved on from being 'virgin soil' led in the late 1930s to greater metropolitan and colonial interest in tuberculosis in India, which had previously been ignored by Cummins and others. Now it was seen as a country from which lessons might be learned for Africa, though within India it was largely political pressures that had prompted the government to act.

TUBERCULOSIS IN BRITISH INDIA

Tuberculosis was 'discovered' by Europeans in India only in the 1840s, but there was never a strong belief that Indians were 'virgin soil' in the same way that Africans had been. Joseph Ewart typified Anglo-Indian medical opinion when he suggested in 1881 that the disease had been present for many centuries and had not been identified sooner owing to the extreme difficulty in obtaining Indian bodies for post-mortem examinations and its confusion with other diseases.[58] However, while India was not regarded as 'virgin soil', it was widely believed that its inhabitants enjoyed a *partial* immunity to the disease, and that this accounted for its seemingly lower incidence among Indian as opposed to European soldiers. According to Ewart, this immunity was not an innate 'racial' characteristic, but the result of healthy living, and specifically of outdoor life and a largely vegetarian diet. The comparative absence of alcohol in Indian diets was another factor. Ewart's emphasis on clean living was typical of many nineteenth-century Indian medical texts, which expressed anxiety over the habits of Europeans and their tendency to intemperance. He was also firmly within the Anglo-Indian medical tradition in placing great emphasis on climate as a factor in the incidence of the disease and in recovery.[59]

This preoccupation with climate distinguished the writings of British-Indian doctors from their contemporaries at 'home', where notions of an inherited 'diathesis' were dominant. Although European doctors thought climate to be significant in the development of a tubercular constitution and in the treatment of tuberculosis, it never occupied the same prominence in their work as it did in India.[60] This climatological view of tuberculosis was not immediately undermined by Koch's announcement of the tubercle bacillus in 1882, but attention began slowly to turn to the bacillus and the conditions under which it spread. From the turn of the century, most of those who wrote on tuberculosis in India also subscribed to the view that the disease was a malady of civilisation. It was widely believed that the overcrowding and stress associated with urban, industrialised life provided the conditions under which tuberculosis could spread, as well as lowering the resistance of individuals to infection and the subsequent development of the disease.

Although there was no way of measuring the incidence of tuberculosis among Indians prior to 1914, since there was no separate heading under which to enter the disease in district and municipal returns, there was nevertheless a sense that the disease was increasing. This was borne out by mortality returns for prisons, the army and the Indian police, and in examinations conducted on new recruits and inmates. By 1910 it was admitted that the disease was now common among these groups.[61] A widely cited study, undertaken by Dr Arthur Lankester immediately after the First World War, drew attention to an apparent increase in tuberculosis in most of India's cities, the highest incidence being in the factory town of Ahmedabad, which recorded a death rate from tuberculosis of 5.9 per thousand in 1919. These figures received additional support from post-mortem examinations, such as those conducted by Leonard Rogers in Calcutta, and from a number of local tuberculin surveys. By 1920 the only areas of India regarded as 'virgin soil' were remote, mountainous regions such as Gilgit and Chitral.

Industrialisation and urbanisation were now clearly identified as the most important factors in accounting for the incidence of tuberculosis in India, but it was thought that settled urban populations would gradually gain immunity to the disease and that tuberculosis in such locations would usually be mild in nature. This assumption appeared to be vindicated by tuberculosis figures during the First World War, which showed that Indian troops drawn from Nepal and isolated hill tracts were more susceptible to tuberculosis than those recruited from the plains and the towns.[62] As in Africa, there was a tendency to compare the course of the disease in Indians to the acute type of tuberculosis found among children in Europe. However, according to the medical missionary P.V. Benjamin, most Indian tuberculosis cases exhibited a distinctive pathology, being primarily of the exudative type, yet with a tendency to fibrosis and localisation. Indian tuberculosis, therefore, was typically somewhere between the European and African forms of the disease, since Africans tended to suffer from an acute disseminating form, without the fibrosis that arrested the disease in Europeans.[63]

British and African authorities on colonial tuberculosis may have ignored India, but Anglo-Indian doctors followed events and opinion elsewhere and found many parallels with their experience. For example, they accepted the assumption that colonial peoples would become progressively immune as urbanisation gathered pace.[64] However, with echoes of ideas current in South Africa, in 1937, the Director General of the Indian Medical Service, Sir Cuthbert Sprawson, observed that urban populations in India had yet to acquire immunity from tuberculosis, owing to the fact that many workers returned to their villages after a short period of work in the towns. Immunity depended crucially upon stable populations and was undermined by migration. There were some areas in which the disease had become endemic and apparently less acute, and curiously these were rural areas of the Punjab and the North West Frontier.[65] Sprawson gave no explanation for endemic tuberculosis in these areas, though it is worth noting that they were the main recruiting grounds for the Indian Army, and that tuberculosis may well have been introduced by returning soldiers.[66]

Although the Indian tuberculosis literature stressed the social nature of the problem, other factors were not excluded from discussion. One study claimed that the greater incidence of the disease among Indians as opposed to British and Americans was due neither to innate differences, nor to acquired immunity, but to the influence of climate and lack of exercise. Prolonged exposure to the South Indian climate was said to reduce lung capacity and hence lower the ability of Indians to resist infection.[67] Other writers on Indian tuberculosis also stressed the role of climate and the peculiarity of Indian conditions. Leonard Rogers, for example, found that the incidence of tuberculosis in Bengal was coincident with high rainfall and humidity.[68] Such views still carried weight in India in the 1920s and were congruent with the climatological bias of earlier British Indian medicine, but were by then against the grain of international opinion.[69]

In India as elsewhere, the 1930s brought a more 'racial' turn in writing on tuberculosis. The Danish missionary doctor C. Frimodt-Möller made the point obliquely, saying that 'economic, social and hygienic factors play a far less important part in producing the severe exhaustive type of pulmonary tuberculosis met in India than is generally supposed'.[70] Although he noticed no marked differences among Indians themselves, his assistant at the Union Mission Sanatorium believed that susceptibility to tuberculosis seemed to increase as European blood became attenuated by inter-racial marriages, with mixed race 'Europeans' being more susceptible than Europeans, though less so than Indians.[71]

However, such speculations never detracted from the overriding emphasis of the Indian literature on the conditions that attended urbanisation and industrialisation, and the spread of 'civilisation'. Yet tuberculosis was not foremost on the medical agenda, as it was in Europe, for, unlike cholera, malaria and other epidemic diseases, it did not directly effect the government and economy of British India. Before 1910 only its high incidence in Bengal jails attracted the attention of the British authorities, but thereafter Indians themselves began to point to the increasing incidence of tuberculosis among the population at large.[72] At the second All-India Sanitary Conference at Madras in 1912, Dr Chandra Sakhar lamented that the disease had been neglected by both doctors and patients. His answer to its growing incidence was the improvement of general sanitation in Indian towns and villages, mass education in the basics of hygiene, facilities for early diagnosis and treatment and the establishment of consumption hospitals and sanatoria.[73]

Few medical officers and government administrators would have disagreed with the first three of Sakhar's proposals, for general sanitation, education and the provision of basic treatment at dispensaries, had been the basis of British Indian medical policy since the 1830s.[74] However, the demand for tuberculosis hospitals and sanatoria was far more controversial as it implied considerable state expenditure on institutions whose value was disputed. Lt. Fox of the IMS, who spoke after Sakhar at the 1912 conference, agreed that sanatoria were too expensive for a country such as India and recommended public education through existing channels and the establishment of tuberculosis societies.[75] The first such society – the King George V Anti-Tuberculosis League – was established in Bombay in 1912. The League, which was led by several prominent citizens of Bombay, opened its first 'information bureau' in 1913, with eleven more dispensaries planned for the city's labouring poor. It was also proposed to attach a tuberculosis department to existing free municipal dispensaries. The long-term aim was to disseminate information about the disease and about elementary hygiene, but the dispensaries also had facilities for bacterial examination and basic treatment.[76]

The failure of such organisations to secure substantial funds from either government or private philanthropists practically crippled measures against tuberculosis in India. An example of this was the fate of the anti-tuberculosis campaign in Bengal, where a sanatorium for the free treatment of the poor and middle classes was suggested in 1908. A site was selected but the Bengal government decided that the estimated expenditure would impose too great a financial burden. In 1913 the Calcutta Corporation made a similar proposal which came to nothing because the Bengal government declined to make a contribution towards the expense. When funds were finally made available for a sanatorium from an Indian philanthropist in 1935, the government felt unable to let the scheme go ahead because of opposition from local (Indian) residents, who feared that a sanatorium might spread disease.[77]

Despite the special attention given to sanatoria in some quarters, the dominant approach was to pursue education and, to a lesser degree, to provide treatment through dispensaries. This was the approach endorsed by government and by the main voluntary organisations in India. At a meeting held under the auspices of the Overseas League and the East India Association in London in July 1938, the Medical Adviser to the Secretary of State, Sir John Megaw, laid special emphasis on 'educational persuasion'. He saw this as part of the general medical policy so far developed by the government of India; indeed, he thought that there was 'much to be said for directing propaganda against all infectious diseases'. Megaw also favoured domiciliary treatment rather than sanatorium care, claiming that 'ten to twenty patients could be treated in their own homes for the cost of a single patient in a modern sanatorium'.[78]

The Vice-Regal Tuberculosis Association of India was similarly inclined. Although the Association recognised the need for more sanatoria, it felt that dispensaries should occupy 'the front place in the organisation for combating the disease'. The emphasis was once again on education, though by the late 1930s greater efforts were being made to train Indian medical and lay workers to carry out these tasks.[79] The growing delegation of tuberculosis work to Indians was part and parcel of a gradual devolution of medical policy and practice between the wars, and one which distinguished India's medical experience from that of colonies in Africa.[80]

Such training was vitally important if the tuberculosis campaign was to meet one of its main objects, that of penetrating the *zenana*, the parts of high-caste Indian homes in which women were kept secluded. This *purdah* system had long been the butt of criticism from sanitary campaigners, and organisations such as the Dufferin Fund had been established towards the end of the nineteenth century in order to supply health visitors and medical aid for women. The apparently greater incidence of tuberculosis among Indian women recorded by public health visitors provided new ammunition for their assaults on the *purdah* system and on the institution of child marriage, for early seclusion meant prolonged exposure to infection in the allegedly overcrowded and insanitary conditions of the *zenana*.[81] *Purdah* was also a convenient scapegoat at a time when tuberculosis was firmly equated with changes wrought by British rule. According to some doctors, such as Arthur Lankester, tuberculosis was not necessarily the 'price of progress' but a disease of the *improperly* civilised.[82]

Lankester reflected the dominant view that tuberculosis in India was primarily the result of ignorance and that education was the key to preventing its spread. However, by the 1930s, there was a growing number of doctors who challenged the orthodox approach to tuberculosis control in British India. Not the least of these was the Director General of the IMS, Sir Cuthbert Sprawson, who in 1937 highlighted the lack of specialist tuberculosis hospitals in India, and the fact that most general hospitals were not even equipped with specialist wards. The need for more such provisions for treatment was crucial, according to Sprawson, since the severity of most Indian tuberculosis cases made out-patient treatment impractical.[83] Calls for more sanatoria also came from the voluntary sector, notably religious missions.[84]

As India moved towards independence, calls for government action against tuberculosis became stronger and more insistent: there was a sense that the British had failed in their responsibilities as a colonial power. Just after the transfer of power in 1947, it was claimed that India needed half a million beds for tuberculosis patients, whereas it had only 2 per cent of this number, and 4,400 clinics instead of the 120 then in existence. Existing facilities were also inadequate as a basis for any vaccination programme with BCG, which required well-organised clinics and a good laboratory service in which to produce the vaccine and tuberculin for skin testing.[85] The British administration had clearly failed to pick up the gauntlet thrown down by Cummins at the Empire Conference in 1937, when he made unfavourable comparisons between the lethargy of British colonial administrations and the more impressive efforts made by the French.[86]

By the time of independence in 1947, tuberculosis was the second largest cause of mortality in India, but it was still a 'Cinderella' disease by comparison with malaria, cholera and other perceived scourges of the subcontinent. It lacked both the 'glamour' necessary to sustain political and scientific interest and the economic impact necessary to ensure official intervention. Increasing tuberculosis infection among Indians, and other colonial peoples, became an index of the limitations of colonial rule and was viewed with concern by British doctors and indigenous critics alike. Although there was substantial agreement over the causes of tuberculosis, the question of how to control the disease was never resolved under British rule. The extensive provisions envisaged by reform-minded doctors were incompatible with both the financial position of colonial governments and (sometimes) the feelings and priorities of the indigenous population, as the unpopularity of tuberculosis sanatoria among Indians demonstrates. The centrality of sanatoria in policy discussions also signalled the growing influence of clinicians and hospital medicine as against the earlier dominance of military and sanitary medical officers. With this went a shift of emphasis from the conditions in which tuberculosis spread to the disease in bodies, and the rights of individuals to treatment and protection. It would not be unreasonable to link this to the political changes in India and the 'Indianization' of medical services. In other words, civilisation was constituted not only in terms of social and environmental conditions, but also in terms of the level of the welfare and protection offered to subjects of the British Empire.

CONCLUSION

The history of tuberculosis in early twentieth-century Africa and India that we have presented here challenges many common assumptions about migrants, minorities and health. Contemporaries certainly saw the rising incidence of the disease as a consequence of the activities of expatriate colonialists, but their responsibility lay not in importing infection but in spreading disease-making conditions. The principal reason for this was that these 'migrants', though a minority in terms of population, were anything but marginal politically, economically and socially. As colonial rulers, functionaries or entrepreneurs they had used Western material and social technologies to transform colonial cultures and environments, albeit unevenly and with many unintended consequences. One such was the tuberculisation of the indigenous populations of Africa and India, especially in urban areas and in association with commercial and industrial activity. However, the spread of this disease was said by British and colonial medical experts to be double-edged; they anticipated high mortality in the short and medium term, but in the long term it was likely to be beneficial as a fully tuberculised society was one with great resistance to infection and to fatal tubercular disease. Paradoxically, individuals (and populations) who were infected seemed (potentially) healthy and strong, while those uninfected seemed (potentially) sick and vulnerable.

While such points are interesting, our main argument has been to show how 'tropical', 'primitive' or 'colonial' tuberculosis was constructed and acted upon as a disease of civilisation. The spread of the disease was not linked to population movements, nor the migration of individuals. Interestingly, the rise of tuberculosis in the tropics was never linked to any earlier exchange of pathogens recently discussed by Alfred Crosby.[87] Overall, the problem of colonial tuberculosis was seen as directly analogous to the problem in Europe and North America – in other words, it was a 'social disease'. A large part of the explanation for this is that there was a single, Empire-wide, if not international, community of tuberculosis experts concerned with this disease and its control. This is not to deny any local autonomy, nor to play down the significance of perceived differences between societies and cultures with regard to health. Rather, it is to make the point that approaching colonial medicine in terms of models of centre and periphery is unhelpful. The discourses on colonial tuberculosis between 1900 and 1940 show more than just one-way traffic in personnel, ideas and policies, but changing sources of knowledge, authority and influence within a single discourse.

The issue of racial immunity, resistance or susceptibility was a constant reference point in discussions of tuberculosis and Empire. The epidemiology and pathology of tuberculosis helped construct and reinforce the importance of cultural rather that racial (biological) differences. The 'virgin soil' theory, with its emphasis on acquired immunity, did not impute any significant influence to racial differences. The important word here is 'significant', for while racial ideas were evident in the medical and non-medical writings of many experts, these were never given a determinant role; they were third or fourth order factors, after social and environmental conditions, and exposure. However, the 'virgin soil' theory none the less reinforced wider ideas of racial difference and inferiority by its continued references to 'primitives' and by promoting the idea that 'primitive' people lacked physiological 'toughness'. Yet this was not about constructing the 'primitive' as totally 'other', the point was to connect the 'civilised' with 'primitives' but to stress the huge physiological, historical and cultural gulf between them. The idea that Africans were the immunological equivalent of European children was resonant with anthropological, psychological and religious views of Africans and Indians as childlike, or adolescent. There is, however, little or no direct evidence to suggest that the idea of 'virgin soil' was gendered; indeed, in the 1930s it was most commonly applied to male mine workers. That said, the association of 'virgin soil' with children, its setting in terms of social evolution and its associations with vulnerability and physiological weakness are resonant with the cluster of 'primitive, child, woman' identified by Megan Vaughan.[88]

While it was accepted that imperialism created the conditions for tuberculosis to become a major 'tropical disease', before 1940 colonial rulers and medical services failed to act on the warnings given by Cummins and later by local agencies. No agency really considered the possibility of keeping the disease out or containing established foci. There were many reasons why so much discussion produced so little action. First, Indian and colonial medical services (and indigenous peoples) had other disease-control priorities and programmes. Second, being framed as a disease of civilisation meant that tuberculosis was a problem to be settled in historical time, not by immediate medical or sanitary intervention. The 'virgin soil' theory reinforced this idea, as effective natural immunity would take generations to develop in communities. Progress was bound to be slow, as social evolutionary assumptions, still popular between the wars, made it seem inevitable that the European path of civilisation and tuberculisation had to be followed in India, Africa and elsewhere. In France and the French Empire there were hopes that the use of BCG might substitute for, or short-cut, the 'natural' process of tuberculisation, but the British government and its experts were hostile to the use of the vaccine at home let alone abroad. After 1945 there were new hopes and new agencies, especially when the WHO took up the challenge of tuberculosis. However, as an endemic, 'social disease', the control of tuberculosis did not lend itself to 'vertical' campaigns of eradication favoured by international and other health agencies in the 1950s.

Nearly half a century on, there is no indication that the spread of tuberculosis in the Third World is slowing down. Tuberculosis can still be regarded as a disease of civilisation, though this can no longer be solely linked with urban, industrial societies; there is now more of a case to be made for its linkage to poverty and social inequalities, both nationally and internationally.

NOTES

We would like to thank David Cantor and Harriet Deacon for their valuable comments on an earlier draft of this chapter. A version of this chapter was read at the Symposium on 'TB: Then and Now', at the University of California, San Francisco, April 1995. Professor Guenther Risse kindly invited us to attend the meeting and we profited greatly from the discussions there. Finally we wish to thank the Wellcome Trust for their support of our work.

1 R.W. Philip, 'Tuberculization and detuberculization', in R.W. Philip, *Collected Papers on Tuberculosis*, London, 1937, pp. 171–92. This chapter was originally published in the *British Medical Journal* in 1912. The difference between 'infection' and 'disease' was crucial as by the early decades of this century the great majority of those infected were able to contain or see off the bacillus, and not develop lesions or suffer the disease syndrome.

2 After 1945, attempts were made by the National Association for the Prevention of Tuberculosis, Britain's leading voluntary anti-tuberculosis organisation, to make the control of colonial tuberculosis a new goal. Their domestic mission had been overtaken by the National Health Service and streptomycin, but their attempted move to Empire was thwarted by the growing work of the United Nations and its agencies and by the end of Empire. See: S.L. Cummins, *Empire and Colonial Tuberculosis*, London, 1945; idem, *A New Empire and Colonial Vista*, London, 1945.

3 F.B. Smith, *The Retreat of Tuberculosis*, London, 1988; L. Bryder, *Below the Magic Mountain: A Social History of Tuberculosis in Twentieth Century Britain*, Oxford, 1988.

4 'Although tuberculosis is undoubtedly a communicable disease, it is yet certain that, short of actual inoculation, the bacillus rarely, if ever, infects the human body unless two conditions . . . also be present; that is, unless there is a susceptible body to receive it and the surroundings be such as to enable it to preserve its virulence.' A. Ransome, *Transactions of the Clinical Society of Manchester*, 16 October 1906.

5 The only form of tuberculosis suffered by infants (0–1 year) was *Tabes mesenterica*.

6 M. Worboys, 'The Sanatorium Treatment for Consumption in Britain,

1890–1914', in J.V. Pickstone, ed., *Medical Innovations in Historical Perspective*, London, 1992, pp. 47–71.

7 On Cummins' life and work see Obituary Notices, *BMJ*, 1949, 1, p. 1054 and *Lancet*, 1949, 1, pp. 983–4.

8 L. Bryder, 'The King Edward VII Welsh National Memorial Association and its Policy Towards Tuberculosis in Wales, 1910–1948', *Welsh Historical Review*, 1986, 13/2, pp. 194–216.

9 S.L. Cummins, 'Tuberculosis in the Egyptian Army', *British Journal of Tuberculosis*, 1908, 2/1, pp. 35–46.

10 S.L. Cummins, 'Primitive Tribes and Tuberculosis', *Transactions of the Royal Society for Tropical Medicine and Hygiene*, 1912, 5, pp. 245–55.

11 L. Colebrook, *Almroth Wright: Provocative Thinker and Doctor*, London, 1954; M. Worboys, 'Vaccine Therapy and Laboratory Medicine in Edwardian England', in Pickstone, *Medical Innovations*, pp. 84–103.

12 Cummins, 'Primitive Tribes', p. 252.

13 Ibid. Some physicians cited the Law of Römer: 'Where tuberculosis is a rare disease the cases that occur will be acute and fatal. Where the disease is common the type will be chronic and relatively benign.'

14 *BMJ*, 1922, 2, p. 208.

15 *BMJ*, 1898, 2, p. 948.

16 M. Fishberg, *Pulmonary Tuberculosis*, Philadelphia, 1919, p. 67; G.E. Bushnell, *A Study in the Epidemiology of Tuberculosis, with special reference to the Tuberculosis of the Tropics and of the Negro Race*, London, 1920, p. 210. Also see: R. Wilson, 'Is the Prevalence of Tuberculosis Among Negroes Due to Race Tendency?', *Proceedings of the 6th International Congress on Tuberculosis*, Volume 3, Washington, 1906, pp. 454–61. Teller contends that in the Progressive Era (1900–20) 'the dominant opinion was that the environment outweighed heredity as a cause of resistance to tuberculosis'. M.E. Teller, *The Tuberculosis Movement: A Public Health Campaign in the Progressive Era*, New York, 1988, p. 98.

17 L.F. Flick, 'Tuberculosis in the Irish Race', *Proc. 6th Int. Cong.*, pp. 473–5; A. Kraut, *Silent Travelers: Germs, Genes and the 'Immigrant Menace'*, Baltimore, 1994.

18 See discussion of Cummins, 'Primitive Tribes', p. 271.

19 Bushnell, *Epidemiology of Tuberculosis*, p. 210.

20 A. Lankester, *Tuberculosis in India: Its Prevalence, Causation and Prevention*, London, 1920. Philip spoke of 'incomplete and ill-informed civilisation', 'Tuberculization', p. 174.

21 *BMJ*, 1920, 1, pp. 111–12.

22 See the summary in S.L. Cummins, *Primitive Tuberculosis*, London, 1939, pp. 83–94.

23 R.B. Wild, 'Some Racial Problems, Social Evils and Modern Crusades', *Lancet*, 1920, 2, p. 52.

24 S.L. Cummins, 'Tuberculosis in Primitive Tribes and its Bearing on the Tuberculosis of Civilized Communities', *International Journal of Public Health*, 1920, 1, pp. 138–71.

25 K. Pearson, 'The Hereditary Factor in Tuberculosis', *Lancet*, 1920, 2, pp.

891–3. Cummins was prepared to admit a susceptibility might be inherited but not the ability to resist.

26 M. Greenwood, 'The Etiology of Tuberculosis', *Lancet*, 1920, 2, pp. 1165–6.

27 Willcocks argued that Cummins' views were not racial but depended on 'community experience'. C. Willcocks, *Aspects of Medical Investigation in Africa*, London, 1962, pp. 9–10.

28 *Lancet*, 1920, 2, pp. 1024, 1063–4, 1070–1. For similar fears see the review of Bushnell in *BMJ*, 1921, 1, p. 570.

29 S.L. Cummins, 'Tuberculosis in Wales', *BMJ*, 1922, 1, p. 340.

30 M. Vaughan, *Curing Their Ills: Colonial Power and African Sickness*, Cambridge, 1991, p. 99.

31 *Tuberculosis in South African Natives with special reference to the Disease amongst the Mine Labourers on the Witwatersrand*, Johannesburg, 1932. This report was discussed extensively in British medical journals, see: *Lancet*, 1933, 1, pp. 100–1, 251–3, 315.

32 R. Packard, *White Plague, Black Labor: Tuberculosis and the Political Economy of Health and Disease in South Africa*, Los Angeles, 1989.

33 S.L. Cummins, 'Studies of Tuberculosis Among African Natives: General Introduction', *Tubercle*, 1934–5, 16 (Suppl.), p. 13.

34 Louis Cobbett quoted in S. Roodhouse Gloyne, *Social Aspects of Tuberculosis*, London, 1944, p. 88.

35 F.J. Allen, 'Tuberculosis among Native Colliery Workers', *Journal of the Medical Association of South Africa*, 5, 1927, pp. 554–9.

36 See Cummins' review of Allen in *Bulletin of Hygiene*, 1928, 3/4, pp. 309–12.

37 S.L. Cummins, '"Virgin Soil" – and After', *BMJ*, 1929, 2, pp. 39–41. Also see: V.S. Hodson, 'Pulmonary Tuberculosis in the Tropics', *Transactions of the Royal Society for Tropical Medicine and Hygiene*, 1929, 23, pp. 9–11, and S.L. Cummins, 'Bearing of the South African Tuberculosis Investigations on the Problems of Tuberculosis in General', *Transactions of the American National Tuberculosis Association*, 1933, 29, pp. 26–30.

38 Bryder, *Magic*, pp. 184–7.

39 Cummins, 'Virgin Soil', p. 40.

40 L. Cobbett, 'The Resistance of Civilised Men to Tuberculosis: Is it of Racial or Individual Origin?', *Tubercle*, 1924, 6, pp. 577–90; H.H. Scott, 'Tuberculosis in the Tropics', *British Journal of Tuberculosis*, 1929, 23, pp. 179–89; idem, 'Tuberculosis in Man in the Tropics', *Proc. Roy. Soc. Med.*, 1935, 28, pp. 1343–52. Willcocks also saw racial theory and virgin soil theory as alternatives, but went on to say that neither was 'seriously entertained . . . without reference to environmental factors', Willcocks, *Medical Investigation*, p. 10.

41 *Tubercle*, 1936, 17, pp. 1935–6. But see: E.L. Opie, 'Active and Latent Tuberculosis in the Negro Race', *American Review of Tuberculosis*, 1924, 10, pp. 265–74; M. Pinner and J.A. Kasper, 'Pathological Peculiarities of Tuberculosis in the American Negro', *American Review of Tuberculosis*, 1932, 26, p. 463. For the spectrum of opinion in the US in the mid-1930s see: *American Review of Tuberculosis*, 1937, 35, pp. 1–42.

42 One estimate was that reasonable immunity would be acquired in between

100 and 200 years. D.D. Anderson, 'Pulmonary Tuberculosis in a Native Population: The Development of Resistance', *Transactions of the Royal Society for Tropical Medicine and Hygiene*, 1928, 31, p. 470.

43 In the United States, while it was usually argued that differences in susceptibility to tuberculosis were not innate, there was little optimism about any rapid improvement in the mortality rates of African Americans because of the conditions in which they lived and, most tellingly, because of their intellectual immaturity, ignorance and immorality. Cultural racism may have been more potent than biological or scientific racism. See: E. Barkan, *The Retreat of Scientific Racism*, Cambridge, 1992. Also see: M.M. Torchia, 'The Tuberculosis Movement and the Race Question, 1890–1950', *Bulletin of the History of Medicine*, 1975, 49, pp. 152–68.

44 *Report of the 24th Annual Conference of the NAPT*, 1938,120.

45 E. Cochrane, 'Tuberculosis in the Tropics', *Tropical Diseases Bulletin*, 1937, 34, p. 748.

46 A Belgian study published in 1926 supposed that tuberculosis had been introduced into the Belgian Congo (Zaire) by Arab traders long before European contact. Also in 1934 Willcocks began to doubt the historical validity of 'virgin soil' for Africa, *Tubercle*, 1933–4, 15, p. 462.

47 J.W. Winchester, 'Observations on the Mortality from Tuberculosis in the Straits Settlement', *Malayan Medical Journal*, 1934, 9, pp. 182–7.

48 *BMJ*, 1937, 1, p. 988.

49 S. Constantine, *The Making of British Colonial Development Policy, 1914–1940*, London, 1984; Lord Hailey, *An African Survey*, London, 1938.

50 J.J. Vassal, 'The Occurrence of Tuberculosis Amongst Primitive Peoples, Principally in the French Colonies', NAPT, *Transactions of the 14th Annual Conference*, London, 1928, p. 79; H.H. Scott, 'Tuberculosis in the Tropics', *British Journal of Tuberculosis*, 1929, 23, pp. 179–89.

51 *British Journal of Tuberculosis*, 1937, 31, pp. 252–8.

52 *East African Medical Journal*, pp. 129–38. E. Cochrane, *Transactions of the 24th Annual Conference*, London, 1938, p. 153. W.H. Smith, 'Pulmonary Tuberculosis in Africans', *East African Medical Journal*, 1939, 15, pp. 318–28.

53 NAPT, *Transactions of the 24th Annual Conference*, London, 1938, p. 140.

54 H.N. Davies, 'The Work of the Tuberculosis Unit in East Africa', *Tubercle*, 1938, 20, pp. 76–88.

55 *BMJ*, 1937, 1, p. 988.

56 Ibid. In Capetown John Garlick had adapted the Papworth idea to South African and native conditions.

57 E. Cochrane, 'The Control of Tuberculosis in the Tropics', *Bulletin of Hygiene*, 1937, 12, p. 742.

58 Joseph Ewart, 'Scrofula, Tuberculosis, and Phthisis in India', *Medical Times and Gazette*, June 1911, 1881, p. 643.

59 Ewart, 'Scrofula', p. 645.

60 There was some contact between Ewart and the respected German physician Hermann Weber, who stressed the role of climate in the treatment of tuberculosis. See H. Weber, 'The Hygienic and Climatic Treatment of

Chronic Pulmonary Phthisis', *BMJ*, 1885, 1, pp. 517–22, 575–6, 641–3, 688–90, 725–7.

61 D.G. Crawford, 'Tubercle of the Lung in the Hughli Jail and the Hughli Police', reprint from *Indian Medical Gazette*, July 1910, p. 65, Crawford Collection, Wellcome Institute for the History of Medicine, London.

62 Cummins, 'Tuberculosis in Primitive Tribes', pp. 144–6.

63 P.V. Benjamin, 'The Indian People and Tuberculosis', *British Journal of Tuberculosis*, 1937, 31, pp. 235–9.

64 Winchester, 'Straits Settlements', pp. 182–7; 'Tuberculosis in the Tropics – part II. The Control of Tuberculosis in the Tropics', *Bulletin of Hygiene*, 1937, 12, p. 740.

65 Sir Cuthbert A. Sprawson, 'Peculiarities of the Tuberculosis Problem in India', *British Journal of Tuberculosis*, 1937, 31, p. 129. Address delivered to the *Empire Conference on the Care and After-Care of the Tuberculous*, London, 3–5 May 1937.

66 B.L. Kamra, 'Incidence of Pulmonary Tuberculosis in the Punjab Villages', *Indian Medical Gazette*, 1938, 73, pp. 477–8.

67 B.T. Krishnan and C. Vareed, 'The Vital Capacity of 103 Male Medical Students in South India', *Indian Journal of Medical Research*, 1931–2, 19, p. 65; E.O. Mason, 'Normal Vital Capacity of the Lungs in South Indian Women', *Indian Journal of Medical Research*, 1932–3, 20, p. 117.

68 L. Rogers, 'Tuberculosis Incidence and Climate in India', *BMJ*, 1925, 1, p. 256; idem, 'Climate and its Relationship to Tuberculosis', *Tubercle*, 1936, 18, pp. 49–58.

69 Cummins, 'Tuberculosis in Primitive Tribes', pp. 152–3.

70 C. Frimodt-Möller, 'The Tuberculosis Problem in India', *British Journal of Tuberculosis*, 1938, 32, p. 12.

71 P.V. Benjamin, 'The Seriousness of Tuberculosis in India as Shown by a Study of Incidence and Type', *Indian Medical Gazette*, 73, 1938, pp. 540–4.

72 Crawford, 'Tubercle of the Lung', p. 1.

73 *Proceedings of the Second All-India Sanitary Conference, Madras, 11–16 November*, 1912, 3, pp. 284–94.

74 M. Harrison, *Public Health in British India: Anglo-Indian Preventive Medicine, 1859–1914*, Cambridge, 1994.

75 Lt. Fox, 'Tuberculosis and its Relation to Public Health', *Second All India*, pp. 294–300.

76 J.A. Turner, 'The Anti-tuberculosis Campaign in Bombay, India', *British Journal for Tuberculosis*, 1915, 9, pp. 51–5. These plans required more extensive resources than the League had at its disposal, its annual income being only £2000.

77 A.C. Ukil, 'Anti-tuberculosis Work in Bengal', *Indian Medical Gazette*, 1938, 73, pp. 525–39.

78 'Tuberculosis: A Key Problem of India', *BMJ*, 1938, 2, p. 35; 'India: The Tuberculosis Campaign', ibid., p. 1173.

79 'Fighting Tuberculosis in India', *BMJ*, 1939, 2, pp. 403–4.

80 S.L. Cummins, 'Tuberculosis and the Empire', *British Journal of Tuberculosis*, 1937, 13, p. 142.

81 R.A. Riste, 'Tuberculosis in the Zenana', *Indian Medical Gazette*, 1938, 73, pp. 551–7.
82 NAPT, *14th Annual Conference*, p. 108.
83 Sprawson, 'Peculiarities', pp. 131–2.
84 Frimodt-Möller, 'Tuberculosis problem', p. 13.
85 P.V. Benjamin, *Transactions of the Commonwealth and Empire Health and Tuberculosis Conference*, London, 1947, p. 32.
86 Cummins, 'Tuberculosis and the Empire', p. 141.
87 A.W. Crosby, *Ecological Imperialism: The Biological Expansion of Europe, 900–1900*, New York, 1986.
88 Vaughan, *Curing Their Ills*, pp. 19–20. Packard, *White Plague*, only briefly discusses tuberculosis in black women and makes no link between gender and the idea of 'virgin soil'.

6

GOVERNMENT POLICY AND THE HEALTH STATUS OF ABORIGINAL AUSTRALIANS IN THE NORTHERN TERRITORY, 1945–72

Lindsey Harrison

•

In the second half of the nineteenth century, there was a rapid expansion of colonial frontiers into the farthest reaches of Australia. The indigenous population was declining rapidly and it was assumed that they were doomed to extinction. Governments, it was argued, had a duty to protect Aboriginal people in their last days and, at the end of the nineteenth century, the policy of restricting them to selected areas was adopted, based on the belief that Aboriginal people became degraded on contact with non-Aboriginal society.

Each of the state governments and the Commonwealth conducted its own Aboriginal policy, but there were few differences between them. The Commonwealth or Federal government was responsible only for the Aboriginal population directly under its control in the Northern Territory, which it administered from 1911 to 1978.[1] By 1911, all states except Tasmania had passed discriminatory and restrictive legislation designed to 'protect' Aboriginal people. In the Northern Territory, the Aboriginals Ordinance came into effect in 1918. As a result of these protectionist policies, Aboriginal people occupied a separate legal category from the rest of the Australian population and enjoyed few civil rights.[2]

In this chapter, I examine the policies and activities of the Commonwealth government towards Aboriginal people in the Northern Territory. I focus on the post-Second World War period when the policy of protection and segregation described above gave way to assimilation. The aim of this new policy was that Aboriginal people, whose culture had always been considered primitive and expendable, would now 'advance' into non-Aboriginal society and become indistinguishable from the rest of the population. The policy change occurred for a number of reasons. The Aboriginal population now appeared to be increasing, so that the belief that Aboriginal people could not survive contact with 'civilisation' had to be abandoned. Further, the war had boosted the economy and had drawn Aboriginal people into employment in towns and cities where they were more visible to the non-Aboriginal population. However, the new policy envisioned generations of change before citizenship for all could be attained. Meanwhile, authoritarian control and close supervision of Aboriginal people continued.

The adoption of assimilation coincided in the Northern Territory with the establishment of Commonwealth government settlements. These settlements were mostly in remote areas and, initially, were designed to stop the drift of Aboriginal people into towns. With the adoption of assimilation, and despite their geographic location, the settlements came to be seen by the government as playing a vital role in training Aboriginal people to 'advance' into non-Aboriginal society. Instead they created dislocation and dependence.

Settlement life produced profound socio-economic changes for the Aboriginal population, affecting access to traditional lands, family and community relations, food consumption habits and health. In this chapter, I concentrate on the changes to the food supply and the impact of this on nutritional status. Settlement residents were initially supplied with dry rations, which provided a monotonous and often inadequate diet. The assimilation policy provided the impetus for mass communal feeding of the settlements from the mid-1950s, with profound and unintended consequences for Aboriginal nutrition. Communal feeding was not only meant to meet nutritional needs, which it generally failed to do, it was also seen as a tool that would assist assimilation by inculcating European eating habits and food preferences, thus making Aboriginal people more 'acceptable' to the non-Aboriginal community.

Official control of the food supply was only gradually relinquished when the cash economy was introduced into Aboriginal communities in the late 1960s. Following the adoption of a policy of self-determination for Aboriginal people in 1972, dietary interventions were again limited, this time to the supplementation of 'at risk' groups such as pregnant women and infants. Throughout these shifts in policy, little attempt was made to assess the acceptability of the various feeding schemes or their success. On the whole, governments assumed that improved health status would inevitably follow from changes in Aboriginal behaviour and saw little need to critically assess the role of their own policies and actions.

The main sources for this chapter are government papers and reports, in particular the published reports of the departments responsible for Aboriginal affairs, whose task, of course, is to present government policy and their own actions in the best possible light. This leads to obvious tensions in official accounts (particularly in the latter part of this period when the extent of Aboriginal ill-health was well known) between the requirement to report deficiencies in Aboriginal welfare for which official bodies were responsible and which had adverse health outcomes (e.g. lack of sanitation, water supply and housing), and the attempt to explain health problems as the result of Aboriginal behaviour, which could not be blamed on government departments (e.g. 'nomadic' ways). The use of these sources means that no Aboriginal voice is heard in this account. This is not meant to imply that Aboriginal people did not have views on what was happening, or that they were passive in the face of attempts to control them and incorporate them into non-Aboriginal society.[3]

In the following sections, I provide some background to the establishment of settlements and the adoption of assimilation. I discuss the practical aspects of provisioning remote settlements and then focus on the deleterious effects of communal feeding on health and social life. Finally I detail the abandonment of this policy and the impact on diet and health of the cash economy.

FROM SEPARATION TO ASSIMILATION

During the period of segregation, the Commonwealth government in the Northern Territory concentrated on proclaiming reserves on unwanted crown land, encouraging missionary activity on or near the reserves and setting up ration depots for old and infirm Aboriginal people. For the most part, the people on the reserves were left to themselves and there was minimal contact with the state. For example, in 1939, when the Aboriginal population of the Northern Territory was estimated to be 13,898, plus 902 'half-castes', only some 998 (7 per cent) were clothed and issued with basic foodstuffs.[4] This policy allowed some Aboriginal communities not in contact with missions to retain their traditional way of life, unlike communities in settled areas of southern and eastern Australia, where most Aboriginal people were confined to small reserves totally under the control of the police, welfare officials and missionaries.

In 1937, a Commonwealth and States Authority Conference on Aboriginal policies adopted the goal of assimilation, which recognised the increasing participation of Aboriginal people in the non-Aboriginal economy. To begin with this policy focused on the 'half-caste' population. In the early years of the twentieth century, governments had been concerned to incorporate 'half-castes' within protectionist and restrictive legislation by broadening the definition of 'an Aborigine'. Usually this meant classifying people on the basis of their skin colour or other physical characteristics. Rigid controls included making sexual intercourse between Aboriginal and non-Aboriginal people illegal in an attempt to decrease the number of 'half-castes'. During the 1930s, a minority of non-Aboriginal Australians, including some anthropologists who had first-hand knowledge of contemporary Aboriginal society, began to protest about the lack of Aboriginal civil rights, though the majority of Australians continued to believe in Aboriginal racial inferiority. None the less, demonstrations by Aboriginal activists and their non-Aboriginal supporters led to a growing public awareness of the depressed conditions of the Aboriginal community, and the policy change was partly a response to this.[5]

In spite of the policy of separation, Aboriginal people had been migrating from the reserves into centres of pastoral, mining and commercial activity. Contact between Aboriginal and non-Aboriginal people in the Northern Territory increased substantially during the Second World War when over 1,000 jobs became available for Aboriginal people in the armed services.[6] When the war ended, the government decided that to control Aboriginal movements and counteract the 'undesirable' influence of towns, they would have to make the reserves more attractive and habitable. To this end, settlements were created in suitable areas, run by the Native Affairs Branch of the Northern Territory Administration. It was intended to train Aboriginal people in crafts and industries and, with the co-operation of the Department of Health, to offer medical services.[7] For the most part settlements were placed in remote areas, with poor communications and few opportunities for employment. Natural water supplies were often inadequate and this meant sinking bores or wells, plus a significant capital outlay. The provision of a safe water supply and other amenities such as sanitation and shelter had still not been achieved in all settlements by the end of the period under discussion.[8]

Despite the pre-war aim of assimilation, most state governments were slow to change their policies during the 1950s, but the Commonwealth government adopted assimilation for all Aboriginal people in the Northern Territory, including 'full-bloods'. Social change would be actively promoted, so that they would become indistinguishable from other Australians in 'manner of life, standard of living, occupations and participation in community affairs'.[9] Intensive efforts were made to promote assimilation from the settlements, which began to be described as key instruments of the policy. Settlements were now regarded as a means of temporary protection during a transitional stage before full assimilation.[10] Paradoxically, controls and restrictions were still seen as the means to achieve this.

The establishment of the settlements and their role as policy instruments of assimilation had disastrous effects on nutrition in the Northern Territory. Government intervention resulted in the dislocation of the Aboriginal economy and in growing dependence on the non-Aboriginal economy and the state. Increasingly, the food supply came to depend on official perceptions of the needs of Aboriginal people. Bureaucracies controlled not only the type and quantity of food available but also the social setting in which it was to be consumed. The system resulted in inadequate nutrient intakes, the effects of which were exacerbated by poor environments and a high incidence of infections. Facilities at missions and settlements were far below the standard acceptable in the rest of Australia. For example, as late as 1976 only 42.3 per cent of the population had piped water and 36.6 per cent had a functioning lavatory in or near the dwelling.[11] There was also a severe shortage of houses, even of the special 'transitional' houses – two-roomed shelters made of aluminium with concrete floors and no amenities.[12] One indicator of the scale of the problem was that the Aboriginal infant mortality rate by the 1960s was similar to that in Third World countries.[13] In 1965, for example, the Northern Territory's infant mortality rate was 142.7 per thousand live births, compared to an all-Australia rate, minus the Aboriginal population, of 18.5 per thousand.

SETTLEMENTS AND THE RATION SYSTEM

When the settlements were first established, their Aboriginal residents were issued with dry rations and vegetable gardens were established to provide fresh produce. The Northern Territory Administration hoped that the provision of food would encourage parents to bring their children to the settlement schools and clinics.[14] However, the logistical problems of provisioning the settlements were considerable. Transporting food by ship or road from Darwin, or by road or rail from the southern states, was expensive and frequently unreliable. If food had to be stored for long periods it deteriorated, particularly in the humid north. The southern region of the Territory was usually in a better position because it was arid and also because rail services were generally regular from Adelaide in South Australia as far as Alice Springs and so fewer stores had to be held.

Supply to the settlements was not the only problem. The Northern Territory Administration reported in 1949 that a survey showed that the diet was poorly 'balanced' due to a lack of vitamins and minerals. To meet the immediate problem, dried milk was obtained, but in the longer term the authorities planned to establish herds of milking goats and increase vegetable production – a difficult undertaking given the intense seasonal variations in temperature and rainfall.[15]

The missions had been facing similar problems long before government settlements existed. The earliest mission in the Northern Territory, Hermannsberg, was established in 1877 and several others were set up before the First World War. Eventually there were four religious bodies involved in missionary activity in the Territory: the Catholic Church, the Lutherans, the Methodist Overseas Mission and the Church Missionary Society. After the Second World War, government subsidies were increased and, in return, the missions agreed to implement the policies of the Native Affairs Branch.[16]

The primary reason for the existence of the missions was to convert the Aboriginal population and not to feed them. It was the practice of the Christian Missionary Society, though not the Methodists, to restrict rations to people who worked for them. This saved money but it was also intended to aid the formation of the work ethic among the Aboriginal population. On the government settlements, for the same reason, unemployed adult men were often required to trade artefacts and crocodile skins for rations.[17] Some settlements bought bush foods from Aboriginal residents for cash to supplement the rations.[18]

The type of diet available at missions was assessed in 1948 by an American-Australian Expedition to Arnhem Land, sponsored by the National Geographic Society, the Smithsonian Institute and the Australian Commonwealth Government.[19] They looked at four mission stations and found that the dependence on shipping for supplies caused problems because of its unreliability and expense. This led to a diet largely restricted to cereals and their products, usually wheat, wheat flour and rice. The situation was exacerbated because rations were found to be the major source of food, since most Aboriginal people spent all but a few weeks of the year at the missions and drew rations from five to six days a week. When the mission supply of food ran out, the Aboriginal people were sent away to find their own. Although the Expedition found that local food was still plentiful in the dry season, the supply of bush foods within one day of the settlements was diminishing. No attempt was made to assess the contribution to the diet of bush foods because the types and amounts gathered varied so greatly. It was found that Aboriginal people who depended on rations ate a monotonous diet low in fat and, though no clinical signs of deficiency were observed, the diet was suspected of being deficient in iron, calcium, ascorbic acid and vitamins A and B for many months of the year.[20] Margaret McArthur, an Australian who worked for the Nutrition Unit of the Institute of Anatomy in Canberra, was the Expedition's nutritionist. She remarked that the Europeans in charge of the missions did not appreciate that an adequate diet was necessary for their Aboriginal charges. They considered an 'inferior' diet was good enough.

McArthur assessed the energy available for consumption in the rations for children aged from 5 to 14 years and found it to be lower than the recommended allowances. The tables of the USA National Research Council of 1948 were used, as Australia did not produce its own standards until 1954 and even then they closely followed the American version. That the children may actually have been malnourished is suggested by the fact that, although they were approximately the same height for age as non-Aboriginal children, their heights for weight were lower.[21] McArthur also compiled a growth curve for infants which showed that, for the first five to six months of life when they were all breast fed, they increased their weight very rapidly but thereafter failed to gain weight at the same rate as non-Aboriginal children.[22] However, because medical care for Aboriginal people was either rudimentary or non-existent at this time, no one knew what a 'normal' growth curve for Aboriginal children should look like. McArthur remarked that, although there was no evidence to support the assumption that Aboriginal children should have the same heights and weights as non-Aboriginal children, the possibility that their failure to grow was the result of inadequate nutrition could not be ignored.

Winifred Wilson who, like McArthur, was from the Australian

Institute of Anatomy in Canberra, carried out a similar but larger dietary survey in the early 1950s, questioning the people responsible for rationing so that a list of all foods supplied during the week could be compiled. Despite the problems of accuracy with this method, it was concluded that the Aboriginal population were seldom overfed and were sometimes short of food. Wilson found that the diet available to the residents of missions and government settlements was inferior to that issued to Aboriginal stockmen who were employed by pastoralists to look after cattle, but better than that of the Aboriginal station workers who provided labour around the pastoralists' homesteads.[23]

One of the most interesting aspects of Wilson's survey was the comparison of apparent Aboriginal food consumption with figures for the non-Aboriginal population in the Territory and the rest of Australia. These figures came from food consumption surveys carried out in 1943 and 1947–8. The mean consumption per head of bread, cereals and flour by the Aboriginal population was approximately twice the average Australian consumption. The consumption of meat was 30 per cent higher, without doubt influenced by the large amounts of meat available to stockmen. The average consumption of milk and milk products, fruit, vegetables, fats and eggs was less than half the average Australian consumption. These figures clearly show the restricted food supply available to the Northern Territory's Aboriginal population at this time. Garden produce and eggs from settlement hens were usually just enough for the non-Aboriginal staff.

Would the diet of Aboriginal people have received greater attention if they had been part of the regular workforce? The evidence of Wilson's survey in the early 1950s suggests that it would, since the rations available to Aboriginal stockmen were better in quantity and quality than those issued to other Aboriginal people.[24] However, a later study by Stevens, who investigated the working conditions of Aboriginal people in the pastoral industry, found a different situation. Only seven out of thirty stations visited by Stevens followed the mandatory ration scale outlined in the 1953 Employment Ordinance that controlled the working conditions of Aboriginal people. In eight cases, stations were unaware that ration scales existed. Only in nine cases did Aboriginal workers receive the same food as the rest of the workforce.[25]

In 1953, the Aboriginals Ordinance was replaced by a Welfare Ordinance, although this was not approved until 1957. Though still discriminatory, this legislation avoided the appearance of discrimination against a particular group of people by using the word 'ward' instead of 'Aborigine'. A person was only to be declared a ward, and therefore under the jurisdiction of the Welfare Ordinance, if they were in need of special care and assistance. In practice, all 'full blood' Aboriginal people, numbering over 15,000, were placed on the Ward's Register by the newly established Welfare Branch which administered both the Ordinance and the settlements.[26] The Northern Territory Administration welcomed the Ordinance, which abandoned protection in favour of a 'positive welfare policy', as representing the most important single step yet taken in the approach to the Aboriginal 'problem'.[27] For governments, the Aboriginal population constituted, and were always considered, a 'problem'.

By the middle of the 1950s it was admitted by the new Welfare Branch that there was high infant mortality in the settlements. A major cause of this was recognised to be malnutrition.[28] The answer was to introduce a communal feeding system, which was seen to have the added advantage of promoting assimilation. The policy went beyond the efficient provision of an adequate diet; it was also used to inculcate European tastes, values and behaviour, thus making Aboriginal people more 'acceptable' to the non-Aboriginal majority.[29] Rowse has emphasised that communal feeding should be seen as a system of control, rather than a nutrition programme. It forcefully imprinted the donor's assumption of superiority and divorced the recipient from the cultural resources that had given meaning to food, and its exchange, in Aboriginal society.[30]

ASSIMILATION AND COMMUNAL FEEDING

Communal feeding began in 1955 with the eventual aim of providing three meals a day, seven days a week, and phasing out the issue of dry rations.[31] By this stage there were thirteen government settlements and fourteen missions. By 1961, dry rationing had all but disappeared on settlements in the northern region of the Territory, though elsewhere implementation of the communal feeding programme remained patchy because of continuing problems with staff and supplies. Aboriginal people were still sent away from some of the settlements at certain times of the year to obtain their own food or were expected to find their own food at weekends, or both. Tatz, a political scientist, considered that this was to save money rather than to encourage Aboriginal people to retain their hunting and gathering skills.[32]

According to the Welfare Branch, food services on the settlements continued to improve during the 1950s and 1960s. However, the system was never popular with the Aboriginal population and those who could avoid it did so. For example, many of the Aboriginal residents of Bagot, a settlement then on the outskirts of Darwin but now overtaken by the city, refused to eat in the communal dining room. This was possible because, living close to Darwin, they could earn money wages and spend them in local shops. The Welfare Branch was puzzled by this behaviour, but thought that resistance to communal feeding was probably based on resentment, because Bagot residents could see that the system was 'not common to the European way of life' with which they were in daily contact.[33] Naturally, the Branch did not comment on the paradox that Aboriginal assimilation was expected to be achieved by methods that actually differentiated them from the rest of the population.

The Commonwealth Department of Health issued ration scales for the settlements, but they were not the straightforward 'guide to catering' they appeared to be. The scales divided the population into twelve theoretical groups requiring diets of different nutritional value; but these reflected administrative categories as much as biological ones. Aboriginal residents were not able to choose with whom they ate, but were grouped according to catering convenience. Children and parents, for example, were normally separated for meals. Adults could be embarrassed and offended when they found themselves in close proximity to people who occupied kinship categories they should avoid, and hence they preferred not to attend.

Moira Rankin, the senior dietician who wrote the introduction to the 1962 revision of the ration scales, stated that the recommended energy allowances were lower for most adult groups than the estimated levels of activity warranted, but it was considered that the energy expenditure of adult Aboriginal people was lower than that of an 'average' non-Aboriginal Australian doing equivalent work.[34] This is a strange comment. It could refer to observed Aboriginal adaptation to low energy intakes or, possibly, it implies genetic differences, but no further explanation is given.

The ration scales also attempted to alter existing food consumption patterns by increasing the recommended protein allowances to levels higher than those quoted in 'Adequate Dietary Allowances for Australians'. Rankin explained that this was because Aboriginal people were being assimilated into the 'civilisation of "average" Australians' whose habitual consumption patterns characteristically provided a higher protein intake than the Dietary Allowances recommended. There was therefore more emphasis in the 1962 scales on 'protein foods' such as meat, cheese, eggs and milk, and decreased requirements for white bread or flour, dried beans, sugar and golden syrup, the foods traditionally given as rations. The changes appear to have been prompted as much by assimilationist ideals as by notions of a 'healthy' diet, in the sense of a diet that satisfies nutrient requirements.

It is doubtful whether these adjustments to the ration scales resulted in a better diet during the period of communal feeding. Tatz reported that in practice the Welfare Branch itself did not conform to the ration scales.[35] On paper, meals served from the communal kitchens in the 1960s provided a higher percentage of essential nutrients than the dry rations had in the 1950s, but there was no guarantee that this food was actually available or, because of widespread non-attendance, that it was adequately distributed.[36]

There were many unintended consequences of the communal feeding policy. By the mid-1970s, for example, Annette Hamilton, an anthropologist, found that the status of women in the settlement at Maningrida in Arnhem Land declined as they became redundant as food producers.[37] Previously most groups had depended for their daily sustenance on what women produced and, in fertile areas, women had produced so much that men worked only sporadically and were able to spend time in artistic and ritual pursuits. Women had been independent in their daily lives. In consultation with other women, they decided where to go, what to gather, how much to collect and made communal child care arrangements. Though they continued to collect food from the bush, a large resident population at Maningrida – over 1,000 people by 1967 from thirteen language groups – meant little was available near the settlement and the women had no transport. Settlement staff, armed with a non-Aboriginal stereotype of men as breadwinners and women at home with children, targeted the available work to men, further eroding female independence. Communal feeding also monopolised the time of women by requiring them to walk to and from the feeding centre with their infants and small children three times a day.[38]

It is not surprising then that communal feeding failed to alleviate nutritional problems and probably exacerbated them. However, this is hard to quantify because information about Aboriginal health was, and always had been, scarce. Exclusion from non-Aboriginal society had to a large extent meant exclusion from health care and from the collection of health data. Disease in the Aboriginal population tended to be seen only as a potential threat to the non-Aboriginal community. By the 1960s these attitudes had begun to change. The consequences of discriminatory policies towards Aboriginal people became visible to an Australian population made more tolerant of difference as a result of post-war migration and influenced by the increased political activity of Aboriginal activists. One of the results of this changing social climate was increasing medical interest in research and data collection. The Northern Territory's Medical Service began to collect comprehensive statistics of Aboriginal births and deaths only in 1965, and this process occurred even later in the states. None the less this was a vital development because these statistics showed the extent to which Aboriginal mortality and morbidity rates were higher than those of non-Aboriginal Australians.

The doctors who investigated the growth patterns of Aboriginal children began to suggest that the growth retardation that they observed was the result not of genetic differences but of malnutrition combined with constant bacterial and parasitic infections.[39] Malnutrition was first mentioned in the Welfare Branch Report for 1957–8, though it was not defined and no figures were given for its prevalence. Previously, outbreaks of scurvy had been reported, as in the 'minor' outbreak at the Tanami rationing depot in 1945. The authorities at that time were aware that the issued rations did not contain anti-scorbutics and put the outbreak down to a lack of bush foods in the area which were normally expected to make up the deficit.[40] In the 1950s the problem was more general and endemic, but was still seen in terms of specific vitamin and mineral deficiencies rather than inadequate food intakes.

In order to monitor growth, the Welfare Branch introduced a system of weight cards into the settlements in the late 1950s. In 1966, Ellen Kettle, a senior nurse with the Commonwealth Department of Health in Darwin, attempted to use these records to construct standard weight and height curves for Aboriginal infants and children. It had been the practice to use the mean weight curve for non-Aboriginal Australian infants, but it was felt that standards based on the actual growth of an Aboriginal cohort would be a more 'realistic' guide. Kettle's standards were based on the retrospective longitudinal weight and height records of 400 Aboriginal infants and children at three Arnhem Land missions, but she was forced to conclude that few of these Aboriginal infants had a 'normal' infancy. She found a high prevalence of infections, hookworm and anaemia, all of which would have affected growth.[41] Subsequent studies used international growth standards that allowed inter-community comparisons and the recognition of the degree of deprivation experienced by the Aboriginal population compared to the non-Aboriginal population. Kettle also found that the introduction of community feeding for infants and small children had very little effect on the pattern of diminished growth rates after the first four to six months of life.

In spite of the evidence of the medical literature, little official comment on malnutrition appeared in government reports during the 1960s and early 1970s. Indeed, they present a picture of substantial progress in Aboriginal health and infant welfare. When malnutrition was mentioned, reasons for its continuing existence on the settlements were found in Aboriginal behaviour. For example, in the last report of the Welfare Division, previously the Welfare Branch, before it was incorporated into the new Department of Aboriginal Affairs in 1972, a list was presented of factors that were said to influence child welfare. As usual, its own actions were not implicated. Widespread chronic malnutrition was seen instead to be associated with prolonged demand breast-feeding and with a lack of awareness among Aboriginal people of food values. One factor was the ability of Aboriginal people 'to do without facilities which most Europeans consider basic to satisfactory family and community living, e.g. enough water for daily personal ablutions and the washing of eating utensils'.[42] The Division did not discuss the absence of water or other amenities on the settlements, or the lack of Aboriginal choice as to satisfactory family and community living. It did, however, report, without comment, an infant mortality rate of 163 per thousand, the second highest on record since 1957.

The ability of the settlements to promote social change on the scale the government required was never achievable, even had it been desirable. Altman and Nieuwenhuysen, both economists then at the University of Melbourne, pointed out the contradictions of official policy, especially the location of government settlements (and missions) in isolated areas, with poor market linkage and often with scarce natural resources and a harsh climate.[43] Stanner, an anthropologist, professed himself at a loss to know on what model of human or social reality such institutions were built, describing them as something between a colonial plantation and a corrective institution.[44]

By the 1960s there was a change in attitudes at all levels of Australian society to improve the disadvantaged position of Aboriginal people and remove discriminatory legislation. Continued denial of basic rights became insupportable and, in 1964, most of the rigid controls on Aboriginal people living in the Northern Territory were repealed. The franchise had been extended to them in 1962 on a voluntary basis; voting for everyone else was compulsory. Discriminatory laws also began to be dismantled in many of the states. A national referendum on constitutional change in 1967 gave the Commonwealth government the authority to make new laws in relation to all Aboriginal people, not just those under its direct jurisdiction in the Northern Territory, and for the first time they were included in the national census. In 1972, following the election of a reformist Labour federal government, self-determination became official policy. Responsibility for the welfare of Aboriginal people was transferred from all the states, except Queensland, to the new Commonwealth Department of Aboriginal Affairs.

SELF-DETERMINATION, THE CASH ECONOMY AND DIET

Aboriginal people had been excluded from industrial awards regulating conditions of employment. In the Northern Territory they came under the special provisions of the 1953 Wards' Employment Ordinance, which set pay rates substantially below those of non-Aboriginal workers. In 1969, the Commonwealth government introduced a Training Allowance Scheme into the Territory. This allowance was intended to foster a greater sense of responsibility and to provide experience in the handling of a monetary wage. The economists Altman and Nieuwenhuysen have pointed out that it became a euphemism for paying low wages for low-status work. None the less, with few other options, many Aboriginal people sought employment through it.[45] The Scheme was phased out by the Labour government between 1973 and 1974 because of the inequity of the wage rates, and some award wage positions were created instead.[46] From this time Aboriginal people who were unemployed and living on settlements became eligible to receive unemployment benefit. However, in 1976 only 2.4 per cent of Aboriginal people received benefits although the unemployment rate was over 30 per cent.[47] This was because unemployment benefit was seen by the Commonwealth Department of Social Security as inapplicable to Aboriginal people living in remote areas, where few employment opportunities existed.[48]

Until the 1970s Aboriginal people were also excluded from the provisions of the mainstream Australian welfare system by their separate legal status.[49] Altman and Sanders have described how this pattern of exclusion was gradually dismantled.[50] In the 1940s pensions and other benefits became available to Aboriginal people living away from reserves and settlements. The welfare authorities were concerned that this would encourage Aboriginal people to move away, so they lobbied to have the pension and benefit eligibility extended to those on reserves, which it was in 1959 except for those Aboriginal people deemed still to show 'primitive and nomadic' tendencies. These benefits were not paid directly to the Aboriginal people, rather they went to the welfare authorities on their behalf, as indeed had child endowment payments since 1941. Only 'pocket money' was given to the Aboriginal population until, at some unspecified point in the future, they could demonstrate their ability to handle money wisely. Payment for work continued to be mainly in kind: accommodation and rations. During the 1960s there was pressure from Aboriginal people and non-Aboriginal advocacy groups to have pension benefits and family allowances paid directly to Aboriginal people.[51] This exclusion of Aboriginal people from the welfare system began to change in 1968 following the constitutional referendum, though most remained dependent on welfare authorities for their basic daily needs until they were given more autonomy under the policy of self-determination in 1972.

In a doctoral study of the effects of the food ration system on the family in central Australia, Rowse considered that, despite the negative social impact of the communal feeding system, the switch to low wages and welfare benefits further increased poverty.[52] The per capita income of Aboriginal communities, and hence their purchasing power, was extremely low. The Welfare Division estimated optimistically that a mere A$4.54 was necessary to provide weekly basic needs, including food, clothes, household requirements, rent and entertainment. At Yuendumu in 1969–70, Middleton and Francis calculated the mean weekly per capita income to be A$5.86, but with a range of A$0.40–A$23.04.[53] In 1970, Peterson, an anthropologist from the Australian National University, visited four communities in central Australia and also found that incomes were low and distribution very uneven. Pensioners, who formed about 10 per cent of the population in each community, received between 20 and 66 per cent of the whole community's income. In three of the communities, less than 37 per cent of the males between the ages of 15 and 65 were earning at any one time.[54] Altman and Nieuwenhuysen reviewed the available literature dealing with Aboriginal annual disposable income in this period and concluded that it was never more than 35 per cent of the Australian average, though this did not take subsistence activities such as hunting and gathering into account.[55]

As soon as cash became available at the end of the 1960s, settlement stores became the major suppliers of food, although the lack of refrigeration and distance from wholesalers meant that many were not able to stock a variety of foodstuffs.[56] The Welfare Division began to charge for meals, and attendance declined still further, even though it was more expensive to buy food than to eat in the communal dining room.[57] Communal feeding was gradually phased out, to be replaced by limited nutrition assistance programmes based in health centres, although schemes for the feeding of infants and pre-school children were the last to disappear. In a report of the Welfare Division in the early 1970s, regrets were expressed about the opposition by some Aboriginal parents, who had probably known no other system, to the closure of the infant feeding centres; ten years earlier the Welfare Branch would have been delighted at this sign of acceptance.[58]

As well as low wages and a reliance on welfare benefits, Aboriginal communities faced inflated prices for goods and services because of high transport costs. The Commonwealth Director of Health for the Northern Territory, testifying before a Senate Standing Committee in 1972, reported the findings of a survey to assess the ability of forty-one settlement families to meet the costs of feeding themselves adequately.[59] He said that eleven families earning more than A$100 per fortnight would have no difficulty in meeting food costs if they spent their money 'appropriately'. Sixteen families, with two or three children and an income of A$50 per fortnight, could manage only 'with consistent work and careful money-handling, both the exception rather than the rule'. Fourteen families, or a third of those surveyed, would have no hope at all as the child endowment was their only source of income. Although rent, clothing and other costs were not taken into account in this survey, the results were felt to be reasonably representative of families with young children. However, the Director considered that the poverty thus revealed, arguably the result of government policies, was not the root cause of poor nutrition amongst Aboriginal people. Instead he pointed to behavioural factors, such as the beer drinking, smoking and the costs of card games. He did admit that improved nutritional status could not occur in the present 'incoherent' socio-economic framework.

With the adoption of self-determination, the Aboriginal population once more experienced social change, but this time in a positive direction. Control of settlements shifted to Aboriginal councils and some groups left to establish outstations on their traditional lands. Self-determination also brought immediate and innovative changes in health policy. There was increased spending on Aboriginal health and a recognition of the need for Aboriginal people to participate in the planning and execution of policies designed for their welfare. Aboriginal communities also took the initiative and established community controlled Aboriginal Health Services.[60] Since these changes took place, Aboriginal infant mortality rates have declined, though they remain higher than non-Aboriginal rates and still reflect disadvantaged material circumstances, a legacy of previous policies. Aboriginal people continue to have a life expectancy of up to twenty years less than the rest of the population.[61]

CONCLUSION

After the Second World War, the Aboriginal people of the Northern Territory experienced rapid changes in their social and economic environment, largely as a result of government policy decisions. In particular, government intervention resulted in the dislocation of the Aboriginal economy, and increasing dependence on the non-Aboriginal economy, especially the public sector. Although missions and government ration depots had contributed to the ending of Aboriginal self-sufficiency before the war, this process accelerated with the establishment of government settlements and the adoption of the assimilation policy. Alterations to the supply and distribution of food amply illustrate the enormity of the changes that took place. The food supply came to depend on official perceptions of Aboriginal nutritional and social needs. Bureaucratic control extended not only to the type and quantity of food available for consumption but also to the setting in which it was to be consumed.

The policy of compulsory mass feeding in the 1950s and 1960s was meant both to aid assimilation and to prevent malnutrition. It achieved neither of these aims and no attempt was made to assess the social impact of the policy. On the whole, governments assumed that improved nutritional status would result from changes in Aboriginal behaviour and were unwilling to consider the role of their own political and economic policy decisions. This type of social engineering is unlikely to occur again in the Australian context, but it vividly demonstrates how any government policy, not just 'health' policy, may affect health in some way. Further, it illustrates that health problems generated by change, such as poor nutrition, cannot be solved if governments act without reference to the values and priorities of the people concerned.

NOTES

1 The Commonwealth Government directed the Northern Territory through a variety of Departments: External Affairs 1911–1916, Home and Territories 1916–28, Home Affairs 1928–32, Interior 1932–52, Territories 1951–68, Interior 1968–73 and Northern Territory (NT) 1973–78.

2 For a detailed exposition of the relevant legislation, see the trilogy of books by C.D. Rowley, *The Destruction of Aboriginal Society*; *Outcasts in White Australia*; *The Remote Aborigines*, Canberra, 1970.

3 Recent historical writing no longer portrays Aboriginal people as helpless victims; see, for example, H. Reynolds, *The Other Side of the Frontier: Aboriginal Resistance to the European Invasion of Australia*, Ringwood, Victoria, 1982. There are some hints of resistance in the official records, particularly in the 1960s. For example, it was reported by the Welfare Branch of the NT Administration (*Annual Report*, 1965–6) that some Aboriginal people had left their employment as a protest against their working conditions. In 1965, there was a ruling that there should be equal pay for equal work in the NT cattle industry by 1968. This radically improved wages for some Aboriginal people, but fewer were hired. K.R. Howe, *Race Relations Australia and New Zealand: A Comparative Survey 1770s–1970s*, Sydney, 1977, p. 66.

4 NT Administration, *Annual Report*, Canberra, 1939–40, pp. 18–19. The definition of an Aboriginal person was based on 'blood' and degrees of blood, e.g. full-blood, half-caste, quarter-caste, etc. In practice this meant that judgements about Aboriginality were made on the basis of physical characteristics. The present definition, by contrast, states that an Aborigine is a person of Aboriginal descent who identifies as an Aborigine and is accepted as such by the community in which he or she lives. The Aboriginal population of the NT according to the 1991 census is 39,287 or 22.6 per cent of the population. Overall, Aboriginal people make up only 1.6 per cent of the total Australian population.

5 Howe, *Race Relations Australia and New Zealand*, pp. 55–6.

6 NT Administration, *Annual Report*, 1944–5, p. 3. Howe points out that, on the military installations where Aboriginal people worked as volunteers, the working conditions (fair treatment, cash wages, good food, clean bedding, showers, toilets, etc.) did much to raise their expectations. Howe, *Race Relations Australia and New Zealand*, p. 89.

7 NT Administration, *Annual Report*, 1947–8, p. 18. For an account of health care provision, see S. Saggers and D. Gray, *Aboriginal Health and Society: The Traditional and Contemporary Aboriginal Struggle for Better Health*, Sydney, 1991, pp. 121–43.

8 NT Department of Health, *An Environmental Survey of Aboriginal Communities 1977–79*, Darwin, 1979.

9 NT Administration, *Annual Report*, 1958–9, p. 40. The Commonwealth government was well ahead of the states in its implementation of assimilation, which was only officially defined to include all Aboriginal people in 1961 at a Native Welfare Conference. In the 1950s, assimilation was seen more in terms of individual Aborigines gaining exemption from the special Aboriginal legislation than all Aboriginal people gaining equality. The Native Welfare Conference of 1965 changed the wording of the policy to imply more choice. Aboriginal people could now 'choose to' attain rather than be 'expected to' attain the same manner of living as other Australians. *Howe, Race Relations Australia and New Zealand*, pp. 67–8.

10 Commonwealth Department of Territories, *Progress Towards Assimilation: Aboriginal Welfare in the Northern Territory*, revised edn, Canberra, 1963.

11 Commonwealth Department of Health, *Northern Division Annual Report*, Darwin, 1976–7.

12 For a detailed discussion of housing policy see M. Heppell, ed., *A Black Reality: Aboriginal Camps and Housing in Remote Australia*, Canberra, 1979. After 1967, grants for housing became available from the Office of Aboriginal Affairs, the forerunner of the Department of Aboriginal Affairs and separate from the existing NT Aboriginal welfare administration. The Welfare Division reported that 'attitudes' among Aboriginal people were not conducive to the proper maintenance of a dwelling. *Annual Report*, 1971–2, pp. 13–14.

13 See L.R. Smith, 'Aboriginal Vital Statistics: An Analysis of Trends', in Commonwealth Department of Health, *Aboriginal Health Bulletin, No. 1*, Canberra, 1980, pp. 9–20. Smith looks at statistics from 1965–78. The present Aboriginal infant mortality rate in the NT, though much improved, is still 3.9 times the overall Australian rate. See N.J. Thomson, 'Recent trends in Aboriginal mortality', *Medical Journal of Australia*, 1991, 154, pp. 235–9.

14 T. Rowse, *White Flour, White Power?: Colonial Authority, Rationing and the Family in Central Australia*, Unpublished PhD Thesis, Sydney University, 1989.

15 NT Administration, *Annual Report*, 1948–9, p. 19.

16 NT Administration, *Annual Report*, 1947–8, p. 18.

17 NT Administration, *Annual Report*, 1956–7.

18 Welfare Branch, *Annual Report*, 1958–9.

19 C.P. Mountford, *Records of the American–Australian Scientific Expedition to Arnhem Land*, Melbourne, 1956, vol. 1, *Art, Myth and Symbolism*, and 1960, vol. 2, *Anthropology and Nutrition*. R.L. Specht and C.P. Mountford, eds, *Records of the American–Australian Scientific Expedition to Arnhem Land*, Melbourne, 1958, vol. 3, *Botany and Plant Ecology*. R.L. Specht, ed., *Records of the American-Australian Scientific Expedition to Arnhem Land*, Melbourne, 1964, vol. 4, *Zoology*.

20 M. McArthur, 'Report of the Nutrition Unit', in Mountford, *Records of the American–Australian Scientific Expedition to Arnhem Land*, vol. 2, pp. 1–143.

21 Ibid., p. 139.

22 Ibid., p. 21. At the end of the 1970s, Cockington was able to show that the growth of Aboriginal children was similar to that of non-Aboriginal children when their housing and amenities were of the same standard. R.A. Cockington, 'Growth of Australian Aboriginal Children Related to Social Circumstances', *Australian and New Zealand Journal of Medicine*, 1980, 10, pp. 199–208.

23 W. Wilson, 'A Dietary Survey of Aborigines in the Northern Territory', *Medical Journal of Australia*, 1953, 2, pp. 599–605. Aboriginal people provided much of the labour in the pastoral industry in the NT. See R. Berndt and C. Berndt, *End of an Era: Aboriginal Labour in the Northern Territory*, Canberra, 1987.

24 F. Stevens, *Aborigines in the Northern Territory Cattle Industry*, Canberra, 1974, p. 90. The material was collected in 1965, 1966 and 1968.

25 Ibid., p. 84. Even where the food rations were the same, Aboriginal workers were often segregated from non-Aboriginal workers at meal times.

26 NT Administration, *Annual Report*, 1956–7, p. 34. The Welfare Branch had carried out the first census of Aboriginal people in the NT in 1955 in order to place them on the Register.

27 NT Administration, *Annual Report*, 1953–5, p. 37.

28 NT Administration, *Annual Report*, 1957–8, p. 33.

29 Welfare Branch, *Annual Report*, 1958–9, p. 10.

30 Rowse, *White Flour, White Power?*, pp. 172–5.

31 Ibid., p. 38. In addition, there were still six ration depots operating in remote areas for the aged and infirm and many Aboriginal people continued to live in the towns 'fending for themselves', according to the Welfare Branch *Annual Report* of 1958–9. By the end of the period under review, the number of government settlements had increased to 20. The scale of building and the infrastructure required meant that the settlements became an important industry. By the early 1960s, there were more jobs available at the settlements than there were in the pastoral industry. Rowse, *White Flour, White Power?*, p. 166. See also H. Sinclair, 'Factors Affecting Aboriginal Nutrition', *Medical Journal of Australia*, 1977, 1, Special Supplement 8, pp. 1–4.

32 C.M. Tatz, *Administration in the Northern Territory of Australia*, Unpublished PhD Thesis, Australian National University, 1964, p. 157.

33 Welfare Branch, *Annual Report*, 1961–2, p. 58.

34 M.J. Rankin, Introduction, *Ration Scales for Australian Aborigines for Use in the Northern Territory*, Commonwealth Department of Health, typescript, 1962, pp. 1–4.

35 Tatz, *Administration in the Northern Territory*, pp. 155–6.

36 M.W. Corden, 'The Dietary Situation at Yuendumu and Papunya', in Commonwealth Department of Health, *Some Observations on the Diets and Nutrition of Aboriginal People in Central Australia*, typescript, 1973, pp. 10–48. Margaret Corden was the NT-based dietician of the Commonwealth Department of Health from 1955 to 1960.

37 A. Hamilton, 'Aboriginal Women: The Means of Production', in J. Mercer, ed., *The Other Half: Women in Australian Society*, Ringwood, Victoria, 1975, pp. 167–78. It was reported by the Welfare Branch,

Annual Report 1958–9, p. 11, that an investigation had been commenced by two survey officers, with a view to determining a training programme to 'motivate' Aboriginal women to want the sorts of things European housewives wanted.

38 If attendance dropped at infant feeding centres, women would be 'reminded' by non-Aboriginal staff that they should attend. R.M. Middleton and S.H. Francis, *Yuendumu and its Children: Life and Health on an Aboriginal Community*, Canberra, 1976, p. 78. Middleton and Francis, academics at the Australian National University, had been invited by the NT Administration to investigate the social bases of ill-health at Yuendumu, a desert settlement in the southern region of the Territory. This investigation took place between 1969 and 1971.

39 For a review of this literature see P.M. Moodie, *Aboriginal Health*, Canberra, 1973.

40 NT Administration, *Annual Report*, 1945–6, p. 28.

41 E.S. Kettle, 'Weight and Height Curves for Australian Aboriginal Infants and Children', *Medical Journal of Australia*, 1966, 1, pp. 972–7.

42 Welfare Division, *Annual Report*, Canberra, 1971–2, p. 12.

43 J.C. Altman and J. Nieuwenhuysen, *The Economic Status of Australian Aborigines*, Cambridge, 1979, p. 24.

44 W.E.H. Stanner, 'Some Aspects of Aboriginal Health', in B.S. Hetzel, M. Dobbin, L. Lippmann and E. Eggleston, eds, *Better Health for Aborigines?*, St. Lucia, Queensland, 1974, pp. 1–13.

45 Altman and Nieuwenhuysen, *The Economic Status of Australian Aborigines*, p. 44.

46 Australia has a centralised system of wage bargaining in industrial tribunals at both state and federal level. The negotiated wages and conditions set down for each occupation or group of workers is called the 'award'. Recently there has been a move towards enterprise bargaining, but the centralised system is still operating and is seen to be particularly important for low paid workers, safeguarding minimum pay and conditions and ensuring some wage rises.

47 D.H. Penny and J. Moriarty, 'Aboriginal Economy: Then and Now', in B. S. Hetzel and H.J. Frith, eds, *The Nutrition of Aborigines in Relation to the Ecosystem of Central Australia*, Melbourne, 1978, pp. 19–24. Commonwealth Department of Aboriginal Affairs, Statistics Section, *Newsletter*, Canberra, 1980, 1/9.

48 J.C. Altman and W. Sanders, *From Exclusion to Dependence: Aborigines and the Welfare State in Australia*, Centre for Aboriginal Economic Policy Research, Australian National University, Canberra, Discussion Paper, No. 1, 1991, p. 5.

49 This exclusion meant that responsibility for Aboriginal people was seen by mainstream government departments to lie with special purpose Aboriginal welfare authorities and not with them. For example, immediate health care on settlements was provided by nurses employed, not by the Department of Health, but by the Welfare Branch or by the missions, which were subsidised by the Welfare Branch. A Native Health Survey Section was established by the NT Medical Service in 1957 with one nurse. Staffing was slow to increase over the first ten years but, in the late

1960s and now called the Rural Health Section, it began to grow rapidly and numbered 30 nurses in 1972. The NT Department of Health started to complain about its lack of control over settlement nursing staff. Commonwealth of Australia, Senate Standing Committee on Social Environment. Reference: Aborigines and Torres Strait Islanders, 1971–6, *Official Hansard Transcript of Evidence*, vol. 1, p. 325.

50 Altman and Sanders, *From Exclusion to Dependence*, pp. 1–7.

51 Corden 'The Dietary Situation at Yuendumu and Papunya', p. 43, reported that she visited both Yuendumu and Papunya in 1956 and 1960 (the Papunya community lived at Haasts Bluff in 1956) and then again in 1972. The greatest change over that period affecting dietary intakes was the payment of pensions and child endowment to individuals and the consequent growth of the retail stores. Most settlements had stores controlled by the Welfare Branch by the mid-1950s, where residents could spend their 'pocket money', either the small portion of the pension that was passed on to individual recipients or from employment. According to Rowse, *White Flour, White Power?*, pp. 160–6, it was clear by the 1950s that cash was the preferred method of payment as far as Aboriginal people were concerned. However, retail stores started to develop further only after 1968–69, when all Aboriginal people began to receive the direct payment of pensions and family allowances and when the Training Allowance Scheme was introduced.

52 Rowse, *White Flour, White Power?*, p. 176.

53 Middleton and Francis, *Yuendumu and its Children*, p. 74.

54 N. Peterson, 'Aboriginal Involvement with the Australian Economy in the Central Reserve during the Winter of 1970', in R.M. Berndt, ed., *Aborigines and Change: Australia in the 70s*, Canberra, 1977, pp. 136–46.

55 Altman and Nieuwenhuysen, *The Economic Status of Australian Aborigines*, p. 51.

56 For a discussion of community stores and their management, see E.A. Young, 'Aboriginal Community Stores: A Service "For the People" or "By the People"', in P. Loveday, ed., *Service Delivery to Remote Communities*, Darwin, 1982, pp. 62–8.

57 Sinclair, 'Factors Affecting Aboriginal Nutrition', pp. 1–4.

58 Welfare Division, *Annual Report*, 1971–2, p. 13. At Areyonga, for example, infant meals were still provided because 'regrettably' the women now expected this service. At Papunya, efforts were made to counteract an 'expectation' held by some parents that it was the government's responsibility to care for Aboriginal children.

59 Commonwealth of Australia, Senate Standing Committee on Social Environment Reference: Aborigines and Torres Strait Islanders, 1971–6, *Official Hansard Transcript of Evidence*, vol. 1, pp. 315–54.

60 Saggers and Gray, *Aboriginal Health and Society*, pp. 144–66.

61 N. Thomson and N. Briscoe, *Overview of Aboriginal Health Status in the Northern Territory*, Australian Institute of Health: Aboriginal and Torres Strait Islander Health Series, No. 2, Canberra, 1991. For a detailed discussion of Aboriginal nutrition, see L. Harrison, 'Food, Nutrition and Growth in Aboriginal Communities', in J. Reid and P. Trompf, eds, *The Health of Aboriginal Australia*, Sydney, 1991, pp. 123–72.

7

FROM VISIBLE TO INVISIBLE

The 'problem' of the health of Irish people in Britain

Liam Greenslade, Moss Madden and Maggie Pearson

Irish people make up the largest ethnic minority group in Great Britain. Yet despite this, and particularly from the point of view of research and practical initiatives in health and health services, they remain a peculiarly 'invisible' minority. On the whole, both the study of health amongst ethnic groups and the implementation of health initiatives amongst ethnic minorities have overlooked the Irish. It seems to have been tacitly assumed that their social conditions, culture and lifestyle are not substantially distinct from those of the majority of the white community. The assumption that the white ethnic group is homogeneous not only belies well-established evidence of significant and enduring social class inequalities in health, but also assumes a degree of assimilation by white minorities into the majority white community that is not reflected in hard data.[1]

In the past two decades, the limited amount of research that has been conducted that considers the Irish as a distinct ethnic group, has revealed some possibly unexpected facts about their physical and mental health. Amongst other things, this research has shown that:

- Irish-born men aged between 15 and 64 have the highest death rates of any immigrant group in England and Wales;[2]
- Irish-born men constitute the only immigrant group with whose health is worse in this country than in their homeland;[3]
- Irish-born women have the highest rates of mental hospital admission of any group in England.[4]

Despite this evidence, it is a matter for debate why these findings, and others in the past decade, such as the observation that the Irish experience higher rates of suicide and attempted suicide, have prompted little subsequent and systematic study that might elucidate the circumstances underpinning this apparently acute poor health and distress and its management by the community.[5] The health experience of the Irish in Britain has not received the same attention as that of other ethnic minority groups.

In this chapter we take this poor health and apparent distress in the Irish community as the point of departure for an exploration into the historical background of the health of the Irish in Britain, and an update of the community's present situation. We use recent data sources to establish health profiles, interpreted in the light of socio-demographic circumstances, which aim to remove the cloak of invisibility that covers the health experience of the Irish in Britain. In the next section we draw on Census and General Household Survey (GHS) data to construct a socio-demographic profile of the Irish-born British population, and in the following section draw on GHS data alone to reveal something of their health experience.

HISTORICAL CONTEXT

The health of Irish people in Britain has not always been cloaked in invisibility. In the middle decades of the nineteenth century, the Irish were regarded as a significant factor contributing to public health problems in many parts of the country. The following report of conditions in the City of Liverpool was published in 1847:

> The return shows a great increase in the mortality of this district (the North end), which is without doubt solely attributable to the many thousands of Irish paupers who have landed here within the last three months . . . Everything which humanity could devise and money carry out for their cases has been adopted by the Select Vestry but so many thousand of Irish are continually pouring in, and their habits are so disgustingly filthy, that little can be done as yet to stay the great mortality among them.[6]

The consequences of Irish ill-health in the nineteenth century, and official attitudes towards that ill-health, are perhaps best summed up in the following extract from the Liverpool Medical Officer of Health's Report of 1850:

> During that calamitous season we had to deplore the loss of many respectable and useful citizens. Among them may be enumerated

> the Roman Catholic clergymen, a Missionary Minister to the poor, ten medical practitioners, a number of relieving officers and others whose duties brought them into contact with Irish paupers, and many hundreds of English residents in comfortable circumstances, most of whom might have been alive had Liverpool not been converted into 'a City of the Plague' by the immigrant Irish.[7]

Although the circumstances in Liverpool at this time can be seen as somewhat special and extreme, the pattern was repeated throughout the major cities of England and Scotland during the middle decades of the century. Irish peasants and paupers escaped from famine to settle in overcrowded rooms and poor lodging houses or 'made their beds with a stone for a pillow' on the streets of Glasgow, the Potteries, London, Manchester and Edinburgh.[8]

The picture of the Irish painted in public health reports and newspapers of this period was not, therefore, flattering. While much concern was expressed regarding the poverty of their conditions and its association with disease, as much was said about Irish people's habits as an explanation of their position. Reports mention their 'primitive customs' regarding the treatment of the dead, drunkenness, unrestrained sexuality, criminality and fecklessness.[9] In this period, the health of the Irish was subject to considerable surveillance and monitoring within Britain as they were seen to be a source of infestation and a hazard to health. Appreciation of the severity of their conditions, when contrasted with those of the indigenous urban poor, contributed to the introduction of public health and housing policies. Ironically enough, it was the Irish themselves, forming a large part of the pool of casual labour, who found employment building the drains, sewage systems and other public works that arose because of the fear of epidemic.[10]

THE PRESENT CONTEXT

Post-war migration to Britain

Whilst the migration of Irish people to England has never since matched the influx seen during the middle of the last century, proportionately at least, there have been considerable flows of migrants across the Irish Sea in the intervening years. These flows declined somewhat during the 1970s period of favourable economic conditions in Ireland, increased in the mid-1980s, and declined again in the

1990s. For example, it has been estimated that the annual migration from Ireland in the late 1980s into London alone was of the order of 40,000, while the 1991 Census shows that one-year migrants from the Republic to Great Britain numbered 12,429 and those from Northern Ireland totalled 2,669.[11] Despite this decline, and despite the Irish comprising a relatively small proportion of the total migrants within the previous year, the numbers are still substantial, and can be expected to fluctuate both up and down into the future.

Current migrants join an ageing group of Irish people who emigrated during the 1940s and 1950s. Arriving predominantly from the rural parts of Ireland, these earlier migrants sought work mainly in the unskilled and semi-skilled areas of employment. Their strategy for survival during this period, according to Connor, depended upon 'keeping your head down, your mouth shut and going about your business without rocking the boat'.[12] Compared with other ethnic minorities, the contemporary invisibility of the Irish that we identify might be explained by their adherence to this strategy. It might be said that by drawing a veil over their difference, they facilitated their apparent assimilation into the host community. Not wishing to be seen as encroaching upon the position of the indigenous working class, individually and communally the migrant Irish of the immediate post-war period took a decision to keep out of the spotlight of public policy by doing their work, keeping themselves to themselves and bringing up their children as best they could.[13] However, if we examine the available evidence more carefully, we find that the invisibility of the Irish might be regarded as less of a choice made by them than a part of wider public policy.

A feature of the restructuring of the British economy during the 1950s was its dependence upon the importation of labour from its current and former colonies. With the exception of the Irish, this labour consisted predominantly of black workers. Envisaging a series of cultural and economic problems associated with an influx of ethnically different workers, the immigration policy outlined by the British government during the 1950s was intended to ameliorate the political difficulties surrounding immigration control in both the present and the future. As Connor has pointed out, the Eden administration of 1955 was faced with something of a dilemma.[14] A way had to be found of controlling immigration that would not impede the free flow of labour across the Irish Sea, but at the same time would not appear overtly colour prejudiced. The answer was given in the Cabinet reports of 1955:

> The only way out of this dilemma would appear to be to argue boldly along the lines that the population of the whole British Isles is for historical and geographical reasons essentially one and . . . has always been treated as such.[15]

The 'boldness' of this argument, given historical and political indications to the contrary, must be regarded as remarkable. None the less, with the problems of black immigration uppermost in its mind, the Eden Cabinet opted for a strategy that would effectively cloak the Irish with invisibility. The Irish migrants were apparently willing to adopt the mantle, a willingness common to many migrant groups in an alien culture. However, it might be argued that the Eden Cabinet's policy decision was far more significant than it appears at first sight, and that it had a significant effect in keeping the needs and conditions of Irish people in Britain off the agenda in the areas of strategic planning and policy in housing, education and, most importantly, health.

Socio-demographic circumstances

The socio-demographic profile and circumstances of the Irish population in Britain are very revealing. Our aim here is to gain an understanding, where sources permit, of the circumstances of first- and second-generation Irish in Britain, which will inform and support our interpretation in the following section of data on the health of the Irish population in Britain. In constructing this profile, we have drawn first on the 1991 Census to establish a profile of the Irish-born population (from the thirty-two counties of the Irish Republic and Northern Ireland) resident in Britain, compared with the total British population, and second, on the General Household Survey (GHS) for 1984, 1986 and 1988, which enables an analysis of first- and second-generation Irish populations.[16]

The Irish-born population in Britain

Table 7.1 shows the changes in the last 40 years in the size of the Irish-born population in Great Britain.[17] The decline in the 1970s and 1980s was mainly caused by return migration to, and decreased emigration from, the Republic during the improved economic conditions that prevailed there during that period. In 1991, Irish migrants accounted for about 1.5 per cent of the population of Great Britain.[18]

Table 7.1 The Irish-born population in post-war Great Britain

Census year	*Irish-born population*	*% change*
1951	716,028	
1961	948,320	+32.44
1971	957,830	+1.00
1981	850,397	−11.22
1991	837,464	−1.52

Source: Census, 1951–91

The Irish-born population in Great Britain in 1991 was considerably older than the total British population and, as Table 7.2 shows, almost 60 per cent are aged 45 and over, compared with less than 40 per cent of the British population.

Examination of data from the 1991 Census indicates the socio-economic inequality that Irish people experience in Britain. The unemployment rate amongst the Irish-born population was 11.4 per cent compared with 9.3 per cent for the population as a whole. More detailed evidence of the socio-economic circumstances of the Irish population, available from the GHS, is presented below.

First- and second-generation Irish populations

A profile of the first- and second-generation Republic and Northern Irish-born populations has been constructed from the GHS, which is a nationally representative continuous survey with an achieved sample of approximately 10,000 households containing about 25,000 individuals. The GHS interview includes questions on population and fertility, housing, employment, place of birth of respondent and parents,

Table 7.2 Age of Irish-born and British populations, 1991

Age group	*Irish-born*	*Irish-born %*	*Total popn*	*Total popn %*
0–15	32,529	3.9	10,958,755	20.0
16–44	306,974	36.7	22,888,178	41.9
45–64	315,589	37.7	11,965,278	21.9
65+	182,372	21.8	8,764,629	16.1
Total	837,464	100.0	54,576,840	100.0

Source: Census, 1991

education and health. Questions on smoking and drinking are included in alternate (even) years. We have taken GHS data for the years 1984, 1986 and 1988 and conflated them into one data set. This gives a total of 77,548 respondents, which we have divided into five groups according to their or their parents' birth places. We identified those born in the Republic of Ireland (Republic Irish), Northern Ireland (Northern Irish) and Britain, which we sub-divided into those with one or both parents born in the Republic (Republic-British) or Northern Ireland (Northern Irish-British). The residual group was those born in Britain of two British parents (British-British). It must be emphasised here that, given the history of and current situation concerning Irish migrants in Britain, such a survey of people in households who are willing to talk to interviewers will exclude any homeless people, among whom, in London, the Irish are over-represented. Table 7.3 shows the relative size of these five groups of GHS respondents, disaggregated by sex. The proportion of Irish-born people contacted in these surveys is 1.55 per cent of the total, compared with the 1.58 per cent in England and Wales and the 1.50 per cent in Great Britain reported in the 1991 Census.

Table 7.4 shows the age structure of the five groups. In general, these figures reflect those from the Census, the two Irish-born populations being strikingly older than the population as a whole. The Republic Irish-born population was the demographically oldest of the five groups. British-born respondents show fairly similar profiles whatever their parents' country of origin, although there is a slight over-representation of Republic-British in the second age group. The sex structure of the different populations does not vary remarkably. The first generation migrants have a higher proportion of females in

Table 7.3 Origins of respondents in GHS, 1984, 1986 and 1988

Group	*Male total*	*Male %*	*Female total*	*Female %*	*Total*	*%*
Republic Irish	383	47.46	424	52.54	807	1.04
Northern Irish	181	45.59	216	54.41	397	0.51
Republic-British	892	49.34	916	50.66	1,808	2.33
Northern Irish-British	410	50.12	408	49.88	818	1.05
British-British	35,557	48.23	38,161	51.77	73,718	95.06
Total	37,423	48.26	40,125	51.74	77,548	100.00

Source: GHS, 1984, 1986 and 1988

Table 7.4 Age of respondents, combined GHS, 1984, 1986 and 1988

	0–14 yrs No.	*0–14 yrs %*	*15–34 yrs No.*	*15–34 yrs %*	*35–64 yrs No.*	*35–64 yrs %*	*65+ yrs No.*	*65+ yrs %*	*Total No.*
Republic Irish	11	1.36	121	14.99	523	64.81	152	18.84	807
Northern Irish	16	4.03	113	28.46	210	52.90	58	14.61	397
Republic-British	316	17.48	770	42.59	526	29.09	196	10.84	1,808
Northern Irish-British	168	20.54	247	30.20	282	34.47	121	14.79	818
British-British	14,584	19.78	20,692	28.07	26,554	36.02	11,888	16.13	73,718
Total	15,095	19.47	21,943	28.30	28,095	36.20	12,415	16.01	77,548

Source: GHS, 1984, 1986 and 1988

their numbers than the others, which is expected given the age profiles of these groups.

Marital status is shown in Table 7.5. Those born in Ireland, in both the North and the Republic, are much more likely than other groups to be married, and correspondingly much less likely to be single. These characteristics reflect closely the different age profiles of the five groups. The different proportions of those divorced or separated, and cohabiting, are difficult to interpret safely, particularly given the small incidence of these marital states in the Irish populations.

The household size data for the five groups, which also reflect age distribution to an extent, are presented in Table 7.6. The Irish tend to display slightly higher proportions in single person households, and substantially higher proportions in two-person households. Migrants from Northern Ireland and the British born are less likely than the other groups to live in very large households (5+), whilst the second generation Irish tend to live in the largest households.

Tables 7.7, 7.8 and 7.9 present data indicating the relative economic well-being of the five groups. Table 7.7 shows the net weekly income of the head of household, Table 7.8 shows car ownership figures and Table 7.9 the economic status of the head of household. The data indicate that first-generation migrants from the Republic are more likely to live in poorer households, whereas migrants from the North are most likely to live in a household in the top band. Second-generation Republic Irish households tend to follow the British profile, whilst second-generation Northern Irish show the lowest proportion in the £51–£100 band and the highest in the £101–£200 band. Table 7.8, showing car ownership data, which are commonly used as an indicator of relative affluence, confirms the poor socio-economic circumstances of first-generation migrants from the Republic. In fact, all the Irish groups are less likely than the British-British population to have a car, or several cars where cars are owned. As far as economic status is concerned, the high proportion of the Republic Irish in the retired category, shown in Table 7.9, is an obvious function of their age profile. The substantially higher proportion of this group reported as sick, however, is not so easily explained, and nor are the slightly higher proportions among the Northern Irish and the second-generation Republic Irish. Also difficult to explain for demographic reasons is the high proportion of unemployment among all Irish groups except the Northern Irish.

The data presented indicate that the Irish-born population of Great Britain has been declining in recent decades, but that this rate of

Table 7.5 Marital status by origin, GHS, 1984, 1986 and 1988

	Single No.	*Single %*	*Married No.*	*Married %*	*Widowed No.*	*Widowed %*	*Div/Sep No.*	*Div/Sep %*	*Cohab No.*	*Cohab %*	*Total No.*
Republic Irish	107	13.26	578	71.62	66	8.18	46	5.70	10	1.24	807
Northern Irish	59	14.86	273	68.77	35	8.82	18	4.53	12	3.02	397
Republic-British	586	32.41	952	52.65	115	6.36	109	6.03	46	2.54	1,808
Northern Irish-British	267	32.64	429	52.44	65	7.95	48	5.87	9	1.10	818
British-British	19,856	26.94	43,144	58.53	6,116	8.30	3,317	4.50	1,285	1.74	73,718
Total	20,875	26.92	45,376	58.51	6,397	8.25	3,538	4.56	1,362	1.76	77,548

Note: Cohabiting not included in 1984 data
Source: GHS, 1984, 1986 and 1988

Table 7.6 Household size by origin, GHS, 1984, 1986 and 1988

	1 No.	*1 %*	*2 No.*	*2 %*	*3 No.*	*3 %*	*4 No.*	*4 %*	*5+ No.*	*5+ %*	*Total No.*
Republic Irish	96	11.9	247	30.6	155	19.2	163	20.2	146	18.1	807
Northern Irish	50	12.6	122	30.7	68	17.1	91	22.9	66	16.6	397
Republic-British	163	9.0	417	23.1	342	18.9	460	25.4	426	23.6	1,808
Northern Irish-British	73	9.2	190	23.8	154	19.3	209	26.2	172	21.6	798
British-British	7,515	10.2	19,544	26.5	14,449	19.6	19,853	26.9	12,357	16.8	73,718
Total	7,897	10.2	20,520	26.5	15,168	19.6	20,776	26.8	13,167	17.0	77,528

Source: GHS, 1984, 1986 and 1988

Table 7.7 Net weekly income of head of household

	<£50 No.	*<£50 %*	*£51–£100 No.*	*£51–£100 %*	*£101–£200 No.*	*£101–£200 %*	*>£200 No.*	*>£200 %*	*Total No.*
Republic Irish	157	27.21	177	30.68	201	34.84	42	7.28	577
Northern Irish	37	13.91	78	29.32	110	41.35	41	15.41	266
Republic-British	222	17.26	377	29.32	542	42.15	145	11.28	1,286
Northern Irish-British	92	17.20	139	25.98	229	42.80	75	14.02	535
British-British	8,880	17.23	15,009	29.12	20,951	40.64	6,710	13.02	51,550
Total	9,388	17.32	15,780	29.11	22,033	40,64	7,013	12.94	54,214

Source: GHS, 1984, 1986 and 1988

Table 7.8 Car ownership

	0 No.	*0 %*	*1 No.*	*1 %*	*2 No.*	*2 %*	*3+ No.*	*3+ %*	*Total No.*
Republic Irish	324	40.50	334	41.75	121	15.13	21	2.63	800
Northern Irish	139	35.10	173	43.69	69	17.42	15	3.79	396
Republic-British	620	34.46	803	44.64	313	17.40	63	3.50	1,799
Northern Irish-British	295	36.20	359	44.05	126	15.46	35	4.29	815
British-British	21,699	29.52	34,116	46.41	14,568	19.82	3,131	4.26	73,514
Total	23,077	29.84	35,785	46.28	15,197	19.65	3,265	4.22	77,324

Source: GHS, 1984, 1986 and 1988

Table 7.9 Economic status of head of household

	Working *No.*	*Working* *%*	*Seeking work* *No.*	*Seeking work* *%*	*Sick* *No.*	*Sick* *%*	*Retired* *No.*	*Retired* *%*	*Other* *No.*	*Other* *%*	*Total* *No.*
Republic Irish	447	59.80	459	7.90	38	5.09	158	21.15	45	6.02	747
Northern Irish	238	70.83	17	5.06	11	3.27	53	15.77	17	5.06	336
Republic-British	1,122	68.37	123	7.50	55	3.35	202	12.31	139	8.47	1,641
Northern Irish British	439	68.27	46	7.15	18	2.80	93	14.46	47	7.31	643
British-British	43,139	66.82	3,545	5.49	1,809	2.80	11,273	17.46	4,794	7.43	64,560
Total	45,385	66.81	3,790	5.58	1,931	2.84	11,779	17.34	5,042	7.42	67,927

Source: GHS, 1984, 1986 and 1988

decline seems now to have slowed to almost zero. Whilst the Irish-born population is generally older than the British population as a whole, those born in Northern Ireland are somewhat younger than those from the Republic. Marital status and household size data appear to correlate with, and therefore reflect, age profiles. As far as economic well-being is concerned, the picture is not so clear. The unemployment rate of the Republic Irish born is higher than that of the British as a whole. Northern Irish migrants are more likely to be in work than the British as a whole. Interestingly, second-generation migrants from both parts of Ireland display higher than average rates of unemployment. Republic Irish migrant household heads are most likely to be on lower incomes, while those from the North appear to be better off than the British. These findings are more or less replicated in terms of economic status of head of household, although not repeated so obviously in the car ownership data, where, although the Republic Irish show low ownership rates as we would expect, the Northern Irish do not have the high rates that we might expect would be shown given their income position. Second-generation groups also show lower than expected car ownership rates.

A HEALTH PROFILE OF THE IRISH IN BRITAIN

In this section we present a profile of the health of the Irish in Britain, drawing on data from the GHS, Office of Population Census Surveys (OPCS) and other studies.[19] We discuss differences in the health experiences of the Irish, both first- and second-generation, and the British, in the light of the clear differences in their socio-demographic and socio-economic profiles.

Mortality

We first look at the mortality data for Irish people in Britain available from various sources.[20] One feature of most studies of mortality is that deaths have been analysed on an 'All-Ireland' basis. This aggregate category has been utilised by researchers to avoid inaccuracies from the record of 'country of birth' on a significant number of death registrations as simply 'Ireland'. Whilst the pragmatic response of aggregating deaths among migrants from the Republic of Ireland and from Northern Ireland is understandable, it implies a common experience that is not borne out by the available data where country of birth was more specifically recorded. There is evidence, in fact, that mortality rates for people born in the North and the Republic differ quite markedly. Between 1970 and 1972, for example, Standard Mortality Rates (SMRs: i.e. deaths per year per 1,000 population) for people between 20 and 69 born in the two parts of Ireland were as shown in Table 7.10. With the marked discrepancies shown in this table, the mortality data relating to the 'All Ireland' category require cautious interpretation.

The figures shown in Table 7.11, taken from Adelstein et al., show death rates for all causes for male and female Irish immigrants to England and Wales, and for the population born in England and Wales.[21] We can see that for all causes death rates were higher in 1970–2 for Irish migrants between the ages of 15 and 64, than for those born in England and Wales. For men the excess was 22 per cent and for women 16 per cent.

Given the stereotypical image of the Irish migrant, it might be thought that occupation and socio-economic status play an important role in raising migrants' death rates, lower socio-economic status being generally associated with higher mortality and worse health.

Table 7.10 Standard mortality rates for migrants from the Irish Republic and Northern Ireland

	Males	*Females*
Irish Republic	132	128
Northern Ireland	102	92

Source: A.M. Adelstein, M.G. Marmot, G. Dean and S. Bradshaw, 'Comparison of Mortality of Irish Immigrants in England and Wales with that of Irish and British Nationals', *Irish Medical Journal*, 1986, 79/7, pp. 185–9

Table 7.11 Death rates for all causes by social class, ages 15–64, 1970–2

Male	*I*	*II*	*IIIN*	*IIIM*	*IV*	*V*	*Total*
Irish	96	99	108	122	129	157	122
England and Wales	77	81	99	106	114	137	100

Female	*I*	*II*	*IIIN*	*IIIM*	*IV*	*V*	*Total*
Irish	89	113	109	136	113	136	116
England and Wales	82	87	92	115	119	135	100

Source: as Table 7.10

However, for Irish men a class by class comparison shows higher SMRs in every socio-economic group and for women in all groups except IV. These figures suggest that an 'Irish factor' may be at work influencing the patterns of mortality amongst Irish people in England and Wales. However, looked at from the other side there is also evidence of a 'migrant factor'. Amongst immigrant groups in England and Wales there is evidence that health, or at least life-expectancy, improves, sometimes markedly, on migrating.[22] The experience of the Irish, however, runs counter to this trend.

In Table 7.12 we see that while Irish women experience an extremely marginal improvement in their mortality, their menfolk experience a substantial increase in mortality. Irish men who migrated to England and Wales were 15 per cent more likely to die than those of their compatriots who stayed at home.

Adelstein et al. further address the specifics of the Irish health experience. For the period 1970–2, the principal causes of death amongst Irish men were accidents, poisonings and violence (80 per cent above average), with particularly high risk of homicide, accidental poisoning and falls, cancers of the buccal cavity and pharynx (83 per cent above average), the skin (47 per cent) and the larynx (39 per cent), tuberculosis (145 per cent) and non-acute nephritis (59 per cent).[23] Deaths from liver cirrhosis, peptic ulcers and hypertensive heart disease were 63 per cent, 42 per cent and 35 per cent above average respectively. Amongst Irish women during the same period a similar pattern emerges, although one showing less dramatic shifts from the averages. Deaths due to accidents, poisonings and violence were 35 per cent above average, with high figures for tuberculosis (115 per cent), liver cirrhosis (59 per cent) and peptic ulcers (35 per cent). For cancers, those of the trachea, bronchus and lung exceeded the male figures, being 59 per cent above average, as did cancer of the oesophagus (37 per cent).

Table 7.12 Standard mortality rates for all causes of Irish immigrants aged 20+ years in England and Wales, and Irish population in Republic of Ireland aged 15–74, 1970–2

	Males	*Females*
England and Wales	114	116
Ireland	99	117

Source: Table 7.10

Obviously some of these causes can be related to lifestyle and behaviour, but others, in particular tuberculosis, are probably connected with prevalence in the country of origin. There has been some evidence, for example, that Irish people are more likely to smoke and drink heavily, although this is questioned to some extent in our own figures derived from the GHS, and presented later in this section.[24] However, to date, there has been little systematic attempt to account for or explain the reasons that underlie the causes of early death amongst the Irish. Furthermore, studies reported in the USA indicate that Irish migrants have poorer life expectancy when compared with other migrant groups, such as Italians.[25] In addition, Raftery et al. report that a similar excess mortality applies to second-generation Irish in the UK.[26]

Mental illness

In addition to mortality data, data are available on admissions to psychiatric hospitals in England by diagnosis. A recent study indicated that people born in the Irish Republic had the highest rates of any migrant group to England of first and subsequent admission to psychiatric hospital.[27] For all causes and admissions, people born in the Irish Republic had twice the rate of hospital admission of the English born, and a rate 50 per cent higher than the next highest group. The relevant data here are shown in Table 7.13, in which figures for both the English and Caribbean born are included. The mental health of the latter has been given close research attention, and the figures are therefore included by way of comparison. The considerable discrepancy between the rates for both Irish-born groups and the others in these data is remarkable, but not as remarkable as their

Table 7.13 Age-standardised rates of admission to psychiatric hospital, all diagnoses, population aged 16+ years, England, 1981 (rates per 100,000 population)

Country of birth	*Males*	*Females*	*All*
Irish Republic	1,054	1,102	1,080
Northern Ireland	793	880	838
England	418	583	504
Caribbean	565	532	548

Source: R. Cochrane and S. Bal, 'Mental Hospital Admission Rates of Immigrants to England: A Comparison of 1971 and 1981', *Social Psychiatry*, 1989, 24, pp. 2–11

apparent invisibility, reflected in the scant subsequent investigation into the alarmingly high incidence.[28]

Cochrane and Bal, the results of whose work are summarised in Table 7.14, also report admission rates for principal diagnoses for all admissions for men and women in the same period.[29] Irish people are over-represented in the diagnostic categories of depression and alcohol related disorders. Men and women born in the Republic have admission rates for depression that are over twice those of their English counterparts. For this condition, the rate of admission for women born both in Northern Ireland and in the Irish Republic is approximately twice that of their male compatriots. For alcohol related disorders, men and women born in the Republic of Ireland respectively suffer approximately nine and seven times the rate of the British born, with men and women of Northern Irish origin suffering seven and five times the British-born rate. Published figures for rates of admission by diagnosis do not appear to be standardised by age, which makes comparison and interpretation difficult for a number of reasons. However, there are several striking points that merit comment.

Although the rates for schizophrenia are high, they are perhaps less than expected given the extent of the problem in Ireland. Other studies have shown the Irish to be under-represented in the schizophrenic population in England.[30] Cochrane and Bal included affective psychosis in the category of depression and alcohol psychosis in their category of alcohol abuse. When placed alongside the issue of endemic schizophrenia amongst the indigenous Irish, there is a possibility that these sub-categories have been misapplied in the case of migrants as a result of ethnic stereotyping by English practitioners. There is evidence that Irish men are diagnosed as alcoholic by British psychiatrists in preference to schizophrenic, and that alcoholism in Irishmen can mask schizophrenic symptoms.[31]

The extensive study by Cochrane and Bal compares well, however, with another study in south-east England by Dean et al., which showed admissions for alcoholism to be 5.3 and 2.4 times the expected number for Irish men and women respectively, with schizophrenia admissions being 2.4 and 4 times greater than expected.[32] The latter study also compared admissions with those in the Republic of Ireland. It found that migrant admissions for both diagnosed conditions were significantly lower than might be expected from admission rates in Ireland. Except for a drop in the incidence levels for people from Northern Ireland, the findings reported for Irish people by Cochrane

Table 7.14 Rates of psychiatric hospital admission by country of birth, England 1981

	Republic Ireland Male	*Republic Ireland Female*	*Northern Ireland Male*	*Northern Ireland Female*	*England Male*	*England Female*	*Caribbean Male*	*Caribbean Female*
Schizophrenia+	158	174	103	111	61	58	259	235
Other psychoses	36	50	28	52	16	27	28	40
Depression*	197	410	143	266	79	166	65	152
Neuroses#	62	111	44	80	28	56	6	25
Personality disorder	62	80	50	52	30	35	22	42
Alcohol abuse$	332	133	261	90	38	18	27	9
Drug abuse	13	8	17	8	5	3	13	0

+ including paranoia
* including affective psychoses and depressive disorders
# including 'neurotic depression'
$ including psychosis, dependence and non-dependent abuse

Source: R. Cochrane and S. Bal, 'Mental Hospital Admission Rates of Immigrants to England: A Comparison of 1971 and 1981', *Social Psychiatry*, 1989, 24, pp. 2–11

and Bal show a level of stability during the preceding decade.[33] Overall rates of hospitalisation from people from Northern Ireland and the Irish Republic were more than twice those of the native-born rate in 1971.[34]

Unfortunately, the excessively high and apparently persistent rates of psychiatric hospital admission have prompted little investigation. Only six studies have addressed the question of psychological morbidity within the community as a whole.[35] This dearth of research is more alarming, when at the same time that high rates of incidence were being identified, other research was showing a strong over-representation of Irish-born people in figures for attempted suicide.[36]

Attempts to assess levels of psychological symptoms amongst the non-hospitalised Irish community that might account for the hospitalisation rate have largely been unsuccessful. Neither Cochrane and Stopes-Roe, nor Der and Bebbington could find indicators in the community that might predict the observed hospitalisation rates.[37] Stopes-Roe and Cochrane compared Irish immigrants with those from India and Pakistan (both groups that have considerably lower rates of hospitalisation for mental illness, compared to the Irish or the native born). They found that with psychological well-being, as measured using Langner 22 item scale, the Irish occupied an intermediate position between the two groups, a finding that would not have been predicted from the admission data.[38] McNicholl's study compared Irish migrants who had been referred to statutory alcohol services with a control group who had not.[39] As might be expected, he found that the non-referred group exhibited better psychological adjustment to life in England than the referred group. It is not clear from these reports what is happening in the diagnosis when they are applied to Irish patients. It may be that schizophrenic symptoms in Irish patients are being interpreted in many cases by British psychiatrists as due to alcohol, because of the stereotype of the Irish drunkard, and it may also be that the Irish are at the same time being generally overdiagnosed as mentally ill.

Of these studies, which are not without their methodological and other difficulties, it is the study by Cochrane and Stopes-Roe that is the most comprehensive and that provides the most intriguing results.[40] On the basis of 1971 hospitalisation and census data, reported in Cochrane, it sought to test a series of hypotheses by the comparison of Irish people resident in Ireland, English people resident in England and immigrant Irish people in England who were matched on age, sex and residential area.[41] They found that the migrant group exhibited better psychological adjustment than either of the non-migrant groups, were slightly less socially isolated and more likely to be downwardly socially mobile. This study found no significant relationships between social mobility, urban/rural origin, marital or employment status and levels of psychological symptoms, all of which have been hypothesised at some time or other as playing some role in mental illness amongst migrants.[42] One finding was reported that directly contradicted a stated hypothesis regarding the relationship between psychological stability and acculturation. Namely, in Cochrane and Stopes-Roe's migrant group, there was a distinct tendency for those oriented more towards England and less towards Ireland to have higher psychological symptom scores. They note that, 'It appears that for males at least, maintaining strong ties with the home country is associated with psychological stability.'[43] This finding is supported by the McNicholl study, which found that the non-referred group were significantly more oriented culturally and perhaps socially towards Ireland, even when age was taken into account.[44]

General morbidity

In the GHS, data are available on the self-reported illness or morbidity of both first- and second-generation migrants in Great Britain. Our source for these data is a conflation of a subset of the GHS surveys for 1984, 1986 and 1988.[45] Our aim in this section is to look at the information that can be derived from this source for a number of indicators of general morbidity. We analysed these data by calculating Standardised Morbidity Rates (SMoRs) for each sex, standardised for age and socio-economic group of the head of household. We also calculated total SMoRs, with additional standardisation for sex, in an attempt to account for obvious disparities in sex structure between the Irish and the British-British sub-groups. The method of calculation was exactly that as for Standardised Mortality Rates, using:

$$SMR = \frac{O}{E} \times 100$$

where

O is the observed frequency of occurrence, and
E is the expected frequency of occurrence

E was calculated by applying the probability of occurrence derived from the whole sample to the particular sub-group. It should be noted that in the tables that follow the large numbers of British-British compared to other categories mean that the SMoRs for that group are usually 100.

Table 7.15 shows SMoRs for the incidence of general health being reported as 'not good on the whole' in the twelve months before the survey date. The data presented here are fascinating. It appears that the least healthy group on this indicator are the second-generation Northern Irish females, followed by their male counterparts, whereas the first-generation migrants from both parts of the island are less likely than the total group to report problems with their general health. In the cases of both second-generation groups, the females are noticeably more likely than the males to report worse general health, while in the first-generation groups the Northern Irish females are apparently the healthiest of all groups, according to their own reports.

The data on the prevalence of long-standing illness reported in Table 7.16 show a similar picture. Here the healthiest group again appears to be the first-generation Northern Irish, and the least healthy the second generation from the north. The first-generation migrants from the Republic seem to score worse on this indicator than they did on the general health question; there is also a general trend for men to report substantially more long-standing illness than women.

The SMoRs for 'limiting long-standing illness', that is, whether long-standing illness caused activities to be limited, are set out in Table 7.17. Comparison of the data shown here with that in Table 7.16 is instructive. The group reporting the highest rate of limiting long-standing illness is again the second-generation Northern Irish females, and the healthiest group overall is again the first-generation Northern Irish. There are, however, substantial differences between the sexes within the first-generation Northern Irish group, with these males showing the highest SMoR for any male group, and the females reporting the lowest ratio. In fact, first-generation Northern Irish females are the only female group with a ratio less than 100 (i.e. average) in this table.

The SMoRs in Table 7.18, based on reports of activities 'cut down as a result of illness in the two weeks before the date of the survey' can be taken as an indicator of 'acute sickness'. Here we see a dramatically different picture from that shown in the previous two tables which largely concern chronic illness. The second-generation

Table 7.15 General health 'not good on the whole' in the last twelve months

	Male No.	*Male %*	*Male SMoR*	*Female No.*	*Female %*	*Female SMoR*	*All No.*	*All %*	*All SMoR*
Republic Irish	307	1.33	97	360	1.38	101	667	1.36	99
Northern Irish	136	0.59	96	158	0.61	75	294	0.60	82
Republic-British	552	2.40	91	634	2.44	109	1,186	2.42	102
Northern Irish-British	217	0.94	115	227	0.87	131	444	0.91	124
British-British	21,799	94.73	100	24,647	94.70	100	46,446	94.72	100

Source: GHS, 1984, 1986 and 1988. Data standardised for age and socio-economic group.

Table 7.16 Long-standing illness (adults)

	Male No.	*Male %*	*Male SMoR*	*Female No.*	*Female %*	*Female SMoR*	*All No.*	*All %*	*All SMoR*
Republic Irish	339	1.37	87	376	1.38	97	715	1.38	92
Northern Irish	143	0.58	88	164	0.60	93	307	0.59	91
Republic-British	598	2.42	99	663	2.44	98	1,261	2.43	98
Northern Irish-British	233	0.94	103	231	0.85	112	464	0.89	108
British-British	23,403	94.69	100	25,777	94.73	100	49,180	94.71	100

Source: GHS, 1984, 1986 and 1988. Data standardised for age and socio-economic group.

Table 7.17 Limiting long-standing illness (adults)

	Male No.	*Male %*	*Male SMoR*	*Female No.*	*Female %*	*Female SMoR*	*All No.*	*All %*	*All SMoR*
Republic Irish	339	1.37	94	376	1.38	107	715	1.38	101
Northern Irish	143	0.58	109	164	0.60	83	307	0.59	94
Republic-British	598	2.42	94	663	2.44	104	1,261	2.43	100
Northern Irish-British	233	0.94	108	231	0.85	142	464	0.89	126
British-British	23,403	94.69	100	25,777	94.73	100	49,180	94.71	100

Source: GHS, 1984, 1986 and 1988. Data standardised for age and socio-economic group.

Table 7.18 Activities cut down in the last two weeks

	Male No.	*Male %*	*Male SMoR*	*Female No.*	*Female %*	*Female SMoR*	*All No.*	*All %*	*All SMoR*
Republic Irish	340	1.38	112	366	1.35	116	706	1.36	115
Northern Irish	143	0.58	92	162	0.60	185	305	0.59	149
Republic-British	598	2.42	97	671	2.47	120	1,269	2.44	111
Northern Irish-British	233	0.94	105	232	0.85	114	465	0.90	111
British-British	23,393	94.68	100	25,770	94.74	99	49,163	94.71	99

Source: GHS, 1984, 1986 and 1988. Data standardised for age and socio-economic group.

Northern Irish group now show the highest SMoRs, while first-generation Northern Irish show the greatest ratios, followed by the first-generation Republic group, with the second-generation groups following behind. However, these aggregate ratios mask gender differences, with the males in the Irish groups generally reporting much less incidence than females of acute sickness that affected their activities.

It is intriguing to note the differences between the respondents' views of their long-term health (see Tables 7.16 and 7.17) and their reports of their actual circumstances in the previous two weeks. The groups that reported the best long-term health (first-generation migrants) are those that, in fact, have been the most disadvantaged in health terms in the two weeks before the survey. In particular, the first-generation Northern Irish females, who apparently had the best health in terms of limiting long-standing illness, had a very high SMoR on cut-down of activities in the previous two weeks. We have no immediate explanation for these apparently anomalous findings, but look with interest at the data shown in Table 7.19 on doctor consultations. Here we see a pattern that is not totally dissimilar to those shown in the previous tables. Again, the second-generation Northern Irish women have the highest incidence of morbidity, with an SMoR of 130. Unusually here the males have SMoRs that are consistently below 100, with the exception of the British-British group. It appears that women are more prone to visit the doctor than men, even though the males in some groups report higher than average incidence of limiting long-standing illness and acute sickness.

Several conclusions can be drawn from this group of tables. It appears that Irish men, of both generations, report better health in terms of long-standing illness than their female counterparts, but that some of these men (Northern Irish first-generation immigrants) are more limited than average by these long-standing illnesses. Women report the highest incidence of acute sickness over the previous two weeks and are also more likely to have visited their doctors. Overall, it seems that Irish people in Britain report less long-standing illness than the British, but are more likely to be limited by the long-standing illnesses that they do have. At the same time, they are markedly more likely to have experienced a recent acute illness that limited their activities, but are less likely to have visited their doctors. These findings do not by themselves appear to lead us to any firm conclusions about the health of Irish migrants in Britain. However, the GHS gives us further information.

Table 7.19 Consultation with doctor in last two weeks (adults)

	Male No.	*Male %*	*Male SMoR*	*Female No.*	*Female %*	*Female SMoR*	*All No.*	*All %*	*All SMoR*
Republic Irish	338	1.43	88	376	1.38	101	714	1.40	96
Northern Irish	143	0.60	83	166	0.61	93	309	0.61	90
Republic-British	598	2.52	85	663	2.44	93	1,261	2.48	90
Northern Irish-British	233	0.98	86	228	0.84	130	461	0.91	112
British-British	22,397	94.47	101	25,799	94.73	100	48,176	94.61	100

Source: GHS, 1984, 1986 and 1988. Data standardised for age and socio-economic group.

Smoking and drinking

Given the high rates of psychiatric hospital admissions and death reported by Adelstein et al. from conditions associated with drinking and smoking, coupled with the common identification in literature and the popular media of the Irish with high alcohol consumption, we have also analysed the self-reported rates of drinking and smoking from the GHS.[46] SMoRs derived from these reports are shown in Tables 7.20 and 7.21.

The incidence of drinking any amount at all (see Table 7.20) appears to be lower in all Irish groups apart from the first-generation Northern Irish (both sexes) and the male second-generation Northern Irish. The SMoRs are not substantially different from 100, apart from those for the second-generation Northern Irish females. Evidently, the Irish do not tend to drink according to the myth of the drunken Irishman or Irishwoman – rather the opposite is the case. As far as smoking is concerned, however, we see a very different picture. Here every Irish group has an SMoR that is higher than 100 (see Table 7.21). Indeed, the values are so much higher that the British-British groups, which are so large as normally to dominate the data and thus return SMoRs of 100, in this case show values of 99. There is no particular pattern, however, in these data. The first-generation Northern Irish show a lower propensity to smoke than their Republic contemporaries, who show the highest ratios, whilst this is reversed for second-generation groups. Interestingly, in most cases it is the women who tend to smoke as much as or more than the men. Clearly, the Irish groups have good reason to have higher than average mortality from smoking related diseases. The particularly high SMoRs reported by Adelstein et al. for first-generation Irish females for neoplasms of the trachea, bronchus and lung are not surprising in the light of the data in Table 7.21.[47]

CONCLUSION

Using the Census and GHS, we have presented a socio-economic picture of first- and second-generation Irish immigrants into Britain. First-generation Irish migrants in Britain cannot be treated as a homogeneous group. For example, first-generation Northern Irish migrants tend to be wealthier than the British-British group, in marked contrast to the Republic Irish migrants. Unemployment rates of the Irish born tend to be higher than the national average for the population as a

Table 7.20 Current drinking (reported drinks rather than abstains)

	Male No.	*Male %*	*Male SMoR*	*Female No.*	*Female %*	*Female SMoR*	*All No.*	*All %*	*All SMoR*
Republic Irish	305	1.33	99	360	1.39	93	665	1.36	96
Northern Irish	135	0.59	101	157	0.61	102	292	0.60	102
Republic-British	552	2.41	99	628	2.42	99	1,180	2.42	99
Northern Irish-British	221	0.97	102	281	1.08	83	502	1.03	92
British-British	21,684	94.70	100	24,517	94.50	100	46,201	94.60	100

Source: GHS, 1984, 1986 and 1988. Data standardised for age and socio-economic group.

Table 7.21 Current smoking (reported smokes rather than abstains)

	Male No.	*Male %*	*Male SMoR*	*Female No.*	*Female %*	*Female SMoR*	*All No.*	*All %*	*All SMoR*
Republic Irish	279	1.45	114	281	1.53	125	560	1.49	120
Northern Irish	118	0.61	103	115	0.63	106	233	0.62	105
Republic-British	463	2.41	111	486	2.65	107	949	2.53	109
Northern Irish-British	190	0.99	113	159	0.87	113	349	0.93	113
British-British	18,151	94.53	99	17,324	94.33	99	35,475	94.43	99

Source: GHS, 1984, 1986 and 1988. Data standardised for age and socio-economic group.

whole, and the inactive proportions are higher and the working proportions smaller than those for the whole population. These characteristics are to a certain extent explained by the generally older profile of the Irish born. We have also seen that first-generation Irish migrants have SMoRs substantially higher than those of the British-born population across a number of causes of deaths. They also have high psychiatric hospital admission rates. The situation regarding self-reported ill-health is more complex, with evidence that indicates that Irish migrants are less likely to go to the doctor when ill.

There is a common assumption, long reflected in the exclusion of the Irish from immigration policy, that the Irish are 'not different' from the British population. We have shown that on health and other grounds this is untenable. Marked cultural differences, in areas such as religion, language, dietary and medical practices, have been overlooked as the Irish have been administratively assimilated into British society. The disproportionately high mortality and psychiatric admission rates indicate that a specifically medical-cultural difference obviously exists between Irish migrants and the indigenous population. How might we account for this? A strong influence has been the nature of what may be described as the colonial power relationship into which Irish people have traditionally been inserted on migration to England. On the one hand, the public attention devoted to immigration has concentrated itself on what used to be known as the 'colour problem'. Institutionalised racism directed towards black people was matched by a liberal concern for their health and well-being, the latter stemming from the former. The Irish, on the other hand, although subject to the same kinds of racism over a similar period, were excluded from the same kinds of overt attention.

Despite this exclusion, the material conditions and circumstances under which Irish people have had to live their lives in England have been, in common with other colonial migrants, amongst the worst. Connor's recent analysis of housing conditions amongst migrant groups in London shows that the Irish, along with Bangladeshis, have the lowest rate of owner occupation by head of household.[48] They are over-represented in the private rental sector, and within this sector have the highest proportion of people living in households with shared amenities, and the second highest proportion of people in homes lacking basic amenities, such as a bathroom or a toilet. Such conditions are not conducive to good health. It is therefore not surprising that Irish mortality rates are elevated in each SEG relative to the British-born population.

At the same time, however, we see that the Irish do not report poor health. Indeed, we have shown that they show lower SMoRs than the British on the question of their self-perceived general health and in their much lower tendency than the British to consult with the doctor. There are many possible reasons for this. Perhaps the Irish, for cultural reasons, do not visit a doctor until symptoms are severe, in a sense denying the incidence of illness until it becomes too much to bear on a day-to-day basis. The high incidence of 'activities cut-down' for all categories of Irish in the data does, however, indicate that despite their optimistic report on general health and their relatively less frequent visits to the doctor, the Irish are experiencing illness. There may be a factor here of reluctance to visit the doctor despite recognising the need to do so, again perhaps for cultural reasons, but also possibly because the Irish person in Britain sees the doctor as a figure identified with the British establishment and authority structures. Current work by the authors is investigating, through the use of health diaries, the answers to these and other questions. Whatever the results, it seems clear that there are a range of differences identified in this chapter between the Irish of first and second generations and the host population.

There is an intrinsic practical contradiction between the suppression of the significance of these and other differences, on the one hand, and the active racism that Irish people have traditionally suffered at the hands of the English on the other hand. The suppression of material differences at one level (the administrative) has been balanced by an emphasis on difference at another (the day-to-day social). In the course of this process their particular needs have been ignored. The Irish have become stereotyped as a more stupid, emotional, spiritual, friendly, lackadaisical, drunken and/or violent version of the English themselves. These theoretical distinctions have, however, been ignored for the purposes of practical intervention. The circumstances of the Irish in Britain are closer to that of being black rather than white, yet they do not have the visibility that blackness entails in a racist society. This lack of visibility constitutes the principal practical contradiction suffered by the Irish in Britain. Like all practical contradictions, it does not disappear simply because it fails to be recognised. It is experienced throughout daily life and is manifest in poor health experience.

NOTES

The research on which this chapter is based was funded by the Economic and Social Research Council (Grant no: R000233466).

1 P. Townsend and N. Davidson, *The Black Report: Inequalities in Health*, Harmondsworth, 1982.
2 M.G. Marmot, A.M. Adelstein and L. Bulusu, *Immigrant Mortality in England and Wales, 1970–78*, OPCS Studies on Medical and Population Subjects, No. 47, London, 1984.
3 Ibid.
4 R. Cochrane and S. Bal, 'Mental Hospital Admission Rates of Immigrants to England: A Comparison of 1971 and 1981', *Social Psychiatry*, 1989, 24, pp. 2–11.
5 A. Burke, 'Attempted Suicide Amongst the Irish-born Population in Birmingham', *British Journal of Psychiatry*, 1976, 128, pp. 534–7; V.S. Raleigh and R. Balarajan, 'Suicide Levels and Trends Amongst Immigrants in England and Wales', *Health Trends*, 1992, 24, pp. 91–4.
6 *Times*, 4 May 1847, p. 3.
7 W.M. Frazer, *Duncan of Liverpool: Being an Account of the Work of Dr W.H. Duncan, Medical Officer of Health for Liverpool 1847–1863*, London, 1947, pp. 58–9.
8 R. Swift and S. Gilley, eds, *The Irish in Britain*, London, 1989.
9 R. Swift, 'Crime and the Irish in Britain', in Swift and Gilley, *Irish in Britain*, pp. 163–82.
10 cf., T. Connor, *The London Irish*, London, 1987.
11 Action Group for Irish Youth, *Irish Emigration: A Programme for Action*, London and Dublin, 1988; Office of Population Census and Surveys, *Migration Tables, 1991 Census*, London, 1993.
12 Connor, *London Irish*, p. 18.
13 cf., S. Heath, *Class and Ethnicity: Irish Catholics in England 1880–1939*, Buckingham, 1993, p. 131; K. O'Connor, *The Irish in Britain*, London, 1974, p. 143.
14 Connor, *London Irish*.
15 Ibid.
16 The 1991 Census reports the category 'born in Ireland', which does not allow in all cases the distinction between people born in Northern Ireland and those born in the Republic. Unless otherwise stated, we shall use the term 'Irish-born' to mean people born in the island of Ireland (i.e. the Republic and Northern Ireland).
17 Born in the Republic and in Northern Ireland.
18 L. Greenslade, 'The Irish in Britain in the 1990s: A Preliminary Analysis of the 1991 Census Reports', *Reports on the 1991 Census*, Liverpool, 1993.
19 Marmot, *Immigrant Mortality*, passim.
20 Ibid.; A.M. Adelstein, M.G. Marmot, G. Dean and S. Bradshaw, 'Comparison of Mortality of Irish Immigrants in England and Wales with that of Irish and British Nationals', *Irish Medical Journal*, 1986, 79/7, pp. 185–9.

21 Ibid.
22 Ibid.
23 Ibid.
24 R. Balarajan and P. Yuen, 'Smoking and Drinking Habits: Variations by Country of Birth', *Community Medicine*, 1986, 8, pp. 237–9.
25 I. Rosenwaike and K. Hempstead, 'Differential Mortality by Ethnicity and Nativity: Foreign and Native-Born Irish, Italian and Jews in New York City, 1979–81', *Soc-Biol*, 1990, 37/1–2, pp. 11–25.
26 J. Raftery, D. Jones and M. Rosato, 'The Mortality of First and Second Generation Irish Immigrants in the UK', *Social Science and Medicine*, 1989, 31/5, pp. 577–84.
27 Cochrane and Bal, 'Mental Hospital'.
28 M. Pearson, M. Madden and L. Greenslade, *Generations of an Invisible Minority? The Health of the Irish in Britain*, Liverpool, 1991.
29 Ibid.
30 C. Bagley, 'A Comparative Study of Mental Illness Amongst Immigrant Groups in Britain', *Review of Ethnicities*, 1970, 1, pp. 24–36, and A.W. Clare, 'Mental Illness in the Irish Emigrant', *Journal of the Irish Medical Association*, 1974, 67, pp. 20–4.
31 C. Bagley and A. Binitie, 'Alcoholism and Schizophrenia in Irishmen in London', *British Journal of Addiction*, 1970, 65, pp. 3–7.
32 G. Dean, D. Walsh, H. Downing and E. Shelley, 'First Admissions of Native-born and Immigrants to Psychiatric Hospitals in South East England in 1976', *British Journal of Psychiatry*, 1981, 139, pp. 506–12; Bagley and Binitie, 'Alcoholism and Schizophrenia'.
33 Dean et al., 'First admissions'.
34 R. Cochrane, 'Mental Illness in Immigrants to England and Wales: An Analysis of Mental Hospital Admissions', *Social Psychiatry*, 1977, 12, pp. 23–5.
35 R. Cochrane and M. Stopes-Roe, 'Psychological Disturbance in Ireland, in England and in Irish Emigrants to England: A Comparative Study', *Economic and Social Review*, 1979, 10, pp. 301–20; P.E. Bebington, J. Hurry and C. Tennant, 'Psychiatric Disorders in Selected Immigrant Groups in Camberwell', *Social Psychiatry*, 1981, 16, pp. 43–51; G. Der and P. Bebington 'Depression in Inner London', *Social Psychiatry*, 1987, 23, pp. 73–84; Bagley, 'Comparative Study of Mental Illness'; M. Stopes-Roe and R. Cochrane, 'Mental Health and Integration: A Comparison of Indian, Pakistani and Irish Immigrants to England', *Ethnic and Racial Studies*, 1980, 3, pp. 316–41; D. McNicholl, 'Migration Factors Related to the Psychological Adjustment of the Irish in Britain', unpublished MSc Thesis, University of Leicester, 1990.
36 Burke, 'Attempted Suicide'.
37 Stopes-Roe and Cochrane, 'Mental Health'; Der and Bebington 'Depression in Inner London'.
38 T.S. Langner, 'A 22–item Screening Score of Psychiatric Symptoms Indicating Impairment', *Journal of Health and Human Behaviour*, 1962, 111, pp. 269–76.
39 McNicholl, 'Migration Factors'.
40 Cochrane and Stopes-Roe, 'Psychological Disturbance'.

41 Cochrane, 'Mental Illness'.
42 cf., C. Zwingmann and M. Pfister-Ammende, *Uprooting and After*, New York, 1973.
43 Cochrane and Stopes-Roe, 'Psychological Disturbance', p. 315.
44 McNicholl, 'Migration factors'.
45 The GHS is described in some detail in the previous section of this chapter.
46 Adelstein et al., 'Mortality of Irish'.
47 Ibid.
48 Connor, *London Irish.*

8

ETHNIC ADVANTAGE

Infant survival among Jewish and Bengali immigrants in East London, 1870–1990

Lara Marks and Lisa Hilder

From the end of the nineteenth century to the present day, the survival of the infant has been of substantial interest to health experts, policy makers and the general public in Britain and elsewhere. Debate has continued on the most important influences on infant survival. These range from socio-economic conditions to maternal care, medical provision and genetic inheritance. Such issues have not diminished with the decline in infant mortality in the developed world in the later part of this century. Indeed, the continuing differentials between different social groups, despite the overall decline in infant mortality, have generated even fiercer debates. Increasing in prominence within these discussions has been the role of race and ethnicity in determining infant survival.[1] A burgeoning literature is growing in Britain, America and elsewhere showing heterogeneous infant survival patterns among contemporary infants of different ethnic minorities.[2] Much of this literature points to a complex relationship between ethnicity and health which involves social, cultural and racial considerations.[3]

Many of the studies over the last two decades compare infants of ethnic minorities with the local population without putting these patterns into any historical context. In this chapter we will show, with reference to the East European Jewish immigrants at the turn of the century and Bengali immigrants in the 1980s, that the health of infants among ethnic minorities cannot be understood without reference to the history of their settlement. Indeed, an infant's chances of survival can differ greatly from the time of initial immigration to settlement, when parents are more integrated into their surroundings.[4] In addition, we challenge studies that have presented ethnicity or immigrant status as the explanatory variable in itself, without exploring the ethnic behaviours and values that might underlie the mortality differentials with the indigenous population.

As we shall see, while the Jews and Bengalis of East London experienced very different rates of infant mortality, living in different periods and under dissimilar conditions (particularly in relation to medical knowledge and the facilities for treatment), the rates of infant death in relation to the local population provide an interesting parallel that raises important questions about the impact of ethnicity on infant survival.

MIGRATION

With close proximity to the main ports of London, East London has long been an attractive refuge for immigrant groups, offering cheap accommodation and employment through its casual labour economy. In the years from 1870 to the outbreak of the First World War, East European Jewish immigrants constituted the predominant ethnic minority group within East London, while Bengali immigrants became the predominant ethnic minority in the years between 1970 and 1985. These immigrant populations migrated for different reasons and under different conditions, but they were both in search of better economic prosperity. For the Jews there was the additional element of escaping persecution. As a white ethnic minority, however, the Jews would have had a different experience on arrival to the Bengali immigrants who were more noticeable for their skin colour. Similarly, while the Jews migrated from countries which in many ways had a similar climate to England, though different infrastructure, Bangladeshi immigrants had to make much greater adjustments. The contrast between Bangladesh and Britain could not be greater, climatically, culturally, or in terms of health and social services.

East European Jewish migration[5]

Originally expelled in 1290, Jews began to resettle in Britain from the seventeenth century. Initially those who came were merchants of German, Dutch and Sephardi origin.[6] From the eighteenth century, Ashkenazi[7] Jews began to arrive from Eastern Europe, their settlement growing greatly in the nineteenth century, particularly in the years after 1870.[8] The size and nature of their migration was unprecedented, making them the largest group of immigrants Britain had ever received.[9] Between 1881 and 1905, approximately a million Jews left Eastern Europe, three-quarters of whom came from Russia. Those who migrated to Britain were mostly from Russian Poland, but Galicians and Roumanians also arrived between 1890 and 1902.[10] Between 1881 and 1914, 100,000 to 150,000 East European Jews came to Britain. At the end of the nineteenth century the Russian-Polish, Roumanian and Galician immigrants were the largest group settling in Britain, constituting 65 per cent of the immigrants arriving in the country in 1901.[11] According to the Census of 1901, of the 95,245 Russians and Poles living in the United Kingdom (UK), 53,537 lived in the County of London together with 6,189 Austrians and 246 Roumanians.[12] The majority of these immigrants were Jewish.

Like their predecessors, many of these East European Jews settled in East London. The exact number in East London is unknown as the Census never listed the Jews separately. According to a survey carried out by Charles Booth in 1889, East London accounted for 90 per cent of the Jewish population in the capital, the majority of whom resided in Whitechapel and the immediate areas in the borough of Stepney.[13] Stepney continued to have the highest proportion of foreigners in London through to the turn of the century.[14] In 1911, 83 per cent of London's Russian and Russian-Polish population were living in Stepney and Bethnal Green.[15] Arriving with artisan and commercial skills, many of these immigrants became absorbed into the East End's footwear, tailoring and furniture trades.[16]

Bengali migration

Immigrants have been coming from the Indian subcontinent to Britain for centuries, mainly as sailors, students, professionals and politicians, many of whom returned after completing their mission.[17] Numerically these immigrants were largely insignificant before 1945. From the early 1950s, however, much larger numbers began to arrive from the Indian subcontinent. These immigrants differed from the earlier immigrants in that they arrived as a result of an explicit immigration policy that promised them economic advancement.[18] Substantial numbers of unskilled migrants were attracted to Britain by the economic expansion and shortages of labour in the 1950s; however, many found themselves in the least attractive jobs. Migration reached its peak in the mid-1950s, after which restrictions and new passport regulations were imposed by the Indian and Pakistani governments, reacting to pressure from the British government.

Under these regulations, those with money and skills were favoured, while those who were uneducated and unskilled could no longer travel unless they already had relatives in Britain. This bias was reinforced by the Commonwealth Immigrants Act, 1962, which introduced a voucher system whereby prospective immigrants had to have sponsored UK employment before being allowed entry.[19] Until then, because of their status as Commonwealth citizens, they were able to enter and leave Britain without any official registration.[20] In the period 1955–60, the Home Office estimated a net inflow of 33,070 Indian and 17,120 Pakistani immigrants.[21]

In East London, the overwhelming majority of immigrants originate from the district of Sylhet. Before the partition of India and Pakistan in 1947, this district was included within the jurisdiction of the eastern part of Bengal. After 1971 and the war of independence for Bangladesh from Pakistan, Sylhet became an integral part of Bangladesh. Social and political turmoil in the struggle for Bangladeshi independence prompted further migration. Most of those who settled within East London were unskilled or semi-skilled and had no large capital resources.[22] Estimates of the numbers of Bengalis entering Britain were complicated before the emergence of Bangladesh as a separate country in 1973. Bengali households were categorised separately in the 1981 Census, but these statistics are considered to be under-recordings.[23] In 1981 the Census showed that 48,517 residents of Great Britain had been born in Bangladesh, and that this group showed the most marked concentration of all ethnic minorities, with the London Borough of Tower Hamlets accounting for about a quarter of the national total.[24] Analysis of new arrivals from abroad to Tower Hamlets in 1991, based on notifications by the Health Control Units at ports of entry, shows that immigration from Bangladesh continued and contributed 61 per cent of all entrants in that year.[25]

Migration of women in the two immigrant populations

Initially men constituted the bulk of the immigration among the Jewish and Bengali communities. In the later years of migration, however, women formed a larger proportion of immigrants. Women comprised between 38 and 48 per cent of the Russian and Polish population living in London between 1871 and 1911.[26] Among the overall East European population entering Britain in the years between 1895 and 1902, the percentage of women varied between

26 and 31 per cent.[27] Many of these women either travelled with their husband and family or arrived shortly after. Often they were accompanied by children, who made up between 15 and 26 per cent of the East European immigrants to Britain between 1895 and 1902.[28] Such a high profile of families among the Jewish immigrants showed that their migration was generally a permanent move. This distinguishes them from other migrant groups who were primarily composed of single male wage earners, whose move was often a transitory search for economic gains before returning to their place of origin. Jewish immigrants not only often travelled together as a family unit, they were also greatly dependent on familial financial support both in their departure from Eastern Europe as well as during their period of settlement within Britain.[29]

Among the Bengali population men dominated immigration in the 1950s and 1960s, though most married in Bangladesh and maintained their families there until they were established in Britain. Only in the 1970s did women begin to arrive from Bangladesh in any large numbers, with highest levels between 1981 and 1985. In recent years female and child dependants of Bengali immigrants have been the predominant group. In the 1981 Census, Bengalis stood out from other immigrant groups as having the smallest proportion of its members born in the UK and having the most skewed sex structure, with only 614 females for every 1,000 males.[30] Over the next decade the ratio of males to females shifted towards unity.[31]

After 1975, details collected at birth registration included country of birth, although published statistics have separated Bangladesh and Pakistan only since 1982. The increase in the numbers of births to Bangladeshi-born mothers over the 1980s was notable.[32] The rapid increase in the numbers of women of childbearing age was also reflected in the rise in the annual number of births to women from Bangladesh in the London Hospital in Tower Hamlets between 1974 and 1984. At the beginning of the period Bengali mothers contributed 10 per cent of the births; by 1984 this had risen to just under 50 per cent, and remained reasonably constant at just over 40 per cent up to the end of 1993.[33]

The patterns of migration of women is important when considering the influence of ethnicity on infant mortality, as it is this group who have the most impact on, and indeed directly influence, the number and subsequent care of infants. As we will discuss below, it was the maintenance of ethno-specific behaviours that we suggest favourably modified the environmental risks to infant survival.

Patterns of immigrant settlement within East London and socio-economic conditions

Although arriving at different moments in time, the East European Jewish and Bengali immigrants have occupied many of the same areas of East London. As can be seen from Figures 8.1 and 8.5, Spitalfields and its surrounding area have had the largest congregation of these two groups. Drawn from a map compiled by a house-to-house survey conducted by school inspectors in 1899, to investigate the percentage of Jewish population within East London,[34] and from a map showing the census districts of 1901, Figure 8.1 shows that Jews comprised over 95 per cent of the residents in Spitalfields and over 75 per cent of those in Goodman's Fields, Mile End New Town, Mile End Old Town West and parts of St George North. Figure 8.5 reveals very similar residential patterns among the Bengali population. Compiled from recent maternity records which routinely list the postcode of residence at time of birth and the ethnicity of the mother, Figure 8.5 shows that the proportion of births to mothers reported as a Bengali resident in each ward in the years 1987 to 1990 was concentrated in Spitalfields and in the western wards.

In both the periods in which the Jews and the Bengalis were living in these areas, East London has been noted for its social and economic deprivation and poor health.[35] Indeed today, as in the past, conditions have been noted to be worse in the western areas where the Jews were and Bengalis have recently settled. In particular, the area has been characterised by poor housing, overcrowding and chronic unemployment.[36]

INFANT SURVIVAL

An important measure of health in populations, then as now, is infant mortality. The extreme vulnerability of the infant is reflected in high rates of mortality in adverse conditions. In poorer countries one in four infants still die before their first birthday. Infant survival is determined not only by the conditions under which pregnancy occurs, but also by the immediate environment into which he or she is born. The mortality of the infant reflects its health at birth, the health of its mother, the quality of the environment in which it is cared for, and the access its family has to health services and effective treatment for life-threatening illnesses.

Over this century infant mortality rates in England and Wales have fallen from 154 per thousand live births in 1900 to rates of less than nine per thousand live births in 1993. Indeed, from being a relatively common event (one in ten infants dying before the age of one year), infant mortality is now a rarity. Much of the initial dramatic falls in infant mortality at the beginning of the century were largely due to falls in post-neonatal mortality (i.e. deaths between one and twelve months). The reasons for this decline have been the subject of historical debate, but the consensus is now that improvements in water supplies, housing and general standards of living contributed most to the fall in mortality.[37] Differences in infant mortality rates alone between 1870 and 1990 suggest a substantial absolute improvement. Now as then, infants of immigrant mothers were assumed to be at higher risk of death, not least because of their concentration in deprived areas.

Infant mortality among East European Jewish immigrants

Mortality statistics for the Jewish immigrants are difficult to separate from the general population in East London in the late nineteenth and early twentieth centuries. None the less, a number of contemporary Medical Officers of Health (MOHs) and other investigators commented frequently on the unexpectedly low rates of infant mortality among the Jewish inhabitants of East London.[38] This was particularly surprising given that overall infant mortality was slightly higher in East London than either London as a whole or England and Wales. The high infant mortality in East London was usually attributed to the social and economic deprivation in the area.

To test the assertions made by MOHs about Jewish infant mortality, we have taken rates of infant mortality in registration districts of East London from the Registrar General's Quarterly Returns for the years between 1881 and 1910 and matched them with the map in Figure 8.1. This exercise had to take into account the change in boundaries set by the Registrar General for the collection of the statistics in the late 1880s and again in 1890s. Two areas where Jews constituted between 75 and 100 per cent of the population in 1899, Spitalfields and Mile End New Town, had no change in boundaries up to that date. Goodman's Fields, with between 75 and 95 per cent of its population being Jewish, was expanded in 1892 to include Aldgate where the number of Jews was much smaller. Goodman's Fields was included because no separate statistics remain for Mile End New Town after 1899, when its boundaries changed, and this has made it impossible to

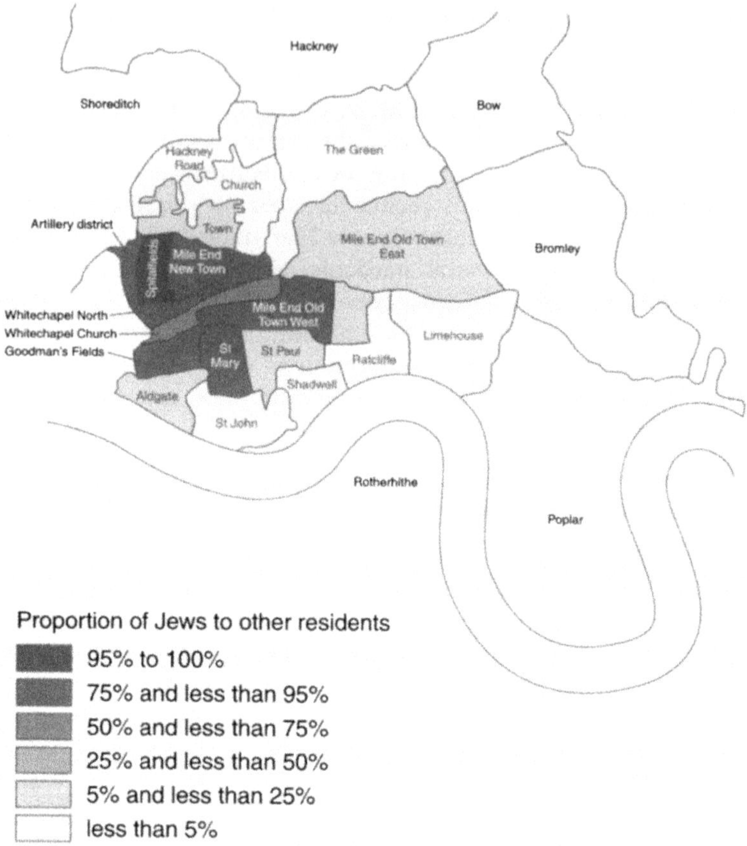

Figure 8.1 Proportion of Jewish immigrants to other residents in East London, 1899

Note: Proportion of Jewish residents not known for St John, Bow, Bromley, Poplar
Source: Adapted from map by George Arkell, prepared for C. Russell and H.S. Lewis, *The Jew in London*, 1901; boundaries adapted from map of sub-ward boundaries of the Metropolis, 1843. The map was compiled from information gathered by the visitors of the London School Board

compute the trend of infant mortality for this area after the 1890s. The infant mortality rates for these districts with a high proportion of Jewish residents were compared with rates from Limehouse and Bethnal Green East, where Jews constituted less than 5 per cent of the population. Before 1889, Bethnal Green East was part of the area known as the Green, and although the population size changed, this probably did not alter the number of Jewish residents found there.

Figure 8.2 shows the three year moving average rates of infant mortality rates for these areas between 1885 and 1910. Rates in the first 15 years appear to be higher in Jewish areas than in the non-Jewish ones, correlating with large-scale in-migration.[39] In 1903, Mr Joseph claimed in his evidence to the Royal Commission on Alien Immigration that infant mortality was especially high among the new immigrants because of the persecution and extreme poverty they had suffered both before arriving in Britain and during the initial period of settlement.[40] A shift is apparent in the rate of decline in infant mortality, starting sooner and proceeding more rapidly in the predominantly Jewish areas compared to those where Jewish immigrants made up less than 5 per cent of the population.[41] This decrease in infant mortality in the Jewish areas in the 1890s was even more surprising given that the trend in England and Wales and London as a whole was a rise in mortality in these years.[42]

Lower rates of infant mortality among Jewish immigrants were not confined to East London.[43] Jewish infants had a much greater chance of survival than their non-Jewish counterparts in Asia, Eastern Europe, Western Europe and North America.[44] This advantage stretched back to the mid-nineteenth century and continued well into the twentieth century, reflecting the earlier decline in mortality of Jewish infants in the nineteenth century compared to other groups.[45] In the United States (US) the low rates of Jewish infant and child mortality contrasted with the higher rates found among Italian and Polish immigrants who arrived during the same period.[46]

The major causes of infant death in this period were infectious diseases, principally of respiratory and digestive systems. Contemporary reports showed that the incidence of diarrhoea and respiratory infections was much lower among Jewish infants.[47] Support for this view is given in Figure 8.2, which shows a rapid decline of infant deaths in the Jewish areas of East London in the late 1890s, a time when overall infant mortality was rising as a result of the increased prevalence of diarrhoea in a series of hot summers.[48] Diarrhoea accounted for nearly a quarter of all the infant deaths in the Borough of Stepney in 1901, and was one of the leading causes of deaths for infants nationally in the nineteenth century.[49]

While age-specific statistics do not exist for Jewish immigrants in East London, it would appear from studies elsewhere in the world that the lower rate of infant mortality amongst the Jews was largely accounted for by a reduction in post-neonatal mortality. Deaths in infants in the neonatal period (birth to one month) did not substantially

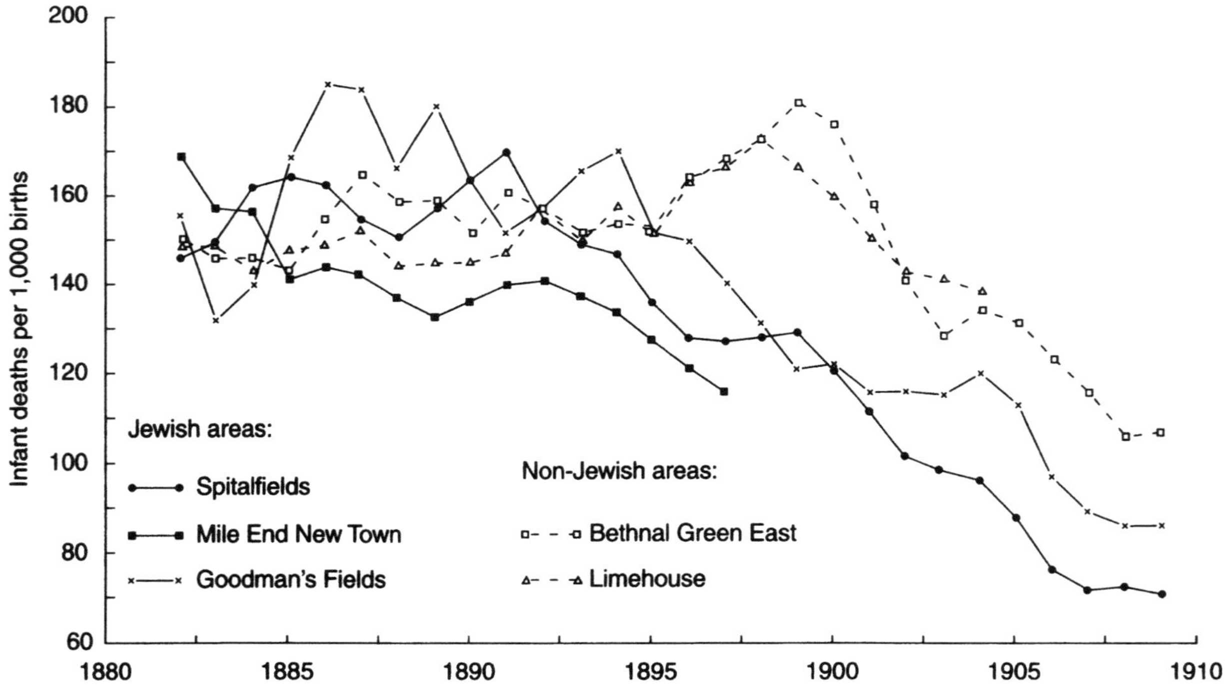

Figure 8.2 Infant deaths in selected sub-districts of East London, 1880–1910, over rolling average of three years

Source: Registrar General, *Quarterly Returns of Births and Deaths for England and Wales*, London, 1880–1910

fall until much later in the twentieth century. Comparisons of age-specific infant mortality rates for Jews and non-Jews recorded in Budapest, Amsterdam and the US in the early twentieth century are given in Figure 8.3, which shows reductions in both the neonatal (to the left of the axis) and post-neonatal components (to the right of the axis) of the infant mortality rate (represented by the total length of the bar). Infant mortality was lower overall for Jewish infants, the largest difference evident in the mortality in the post-neonatal period.[50]

Given that environmental conditions in Budapest were probably much worse than those found in the majority of American cities during these years, these findings suggest that something common to Jews provided a relative advantage in the face of very different environments. This was most pronounced in the US. The between-country differences in rates of infant mortality shown in Figure 8.3 should be treated cautiously, as they may reflect national differences in the way in which statistics were collected.

Infant mortality among Bengali immigrants

In the last quarter of the twentieth century, infectious diseases have played a minor role in infant mortality patterns in Britain, having been superseded by congenital abnormalities as the main cause of death. In early infancy, particularly the neonatal period, the majority of deaths are attributable to congenital malformation, prematurity and the effects of asphyxia during birth. Deaths in the post-neonatal period are now ascribed predominantly to the Sudden Infant Death Syndrome (SIDS), which indicates the sudden death of an otherwise healthy infant whose death cannot be associated with a pathological cause at post-mortem.

How are these factors reflected in the patterns of infant mortality found among Bengali infants? Before 1982, in official statistics reporting rates of infant mortality for births to immigrant mothers, the infants of Bengali mothers were included with those from India. This group was characterised by higher perinatal mortality (stillbirths and deaths in the first week of life) and higher infant mortality rates overall.[51] One study, using linked birth and death registration records for England and Wales for a national cohort of infants born in 1982 to 1985, showed, however, that SIDS was much lower among Asian infants, particularly Bengali ones, which had an important impact on their overall rates of post-neonatal mortality.[52]

On the basis of the number of births and age-specific rates of infant

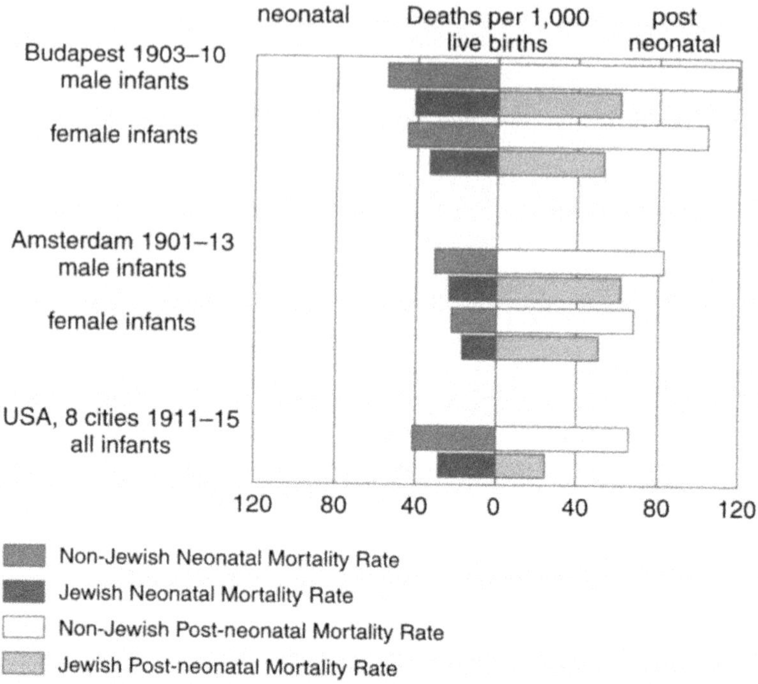

Figure 8.3 Relative age-specific mortality among Jewish and non-Jewish infants in Budapest, Amsterdam and the USA, 1901–15

Source: U.O. Schelz, *Infant and Early Childhood Mortality Among Jews of the Diaspora*, Jerusalem, 1971, p. 38, Table 4

mortality reported by the Office for Population Census Statistics since 1982, Figure 8.4 contrasts the mortality rates of infants of mothers born in Bangladesh with those for infants of mothers born in the UK. Neonatal and post-neonatal mortality rates are separated by the axis. It is evident from Figure 8.4 that the relative disadvantage of Bengali neonates (birth to one month) at the beginning of the period changes abruptly after 1984 as rates fall to a level slightly below that for neonates of mothers born in the UK in all years, the only exception being in 1988. Post-neonatal mortality rates show better survival of infants of mothers born in Bangladesh in all years except 1985.

The same pattern can be shown for East London using linked obstetric and vital registration records relating to births to residents of Tower Hamlets, City and Hackney and Newham in the years 1987 to 1990.[53] Figure 8.5 shows the concentration of Bengali births in

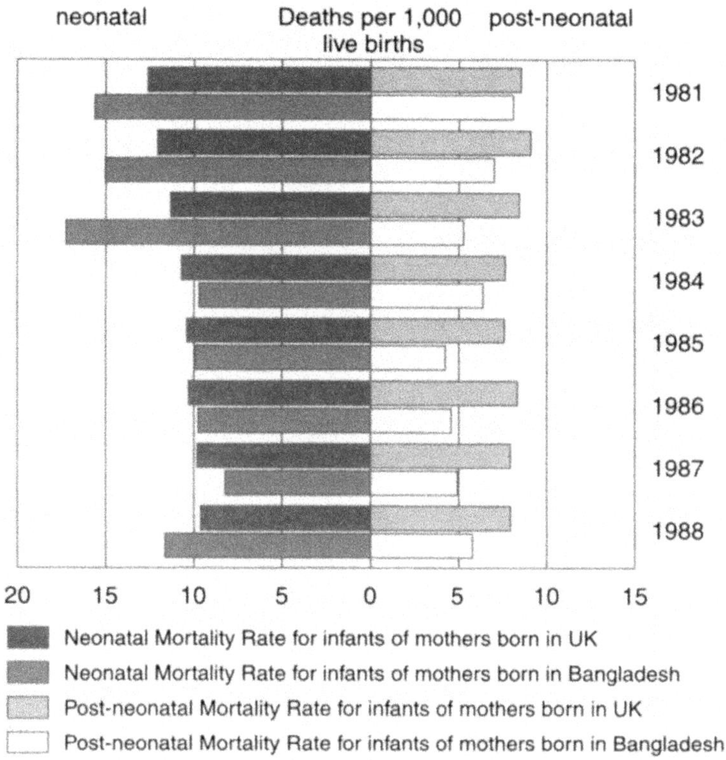

Figure 8.4 Relative age-specific mortality of infants in East London by country of birth of mother (UK and Bangladesh), 1981–8

Source: OPCS DH 3, Nos. 13, 14, 15, 17, 18, 20, 21, 22, London, 1982–90

these areas. Self-reported ethnicity was recorded by midwives at registration for antenatal care. The mortality rates for infants born to Bengali mothers was 6.9 per thousand live births, compared with 9.4 per thousand for infants born to mothers of Anglo-European origin. The aggregated national mortality for the same years was 8.6 per thousand, which shows that, while in East London Bengali post-neonatal infants do better than the national average, infants of neighbouring indigenous families on the whole do worse.

Unfortunately no published data has been found relating to the experience of Bengalis who migrated elsewhere. Studies of immigrant communities in Europe and North America, however, have identified infants of immigrants who tend to fare worse, such as the Hispanics in

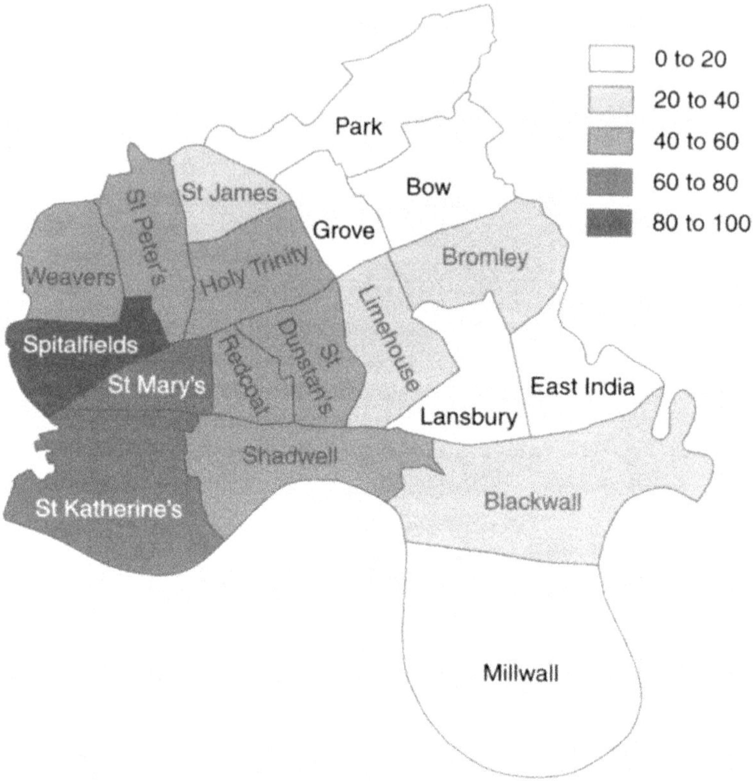

Figure 8.5 Percentage of births in each electoral ward in East London to mothers of Bangladeshi origin, 1987–90

Source: London Hospital Obstetrical Records, 1987–90

the US, Turkish immigrants in Austria and North African immigrants in France. Yet there have also been reports of improved survival of infants of Indo-Chinese mothers in the US, and improved post-neonatal survival of Koreans in Hawaii.[54]

Unlike neonatal mortality, which is more strongly associated with prematurity, congenital malformation and the quality of maternal care, post-neonatal mortality, both in the past and today, is more sensitive to social and environmental factors, especially deprivation and poor sanitary conditions.[55] Given that both the Jewish and Bengali immigrants lived in some of the poorest and overcrowded conditions within East London, we would expect much higher levels of infant mortality than the above evidence portrays. The observed reduction in infant mortality suggests that factors other than environmental conditions prevail.

ETHNICALLY DETERMINED BEHAVIOURS THAT IMPACT ON INFANT MORTALITY

How the Jewish and Bengali populations adapted to their new surroundings and what impact this had on their standards of health and that of their children depended on the social and economic conditions that they had left behind them and those that greeted them on their arrival. The attitudes and behaviours they brought with them and the degree to which these were maintained on settling into East London were also important.[56] While more overt practices such as dress, language and religion serve to distinguish ethnic groups, these point to the fact that other hidden, culturally determined practices, are followed. Family formation, childbearing, hygiene and dietary practices, together with wider networks for social and economic support, are also likely to have an impact on mortality rates.

Jewish practices that could improve infant survival

The principal causes of death among infants at the turn of the century, be they diarrhoeal or respiratory diseases, had a greater chance of spreading where there was poverty, bad sanitation, overcrowding and poor housing. Yet the Jewish immigrants in East London were not living in better circumstances than their neighbours.[57] Their lower rates of infant mortality from infectious and respiratory diseases are therefore puzzling. Hardy has argued that one reason for the lower rates of infectious disease among the Jews was that the Mosaic law instructed for the isolation and disinfection of infectious patients. None the less, as she points out, it is impossible to judge the extent to which such precautions were practised in everyday life.[58] Similarly, the isolation of the infected patient away from the rest of the family would have been especially hard to carry out in the overcrowded and cramped housing of East London. In one respect, however, the Jewish immigrants had the advantage that the established Jewish communal body, the Jewish Board of Guardians, was very active in improving sanitary conditions in the dwellings of Jewish immigrants and in instituting pioneering precautions to help isolate infectious cases such as tuberculosis.[59]

Other religious and cultural traditions that were likely to protect Jewish infants were those concerned with diet and hygiene.[60] The stress that Jewish teachings placed on personal hygiene and cleanliness, and the intricate preparations around food, would have guarded against infantile diarrhoea, which was strongly linked to the type of food an infant received and the conditions under which it was prepared. Infants who were bottle-fed generally had a poorer chance of survival than those who were breast-fed.[61] Those receiving breast-milk not only gain the mother's antibodies for fighting infections, but are better protected from the bacteria that often contaminate bottle-fed milk. At the turn of the century, contamination of food was difficult to avoid in working-class homes, as many had no piped water supply or mains sewerage, and had limited space for food storage. It was often very difficult to guard milk against the 'bacterial organisms (in particular some strains of *Escherichia coli*) which, although not harmful to the more developed digestive system of older children and adults, could produce diarrhoea attacks in infants'.[62]

While Jewish mothers in the working-class housing of East London would have experienced the same problems in the preparation and storage of food as their neighbours, they could counterbalance some of this by the skills that they acquired through the Jewish rituals associated with kosher food. These not only weighed heavily against the consumption of infected food,[63] but also necessitated the separation of milk and meat utensils and called for a high degree of cleanliness of implements.[64] Children of Jewish immigrants in London recall that young babies were never given any water or milk without it having been boiled first,[65] thus reducing the likelihood of infection. Jewish religious teaching also demanded hand-washing before and after meals.[66] Visitors in East London frequently commented that Jewish homes were cleaner than others in the area, which many contemporaries attributed to the Jewish dietary and hygienic laws.[67]

The practice of supplementary feeding among the Jewish immigrants may also have been protective. Contemporary observers claimed that Jewish immigrant mothers commonly supplemented breast-milk with a large variety of extra foods.[68] At the turn of the century, Jewish children stood out in having very low rates of rickets, which results from the lack of vitamin D. This vitamin is produced by the body from precursors in the skin in response to exposure to sunlight. In countries where days are short and protection from the cold requires extensive covering of skin, dietary sources become more important. In 1902, 50 per cent of children in poor schools in Leeds were found to have rickets, while in Jewish schools the figure was only 7 per cent.[69] Unlike the diet of many of the local residents in East London, a high proportion of the Jewish diet involved fish, milk, eggs, fruit and vegetables, all foods containing vitamin D and also vitamin A.

It has been suggested by Hardy that those suffering from rickets often did not have the strength and stamina to withstand the effects of infectious diseases. Contemporary observers noted the link between rickets and the survival of young children with measles and whooping cough.[70] Although not yet conclusive, current research on respiratory disease has begun to show that there might be a link between a deficiency in vitamin A and an increased morbidity from respiratory infection and overall mortality among young children.[71]

Infants may have benefited also from the relative absence of alcohol among the Jewish population living in East London.[72] This stood in apparent contrast to the local population, where the public house reputedly dominated the social scene, especially among men.[73] At the turn of the century many observers pointed to alcoholism as one of the causes of high infant mortality. While many of these arguments can be seen as middle-class reformers' disparaging criticism of the working class, there is none the less good evidence that chronic alcohol use by women while pregnant is detrimental to the developing foetus, and to this day excessive alcohol consumption in pregnancy and after continues to arouse concern.

Bengali practices that could improve infant survival

Low rates of infant mortality, and in particular low rates of SIDS, among Bengali infants has stimulated many studies. Using routinely collected health service data from East London, one investigation compared the effect of maternal and birth factors between Bengali and Anglo-European residents.[74] Of the factors examined, smoking and alcohol use during pregnancy appeared to have the greatest impact on infant survival, especially in the later infant period. While both smoking and alcohol consumption are undoubtedly under-reported, the virtual absence of smoking or alcohol use amongst the Bengali mothers contrasts with the 30 per cent of indigenous mothers who report smoking and the 20 per cent who report drinking alcohol. Despite a higher prevalence of infants born weighing less than 2,500g, which remains the single factor that poses the greatest risk of SIDS, infants of mothers born in Bangladesh had more favourable rates of birthweight-specific mortality, reflecting the smaller stature of this population rather than higher rates of pathological pregnancies resulting in poor foetal growth.[75]

All Asian groups in this study demonstrated very low rates of illegitimacy, reflecting the extreme unacceptability of birth outside marriage in these communities and the importance attached to belonging to a family network. The importance of family networks was also reflected in an anthropological study of Bengalis who settled in Cardiff.[76] Using ethnographic techniques, this study built a picture of life within a Bengali household, highlighting in particular the central focus of the infant within the household. Care was shared amongst women in the extended family, and the infant was rarely left in a room alone, even when sleeping. The belief amongst this group that lying babies on their backs promotes a 'culturally valued "rounded" head', may be the key to the lower rates of SIDS amongst these infants. Evidence that the prone sleeping position affects the chances of infant survival, and the apparent success in the UK of the 'Back to Sleep' campaign, follows similar successes in other countries. These campaigns focused attention on reversible risk factors for SIDS: maternal smoking, breast feeding and sleeping position.

ETHNICITY, HEALTH AND THE SELECTION PROCESS

It is generally assumed that the health of immigrants in Britain is poorer than that of the indigenous population. This disadvantage has been ascribed to the higher mortality experienced in their countries of origin, and the language and cultural barriers the immigrants face in gaining access to health care and social welfare particularly in the first years of settlement. Migrants, however, tend to be less vulnerable than these assertions would at first suggest.[77] Many of the East European Jews and the Bengalis who came to Britain were younger, healthier and more economically mobile than the host population. Despite the high rates of unemployment in Spitalfields, the Bengali population was recently found to have low rates of unskilled adults.[78] Indeed, many of the Jews and Bengalis gained acceptance into Britain on the basis of their skills and their ability to contribute to the national economy. Over the century the government has increased restrictions relating to the skills or resources sought and has imposed minimal health requirements.[79] This has resulted in highly selected immigrant populations who tend to be healthy young men and women.

There was, in addition, another selection process operating with

Bengali women: many came to this country as selected brides. Marriages within this community are contractual arrangements between families. The high status of London Bengalis enabled a man's family to choose amongst wealthier families for a bride. Although the strength of sterling and the relative costs of living in Britain tend to diminish the value of family resources in Sylhet, most of the Bengali women came from a background of relative affluence.

Health of the female population of childbearing age

One of the most important components when considering infant health is the health of the mothers. Indeed, the health of an infant is influenced by the age of its mother, the number of previous births she has experienced and, hence, the number of young children she has to look after when the newborn infant arrives. In general, East European Jewish and Bengali immigration women married earlier and had higher fertility rates than indigenous women. No comparative statistics exist for the first years of East European Jewish settlement in East London, but evidence from the Edwardian period shows that the average age for the East European Jewish brides was 23, while the average age of marriage for English women was 26 years.[80] Of the few figures that remain on fertility, it would seem that the first generation of Jewish East European immigrants generally had a higher rate of fertility. According to the Fertility Census of 1911, in Leeds the average number of children born to Russian (Jewish) couples was 3.95, while for English couples it was 2.82.[81] Similarly, among the Bengalis the majority of women came as brides or young wives, and frequently became pregnant soon after arrival. Bengali family size on average was also much higher than the average in the country as a whole. In the early 1990s, 34 per cent of Bengali mothers had fourth or higher order births, compared with only 5 per cent of Anglo-European mothers.[82]

Thus, while many of the immigrant women giving birth for the first time tend to be younger than indigenous women, the large size of their families indicates that many of them went on giving birth to a late age. From this it might be assumed that the health of Jewish and Bengali women and their children are at greater risk than those of the indigenous population. Yet, as we can see in the case of the Bengali immigrants, this does not seem to be the case. Prolonged childbearing has resulted in a distribution of maternal ages that is very different from that seen in the UK in general – with 17 per cent of the Bengali maternity population being over the age of 35, in contrast to 9 per cent of Anglo-European East London mothers. None the less, infant mortality rates for older mothers from the Bengali community have been lower than those observed for Anglo-European women of the same age, and the trend of an increasing rate of infant mortality with maternal age is not apparent.[83] Such evidence suggests that factors beyond the age of the mother and her fertility record were and are more important determinants of infant survival among immigrants.

Health care availability and access

While the religious and cultural practices appear to have been important in protecting the infants of the Jewish and Bengali immigrants, these factors need to be considered alongside the availability and access these immigrants have had to health care provision. We need to consider not only the access that these immigrants had to services, but also the degree to which they were able to communicate and make effective use of services. As already stated, neither of these immigrant populations had English as their mother-tongue, which would have made communication and access to provision difficult. Such problems were not any easier in the case of Bengali women, many of whom had poor literacy skills. Along with the linguistic and educational barriers, there were also the different values immigrants attached to health and their perception of health care provision. Much of this was determined by the type of access that they had to pre-natal and maternity care before migration. In this respect the Bengali population, as the later arrivals and having experienced poor access in their home country, stood out much more than the Jews, partly reflecting the changes that the latter had experienced in UK health care and maternity provision over the century.

At the turn of the century domiciliary midwifery dominated much of the maternity care provided in East London as well as in Eastern Europe. The majority of births took place at home and were attended by traditional midwives who rarely had any formal training. While the infrastructure of maternity care in Eastern Europe was very similar to that of Britain, there were many differences in the type of care provided in Bangladesh from that offered in Britain. Organised maternity care in Bangladesh was not available to most women. Childbirth occurred at home, with the attendance of a female relative, or a traditional midwife who may or may not have had any formal training. There was little secondary or tertiary referral if problems arose, with the result that maternal mortality rates were high – five out of every thousand pregnant women died in childbirth. Thus, women who were newly arrived in this country had little experience of antenatal services or hospital based deliveries. The highly regimented systems of care that have developed in Britain around pregnancy and childbirth were potentially both alien and frightening to many Bengali women.

Despite, or perhaps because of, the various possible handicaps that the immigrants have had when it comes to the access and availability of health care provision, support systems set up by the immigrants for themselves, as well as schemes initiated by the host society, developed to counter these difficulties. One of the most important supports that the immigrants have had access to on an informal level came from the closely knit family networks that existed amongst them. This often involved a large extended family, with fellow immigrants who were not blood relatives, but who migrated from the same village or town. For many immigrants these networks were an important means of social and economic aid in times of crisis, and passed on crucial knowledge on childbearing as well as support in child care. The importance of the closely knit family and the support this provided for Jewish immigrants was continually remarked upon by contemporary observers, who saw this as a crucial determinant in the better records that they had on infant health.

Besides the support of these kinship networks, many of the immigrants also had access to aid through their religious communal agencies. In the Jewish community, welfare agencies were a long-established tradition in both Eastern Europe and in Britain. Based around religious institutions, these bodies not only provided welfare relief, but also provided help for the sick and the infirm, including the lying-in period. Contemporaries frequently remarked on the abundance of such facilities in the Jewish community by comparison with the local population, and their high degree of co-ordination. One of the most important charitable organisations that provided help during childbirth and nursing care was the Sick Room Helps Society established in 1895. Apart from the immediate task of nursing women during their confinements, the Society provided a whole range of social services which included the provision of home helps. These home helps were used to fill in the gaps between the visits of the midwife and nurse and to attend to the usual tasks of the mother, such as housework, shopping and cooking, as well as child care. Such help gave mothers a much valued mental and physical break from some of the chores that were seen as hindering recovery.[84] These home helps were mainly Jewish, unlike many of the midwives and nurses who attended the immigrants. While nurses of whatever religion could undertake the general nursing care, they often did not have knowledge of Yiddish or the Jewish dietary habits which were essential not only for communication but also in the daily routine of care of the patient. From 1913 the Society also set up the Jewish Maternity Home, which provided for hospital deliveries.[85]

Like Jewish women, Bengali women also had access to special forms of support. Health advocacy schemes were initiated as a result of the anxieties in the late 1970s over the high rates of infant and perinatal mortality found among Bengali immigrants and the fact that many of the Bengali mothers were not making use of antenatal services within East London. In 1981, the Maternity Services Liaison Scheme was set up in Tower Hamlets to improve the access of newly immigrant mothers to maternity care. Bilingual women were employed to respond to requests from the community, health professionals and welfare workers. The major part of their work was effecting communication by providing services, including advocacy, support, clarification of information and direct language translations. The provision of information in a culturally appropriate form was seen as a first step in breaking down the barriers that prevented mothers from using services. In the 1990s, the utilisation of antenatal services by women of this community has increased and poor attendance rates have become uncommon. Evaluations of health advocacy schemes indicated the beneficial effect they had in improving the access of immigrants to services.[86]

CONCLUSION

The chance finding of two ethnically distinct groups in the same geographical area at different times, with a similar experience of initial relative disadvantage in infant survival in the early years of settlement giving way to relative advantage compared to the host community, is intriguing. Both groups have strongly maintained ethno-specific identities after settlement in the UK, and many of these have been shown, in the light of present knowledge, to benefit infant health and reduce their mortality. The better reproductive health of immigrants in East London in comparison with their indigenous neighbours, as measured by infant survival, can be explained by the selection of healthy women and a lifestyle that stems from cultural rituals and prohibitions. Although superficially very different, both Jewish and Bengali cultures had a number of similar values: marriage, with its formalisation of support, especially financial; restriction in the use of alcohol and cigarettes; and traditions in food preparation and diet. Likewise, each of these communities evolved support networks to supplement or provide better access to state or charitable services, many of which had a particular focus on mothers and infants. In the wider social context, the role of early social welfare programmes to aid immigrant women in pregnancy must also be considered in the favourable infant mortality displayed in these groups.

Our analysis has demonstrated the value of considering infant mortality in the historical context of settlement. We have argued that cross-sectional studies at the beginning of the migration, when new arrivals stimulate local interest, may present a misleading and antithetical picture of the impact of ethnicity *per se* on infant survival. Initial rates of infant death may reflect to a greater extent the impact of access to services, while rates observed after some years of settlement may better reflect the impact of ethnicity on infant survival. The better survival of both Jews and Bengalis, living in one of the poorest areas in the UK, compared to the whole population is of extra significance as rates for indigenous residents in the same area in each time period were higher than national averages. This suggests that behavioural and lifestyle factors can substantially modify the effects of the environment on infant mortality.

NOTES

1 This is also emphasised in D. Forbes and W. Parker Fisbie, 'Spanish Surname and Anglo Infant Mortality: Differentials over Half-century', *Demography*, 1991, 28/4, pp. 639–60.

2 See V.S. Raleigh, B. Botting and R. Balarjan, 'Perinatal and Postneonatal Mortality in England and Wales among Immigrants from the Indian Subcontinent', *Indian Journal of Paediatrics*, 1990, 57, pp. 551–62. In America, Indo-Chinese refugees from Vietnam, Laos and Cambodia have been shown to have surprisingly much lower rates of infant mortality than non-Hispanic whites and than blacks, and were comparable to other Asian groups. J. Weeks and R.G. Rumbaut, 'Infant Mortality among Ethnic Immigrant Groups', *Social Science and Medicine*, 1991, 33/3, pp. 327–34. Korean infants also have good survival rates. See J.M. Mor, G.R. Alexander, E.C. Kieffer, G. Baruffi, 'Birth Outcomes of Korean Women in Hawaii', *Public Health Reports*, July–August 1993, 108/4 pp. 500–5. Although by no means homogeneous, survival rates among Hispanic infants in America are less favourable, particularly among Puerto Rican

immigrants. See C.A. Stroup-Benham and F.M. Trevino, 'Reproductive Characteristics of Mexican-American, Mainland Puerto Rican, and Cuban-American Women', *Journal of American Medical Association*, 1991, 265/2, pp. 222–6; J.E. Becerra, C.J.R. Hogue, H.K. Atrash and N. Perez, 'Infant Mortality among Hispanics: A Portrait of Heterogeneity', *Journal of American Medical Association*, 1991, 265/2, pp. 217–21, and B. Cohen, D.J. Friedman, C. Mahan, R. Lederman and D. Munoz, 'Ethnicity, Maternal Risk, and Birth Weight among Hispanics in Massachusetts, 1987–89', *Public Health Reports*, May–June 1993, 108/3, pp. 363–71.

3 For the complexities involved in exploring the links between ethnicity and health see S.L. Barron, 'Birthweight and Ethnicity', *British Journal of Obstetrics and Gynaecology*, 1983, pp. 289–90.

4 One study that has attempted to address this issue is Forbes and Parker Fisbie, 'Spanish Surname'.

5 For a more detailed description of the East European Jewish migration and their settlement within East London see L. Marks, *Model Mothers: Jewish Mothers and Maternity Provision in East London 1870–1939*, Oxford, 1994, chapters 1–3.

6 Sephardi Jews were descendants of the Spanish Jews who reached England via Holland. For more information on this early settlement see essays in V.D. Lipman ed., *Three Centuries of Anglo-Jewish History*, Cambridge, 1961; idem, *A History of the Jews in Britain since 1858*, Leicester, 1990, pp. 1–4; T.M. Endelman, *The Jews of Georgian England 1714–1830*, Philadelphia, 1979; idem, *Radical Assimilation in English Jewish History, 1656–1945*, Indianapolis, 1990, chapters 1 and 2.

7 Ashkenazi Jews were descendants of the Jews who originally settled in Germany and then migrated to Eastern Europe (Poland, Lithuania and Russia). They differed from Sephardi Jews in their Hebrew pronunciation, cultural and devotional traditions and language. Sephardi Jews did not speak Yiddish.

8 B. Williams, '"East and West": Class and Community in Manchester Jewry, 1850–1914', in D. Cesarani, ed., *The Making of Modern Anglo-Jewry*, Oxford, 1990, pp. 16–17; idem, *The Making of Manchester Jewry 1740–1875*, Manchester, 1985, p. 1; V.D. Lipman, *Social History of the Jews in England*, London, 1954, pp. 5–9.

9 The largest groups of immigrants who arrived before the Jews were the Huguenots in the seventeenth century and the Irish during the years of the Famine in the late 1840s. Both of these groups also settled in East London. For more information on this see C. Bermant, *Point of Arrival*, London, 1975.

10 C. Holmes, *Anti-semitism in British Society 1876–1939*, London, 1979.

11 Summary of Returns Made to the Board of Trade of Customs, in *Royal Commission Alien Immigration*, PP 1903 IX, Report and Minutes, Appendix, p. 76.

12 *Royal Commission on Alien Immigration*, 22; Lipman, *Social History of the Jews in England*, pp. 89–90.

13 C. Booth, *Life and Labour: Religious Influences*, London, 1902, p. 9; D.M. Feldman, 'Immigrants and Workers, Englishmen and Jews: The

Immigrants in the East End of London, 1880–1906', Ph.D thesis, Cambridge University, 1985, Table 1.8, pp. 26–9.

14 In 1901 a witness estimated that 44 per cent of the population in Whitechapel were immigrants, while the census enumerated it at 37 per cent. The next highest concentration of immigrants was found in St George's-in-the-East, which a witness estimated to be 31 per cent, and the census enumerated at 28 per cent. This was much higher than for the other areas of Stepney which ranged between 3 and 8 per cent. See *Royal Commission on Alien Immigration*, IX I, 22, Table XXXV (c) in Appendix, p. 42. Between 1871 and 1901 the total population in Stepney increased by 24,154, but the number of British-born residents fell by 16,126, representing a decline from 95 to 82 per cent of the borough's total population.

15 Feldman, 'Immigrants and Workers', pp. 26–9.

16 H. Adler, 'Jewish Life and Labour', in H. Llewellyn Smith, *New Survey*, London, 1934, vol. 6, p. 283.

17 For an interesting and more personal insight into the experiences of these immigrants see C. Adams, *Across Seven Seas and Thirteen Rivers*, London, 1987.

18 R. Desai, *Indian Immigrants in Britain*, Oxford, 1963, p. 5.

19 C. Jones, *Immigration and Social Policy in Britain*, London, 1977, pp. 109–12; Desai, *Indian Immigrants in Britain*; Adams, *Across Seven Seas*, pp. 58, 66.

20 J.A.G. Griffith, J. Henderson, M. Usborne and D. Wood, *Coloured Immigrants in Britain*, Oxford, 1960, p. 4.

21 Jones, *Immigration and Social Policy*, pp. 122–6.

22 Adams, *Across Seven Seas*; Desai, *Indian Immigrants in Britain*.

23 D.A. Coleman, 'Some Problems of Data for the Demographic Study of Immigration and of Immigrants and Minority Populations in Britain', *Ethnic and Racial Studies* 1983, 6/1, pp. 103–10. See also J. Eade, 'The Power of the Experts: The Plurality of Beliefs and Practices Concerning Health and Illness among Bangladeshis', unpublished paper presented to a Conference of UK Social Anthropoligists, Institute of Commonwealth Studies, 10–11 September 1991.

24 S.E. Curtis and P.E. Ogden, 'Bangladeshis in London: A Challenge to Welfare', *Revue Europeenen des Migrations Internationales*, 1986, 2/3, pp. 135–49.

25 Department of Public Health Medicine, Tower Hamlets Health Authority, *Tower Hamlets People*, Nov. 1991, 4, pp. 45–8.

26 Feldman, 'Immigrants and Workers', Table 1.8, p. 37.

27 A Summary of Returns made to the Board of Trade of Customs, in *Royal Commission on Alien Immigration*, IX, Report and Minutes of Evidence, Appendix, p. 76.

28 Ibid.

29 Feldman, 'Immigrants and Workers', pp. 38–40.

30 Curtis and Ogden, 'Bangladeshis in London', pp. 135–49.

31 *Census County Report, Inner London: Part 1, 1991*, London, 1993.

32 *Births by Birth Place of Parent, 1985*, OPCS, Monitor Reference FM1, London.

33 A.S. Hilder, 'Short Birth Intervals in Tower Hamlets: A Failure of Post-natal Support?', *Ethnicity and Disease*, 1992/3, 3/2, pp. 137–44, Table 1.

34 This map was originally drawn up by George Arkell who used the same method as Charles Booth for his poverty maps of London. The map appeared in C.S. Russell and H.S. Lewis, *The Jew in London*, London, 1901.

35 For information on the poverty and overcrowding of East London in the late nineteenth and early twentieth century see J.A. Gillespie, 'Economic Change in the East End of London during the 1920s', Ph.D. thesis, Cambridge, 1984, pp. 83–4, 88; G. Stedman Jones, *Outcast London*, London, 1971. A detailed personal account on present conditions appears in D. Widgery, *Some Lives!: A GP's East End*, London, 1993. Using the Underprivileged Area Score, derived from census responses for selected social, economic and environmental factors, one report finds the district the second most deprived in England in 1981. By 1991 the Department of Public Health Medicine claimed Tower Hamlets to be the most deprived district in England; Department of Public Health Medicine, Tower Hamlets Health Authority, *Tower Hamlets People, Health Report, No.1*, Sept. 1988, and *No.5*, 1992/3.

36 *Census of England and Wales, 1901*, Table 12. Houses and Population 1891 and 1901, pp. 33–4. For more detail on the socio-economic conditions in East London at the turn of the century see Marks, *Model Mothers*, pp. 18–21, 60–4; *Tower Hamlets People, Health Report, No. 1*, p. 198.

37 I. Loudon, 'On Maternal and Infant Mortality, 1900–1960', *Social History of Medicine*, 1991, 4/1, pp. 33, 38–9, 72–3. See also R.I. Woods, P.A. Watterson and J.H. Woodward, 'The Causes of Rapid Infant Mortality Decline in England and Wales, 1861–1921', Part I, *Population Studies*, 1988, 42, pp. 343–66 and Part II, *Population Studies*, 1989, 43, pp. 113–32.

38 *Royal Commission on Alien Immigration*, IX, 2, Dr Shirley Murphy, Q.3960, p. 203; Table XVII in S. Rosenbaum. 'A Contribution to the Study of Vital and Other Statistics of the Jews in the UK', *Journal of the Royal Statistical Society*, 1905, 68, p. 528. See also Table 1 in L. Marks, '"Dear Old Mother Levy's": The Jewish Maternity Home and Sick Room Helps Society, 1895–1939', *Social History of Medicine*, 1990, 3/1, p. 62.

39 One contemporary observer noted that many of the Jewish immigrants who arrived in England were initially very weak and had lost many of their infants due to the conditions they had endured before arriving in England. Within a short period of settling, however, many of these immigrants became much stronger. *Royal Commission on Alien Immigration*, IX, Qs.15970–15983. See also G.A. Condran and E.A. Kramarow, 'Child Mortality among Jewish Immigrants to the United States', *Journal of Interdisciplinary History*, 1991, 22/2, p. 239.

40 Mr N.S. Joseph, evidence to *Royal Commission on Alien Immigration*, Qs.15970–15982. High mortality was also found among the infants and young children of those immigrants who travelled to Australia in the nineteenth century. See R. Shlomowitz and J. McDonald, 'Babies at Risk on Immigrant Voyages to Australia in the Nineteenth Century', *Economic History Review*, 1991, 44/1 pp. 86–101.

41 The low rates of infant mortality in Mile End New Town are surprising because of the workhouse in the area, which might be expected to have had an adverse affect on rates of infant mortality. Illegitimacy rates were certainly much higher as a result of the workhouse. In St John, where there was a workhouse, infant mortality rates were abnormally high, as they were in Whitechapel Church and Shadwell which might be explained by the existence of the London Hospital and the East London Hospital for Children and Women in these two areas. The presence of such institutions in these districts, coupled with the abnormally high rates of infant mortality, prevented the use of these districts in this study.

42 Woods et al., 'The Causes of Rapid Infant Mortality Decline', Parts I and II.

43 R. Salaman, 'Anglo-Jewish Vital Statistics', *Jewish Chronicle, Supplement*, 29 July 1921, p. v; A. Ruppin, *The Jews of Today*, London, 1913, p. 79; D. Dwork, 'Health Conditions of Immigrant Jews on the Lower East Side of New York: 1880–1914', *Medical History*, 1981, 25, p. 28. See also *Royal Commission on Alien Immigration*, Mr J. Prag, Q.17877.

44 For full figures on the rates of Jewish infant mortality and the trend since the mid-nineteenth century see U.O. Schmelz, *Infant and Early Childhood Mortality among Jews of the Diaspora*, Jerusalem, 1971, Table 2, pp. 15–27; and Condran and Kramarow, 'Child Mortality', Table 1, pp. 225–6.

45 Schmelz, *Infant and Early Childhood Mortality*, p. 13; Condran and Kramarow, 'Childhood Mortality', pp. 224, 227; Marks, *Model Mothers*, pp. 52–3.

46 Condran and Kramarow, 'Childhood Mortality', p. 223, Table 2, p. 238.

47 *Royal Commission on Alien Immigration*, Qs.327, 3960, 5787, 5788, 21415 and 21417. Schmelz, *Infant and Early Childhood Mortality*, pp. 41–5, Table 5; Ruppin, *The Jews of Today*, p. 77; E. Hart, 'The Mosaic Code of Sanitation', *Sanitary Record*, 1877, 1, pp. 183, 198; J. Critchton-Browne, 'The Prevention of Tubercular Disease', *Journal of the Sanitary Institute*, 1894, 15, p. 455, cited in A. Hardy, *The Epidemic Streets: Infectious Disease and the Rise of Preventive Medicine, 1856–1900*, Oxford, 1993, chapter 9. See also J.H. Stallard, *London Pauperism Among Jews and Christians: An Inquiry into the Principles and Practice of Outdoor Relief in the Metropolis*, London, 1867, p. 13. For a more detailed discussion and breakdown of the incidence of these diseases see Marks, *Model Mothers*, pp. 55–9.

48 Contemporaries noted this in their evidence to the *Royal Commission on Alien Immigration*, Qs.3960, 3963, 5787; see also E.W. Hope, 'Autumnal Diarrhoea in Cities', *Public Health*, July 1899, pp. 660–5. For more information on the historical trends in infant mortality, and the particular rise in the years 1895–1900, see Woods et al., 'The Causes of Rapid Infant Mortality Decline', Part I, pp. 361–2 and Part II, p. 120.

49 Dr D.L. Thomas, *Royal Commission on Alien Immigration*, p. 264. Contemporaries regarded diarrhoea as one of the 'preventable' causes of infant mortality, linking it primarily to bad infant feeding habits. D. Dwork, *War is Good for Babies and Other Young Children: A History of the Infant and Child Welfare Movement*, London, 1987, pp. 49–50; N. Williams, 'Infant and Child Mortality in Urban Areas of Nineteenth

Century England and Wales: A Record Linkage Study', Ph.D. thesis, Liverpool, 1989, p. 30.

50 Stillbirths were also thought to be less among the Jewish population, but there are no statistics to confirm this assertion. Salaman, 'Anglo-Jewish Vital Statistics', *Jewish Chronicle*, Aug. 1921, 26, p. i.

51 See Table 5 in Curtis and Ogden, 'Bangladeshis in London'. This table lists infant mortality rates for infants of Bangladesh- and Indian-born mothers compared with UK-born mothers for the years 1978–80 and 1983.

52 Raleigh, et al., 'Perinatal and Postneonatal Mortality'.

53 A. S. Hilder, 'Ethnic Differences in Sudden Infant Death Syndrome: What We Can Learn from the Experience of Immigrants to the UK', *Early Human Development*, 1994, 38, pp. 143–9.

54 Stroup-Benham and Trevino, 'Reproductive Characteristics'; Becerra et al., 'Infant Mortality among Hispanics' and Cohen et al., 'Ethnicity, Maternal Risk, and Birth Weight'; C. Brezinka, O. Huter, G. Busch and S. Unus, 'Communication, Compliance and Perinatal Risks of Turkish Females in Tyrol', *Geburtshilfe-Frauenheilkd*, 1989, 49/5, pp. 472–6; Weeks and Rumbaut, 'Infant Mortality'; and Mor et al., 'Birth Outcomes'.

55 Loudon, 'On Maternal and Infant Mortality', pp. 33, 38–9, 72–3. See also Woods et. al., 'The Causes of Rapid Infant Mortality Decline', Part 2, pp. 114–15; Schmelz, *Infant and Early Childhood Mortality*, p. 39; Williams, 'Infant and Child Mortality', pp. 23–5.

56 This can be seen most clearly in J. Eade's chapter in this book.

57 Dr Shirley Murphy, *Royal Commission on Alien Immigration*, Q.3960, p. 203. See also H.J. Ashby, *Infant Mortality*, Cambridge 1915, p. 25; *Interdepartmental Report on Physical Deterioration*, PP 1904, XXXII, Dr Eicholz, Q.475. Some idea of the conditions in which some of these immigrants were living can be seen from a report in 1884, which showed many of the Jews to be living in cramped and very overcrowded accommodation that lacked adequate sanitation, *The Lancet*, 3 May 1884. A more detailed analysis of the socio-economic conditions of the Jewish immigrants and their neighbours appears in Marks, *Model Mothers*, pp. 60–5.

58 Hardy, *Epidemic Streets*, chapter 10. See also Hart, 'The Mosaic Code of Sanitation', p. 183.

59 L.P. Gartner, *The Jewish Immigrant in England, 1870–1914*, London, 1973, pp. 150–8; E. Black, *Social Politics of Anglo-Jewry*, Oxford, 1989, pp. 86–90, 101, 165–6.; *Royal Commission on Alien Immigration*, Q.15400; Jewish Board of Guardians, President's Address: Annual General Meeting, 22 March 1937, p. 7, Mocatta Library: box pamphlet BA 28 COH.

60 Condran and Kramarow, 'Child Mortality', pp. 228–33.

61 At the turn of the century numerous medical experts showed that infant mortality rose dramatically in the years of hot, dry summers. *Royal Commission on Alien Immigration*, Qs.21415–17. See also V. Fildes, 'Breastfeeding in London, 1905–1919', *Journal of Biosocial Science*, 1992, 24, p. 64.

62 S. Szreter, 'The Importance of Social Intervention in Britain's Mortality

Decline', *Social History of Medicine*, 1988, 1, p. 31. See also Hope, 'Observations on Autumnal Diarrhoea in Cities', p. 662.

63 For more detail on this see M. Fishberg, 'Health and Sanitation of the Immigrant Jewish Population of New York', *The Menorah*, August 1902, 33/2, pp. 158–90 and Dwork, 'Health Conditions of Immigrant Jews', p. 29. See also *Report of the Interdepartmental Committee on Physical Deterioration*, Q.1173.

64 *Royal Commission on Alien Immigration*, Q.17900.

65 Unpublished letter from Mrs J.J. to L. Marks, 9 February 1992. Over the centuries Jews had continually been noted as a group that escaped the ravages of cholera and typhus epidemics. Such diseases are often spread through contaminated water and raw sewerage. The lower rates of these diseases among Jews indicates that they were probably better protected from such insanitary conditions because of the cultural and religious practice of boiling water and thorough cleansing of eating and cooking utensils. See Gartner, *The Jewish Immigrant in England*, pp. 160–1; *Royal Commission on Alien Immigration*, Q.5105.

66 Personal hygiene was also said to be high among Jewish immigrants as a result of Jewish religious laws which required both sexes to cut their finger and toe nails at least once a week, and for women to attend a ritual bath, the *mikveh*, once a month after menstruating. In addition to the religious rituals, bathing was said to be customary among Jewish immigrants. In New York many more baths appeared with the appearance of the East European Jews, as they did in East London. For detail on New York see Dwork, 'Health Conditions of Immigrant Jews', p. 30 and Fishberg, 'Health and Sanitation', p. 75.

67 Dr Shirley Murphy, *Royal Commission on Alien Immigration*, Q.3960, p. 203; see also Qs.17900, 18311; Salaman, 'Vital Statistics of the Anglo-Jewish Community', *Jewish Chronicle*, May 1921, 27, pp. ii-iii. The degree of cleanliness of the Jewish homes is open to question, as it could largely have reflected the attitude of the observer rather than be based in reality. While many contemporaries commented that the Jewish homes were cleaner than most of the general population, others saw them as more slovenly. *Royal Commission on Alien Immigration*, A.J. Williams p. 9 and Qs.9418, 17512; *Interdepartmental Committee on Physical Deterioration*, Q.475; *Eastern Post and City Chronicle*, 22 November 1884. Such a disparity in views was also present among American observers in this period. See Condran and Kramarow, 'Child Mortality', p. 231 and Fishberg, 'Health and Sanitation', pp. 75–6.

68 R.M. Woodbury, *Causal Factors in Infant Mortality: A Statistical Study Based on Investigation in Eight Cities*, Washington, 1925, p. 114; and Fildes, 'Breastfeeding in London', p. 65.

69 *Interdepartmental Report on Physical Deterioration*, Qs.327, 448, 450, 452, 475, 1168; *Royal Commission on Alien Immigration*, Q.17877. The widespread prevalence of rickets is attributable to the air pollution from the dense palls of smoke from industry and domestic heating arrangements in these years, as well as the types of dwellings people lived in which were not designed to let sunlight in. Hardy, *Epidemic Streets*, chapter 9. See also idem, 'Rickets and the Rest: Diet, Infectious Disease

and the Late Victorian Child', *Social History of Medicine*, 1992, 5/3, pp. 389–412. Air pollution not only blocked out the necessary sunlight, but was also probably an important factor in higher levels of respiratory diseases. Recent research has shown a strong correlation between air pollution and respiratory diseases among young infants and children. See N. Graham, 'The Epidemiology of Acute Respiratory Infections in Children and Adults: A Global Perspective', in *Epidemiological Review*, 1990, 12 pp. 149–78, 157.

70 Hardy, 'Rickets and the Rest' and *Epidemic Streets*, pp. 395–400.

71 Graham, 'The Epidemiology of Acute Respiratory Infections', pp. 161–2. See also M. Mamdani and D. Ross, 'Review Article: Vitamin A Supplementation and Child Survival: Magic Bullet or False Hope?', *Health Policy and Planning*, 1989, 4/4, pp. 273–94.

72 *Royal Commission on Alien Immigration*, Qs.3963, 21753; *Jewish Chronicle*, 19 August 1904; Salaman, 'Vital Statistics', p. v. See also L. Golding, *Magnolia Street*, London, 1932, pp. 129–30.

73 Gambling, however, was not an unknown phenomenon in Jewish homes.

74 Hilder, 'Ethnic Differences in Sudden Infant Death Syndrome'.

75 'Stillbirth and Infant Death: Social and Biological Factors', *OPCS DH3*, Numbers 13,14,15,16,17,19,20,21, HMSO, London.

76 M. Gantley, D.P. Davies and A. Murcott, 'Sudden Infant Death Syndrome: Links with Infant Care Practices', *British Medical Journal*, 1993, 306, pp. 16–20.

77 A.M. Adelstein and M.G. Marmot, 'The Health of Migrants in England and Wales: Causes of Death', in J.K. Cruickshank and D. G. Beevers, eds, *Ethnic Factors in Health and Disease*, London, 1989.

78 *OPCS 1981 Census*, London, 1981, and *OPCS 1991 Census*, London, 1991, data by ward.

79 Such as the Alien's Act of 1905 and the Commonwealth Immigration Act of 1962.

80 Jewish immigrants married earlier than many Anglo-Jews. During the 1880s the average age for bridegrooms was 28.2 among the Anglo-Jews in England, while in Russia the average age was 24.5; for brides the respective ages were 21.3 and 24.1. B.A. Kosmin, 'Nuptuality and Fertility Patterns of British Jewry 1850–1980: An Immigrant Transition?', in D.A. Coleman, *Demography of Immigrants and Minority Groups in the UK, Proceedings of the 18th Annual Symposium of the Eugenics Society, London 1981*, London, 1982, Table VI, and p. 255.

81 Marks, *Model Mothers*, pp. 82–3.

82 Hilder, 'Ethnic Differences'.

83 Tabulations of ethnic and factor-specific rates of infant mortality as well as SIDS mortality were produced in the final report of the project. A.S. Hilder, *Infant Deaths in East London 1987–1990: Ethnic Differences in Infant Mortality*, London, 1992. Report produced for the Foundation for the Study of Infant Deaths.

84 *Jewish Chronicle*, 3 January 1896, p. 9.

85 For more information on the Society and the hospital see L. Marks, 'Dear Old Mother Levy's'.

86 L. Parsons and S. Day, 'Improving Obstetric Outcomes in Ethnic Minorities: An Evaluation of Health Advocacy', *Hackney Journal of Public Health Medicine*, 1992, 14/2, pp. 183–91.

9

GREEK MIGRANTS IN AUSTRALIA

Surviving well and helping their hosts

John Powles

INTRODUCTION

Migrating populations have a particular fascination for epidemiologists and amongst the most studied migrants are a group of ethnic Japanese in Hawaii. They were originally chosen to throw light on how affluence and modernity cause heart attacks, with the expectation that their mortality from 'diseases of affluence' would rise with increasing exposure to the American way of life. Things turned out differently, for although there was some rise in heart disease mortality rates towards that of the host population up until the 1960s, rates then fell in parallel with the decline in rates throughout the US. The death rate from all causes in Hawaiian Japanese around 1980 was some 20 per cent lower than the rates of Japan, which were substantially lower than those in the US.[1] The interesting question is no longer 'how are they harmed', but rather 'what protects them'? Numerous studies have tried, with limited success, to identify the sources – genetic, behavioural, environmental or a combination of these – of their low mortality.[2]

A less well-known group that also enjoys a migrant, or perhaps ethnic, advantage in longevity are the Greeks in Australia. Most of them left rural Greece between the late 1950s and the early 1970s, and they are now seen as exemplars of the Mediterranean 'migrant advantage' in health because of their very low risk of death from heart disease and other causes.[3] This outcome has been contrary to the expectation that a diet of lamb chops and Foster's lager would lead the migrants to succumb to heart attacks at the same rate as their hosts. This has happened to an extent, but more interesting and intriguing is the fact that their risk of death from all causes remains very low. It has been running at 35–40 per cent below that of their Australian-born hosts, which has in itself been in steep decline. In this chapter I explore why Greek migrants in Australia have maintained their 'migrant advantage'. In doing this I shall discuss the complex dynamic in health determinants and health experience set in motion by mass migration from the Mediterranean to Australia. However, I will not consider the full range of factors that determine health, concentrating instead on those that seem relevant to the differences between Greek migrants and their host Australian population.

GREEK MIGRATION TO AUSTRALIA

In 1971, after two and a half decades during which the Australian government sought to add 1 per cent per year to the population by immigration, the proportion of Australians born outside the country was over 20 per cent; only Israel had a larger proportion of immigrants. Of the over 3 million arrivals between 1945 and 1971, those from the British Isles comprised just less than half, while those from the Mediterranean region (taken here to include the eastern Mediterranean and Egypt) comprised slightly more than one quarter. Ethnic Greeks were the second most numerous of this latter group (after Italians) with just under 200,000 arrivals. Many returned home, although the 1986 Census showed that there were still 137,000 Greek-born Australians and 293,000 claiming Greek ancestry.[4]

Although the civil war loosened some ties, the main reason for Greek migration was economic; Australia was presented as a land of opportunity with better prospects for gainful employment, especially to those who had lived in rural areas. Most migrants were sponsored by kin and friends in a process of chain migration and thus entered Australia as part of a social network.[5] However, with few skills that were marketable in Australia, male and female immigrants were forced to accept work in low quality and often arduous manual jobs. Greek women had typically to cope with the 'double shift' of housework plus factory work – the latter often under an unsympathetic if not abusive supervisor.[6] Given their disadvantageous position in the labour market, it might be expected that the morbidity and mortality levels of these migrants would move, not just to the Australian norm, but to the levels of Australian manual workers.[7] With the country of birth recorded both on death certificates and in the census in Australia, it is possible to calculate death rates by country of origin and hence to test this hypothesis.

The results, as indicated already, are surprising. Just as adult male death rates in Greece are among the lowest in Europe, so those among Greek-born Australians are among the lowest of all birthplace groups in Australia. Indeed, in absolute terms, death rates between 45 and 64 are even 44 per cent lower than those of Greece overall (see Figure 9.1).

Surprisingly, there is no clear tendency, with increasing length of residence, for mortality rates to converge towards the higher rates of the host population. The Standardised Mortality Rate (SMR) for ages 15 to 74 (where the value for the total Australian population is 100) was 66 for male Greek migrants of all lengths of residence in 1986, and 64 for those resident for more than fifteen years. For females the corresponding ratios were 72 and 73.[8] This very substantial mortality advantage of the Greek immigrants is present across the major groups of causes: circulatory diseases, cancer and injury, including suicide (see Table 9.1).[9] Of the commoner conditions, only diabetes stands out with a relatively high rate of attributed deaths.[10]

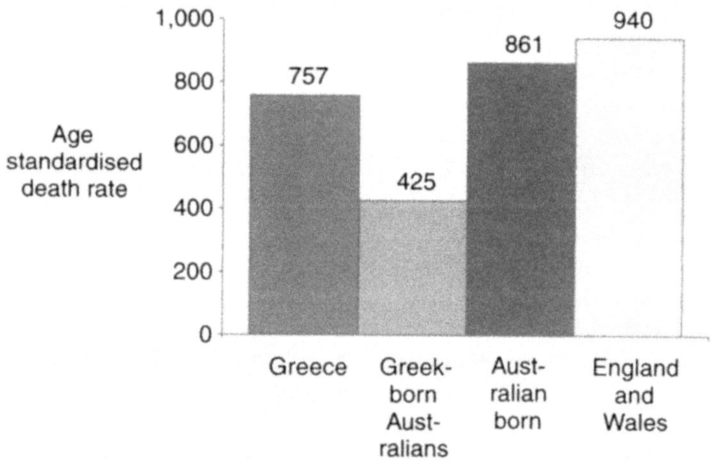

Figure 9.1 Age-standardised male death rates at ages 45–64: Greeks in Greece, Greek-born migrants in Australia, native-born Australians and population of England and Wales, c.1988

Note: Comparable rates for female migrants not available in source, but other estimates provided indicate that female rates will show similar pattern.

Sources: C. Young, 'Mortality, the Ultimate Indicator of Survival: The Differential Experience Between Birthplace Groups', in J. Donovan, E.M. d'Espaignet, C. Merton and M. van Ommergen, *Immigrants in Australia: A Health Profile*, Canberra, pp. 34–70. *World Health Statistics Annual*

Table 9.1 SMRs for major groups of causes, Greek-born Australians, aged 15 to 74, in 1987 to 1989 (ratio of rate to that for total Australian population, set at 100)

Group of causes (International Classification of Diseases, 9th revision)	*Males*	*Females*
Malignant neoplasms (140–208)	61	67
Diseases of the circulatory system (390–459)	62	55
Injury (including suicide) (E800–E999)	59	86
All causes	59	60

Source: C. Young, 'Mortality, the Ultimate Indicator of Survival: The Differential Experience Between Birthplace Groups', in J. Donovan, E.M. d'Espaignet, C. Merton and M. van Ommergen, *Immigrants in Australia: a Health Profile*, Canberra, 1992, pp. 34–70

WHY ARE GREEK MIGRANT DEATH RATES SO LOW?

Five possible explanations may be advanced to explain the low mortality in Greek migrants:

1 an artefact of the data;
2 genes;
3 selection;
4 low exposure to adverse influences on health;
5 high exposure to favourable influences on health.

The first possibility is that the observed phenomenon is due to the nature of the data and its collection. The most serious problem is likely to be that mortality rates are distorted by the number of migrants who return to their homeland to die, though there is no positive evidence for this. Moreover, if such an effect were present, it would be expected that death rates from causes with more warning (such as deaths at higher ages and deaths from causes such as respiratory disease and cancer) would show an artefactual deflation relative to those from causes that are more sudden (such as deaths in middle age and deaths from causes such as circulatory disease and injury). There is no such pattern in the data.

Could the advantage be due to genes? It is unlikely that genetic protection would operate across multiple causes of death and there is no evidence to support such a contention. What of selective migration of healthier persons? This is a much stronger possibility. There are good a priori grounds for supposing that the fit and more energetic select themselves in the first place, on top of which the Australian immigration authorities impose health checks on all immigrants. The effect of screening would be expected to show itself most strongly in the first few years after migration and then fade. Such a pattern is observed in several migrant groups, but is not especially marked among the Greeks.

Lastly, mortality-sparing effects could arise either from lower levels of 'adverse' influences, or from higher levels of 'favourable' influences. The Australian National Risk Factor Studies in 1980, 1983 and 1989 provide data, presented in Table 9.2, both on exposures such as smoking and leisure-time physical activity and on intermediate outcomes such as body weight relative to height, blood pressure and blood cholesterol concentration.[11]

Smoking is a leading 'adverse exposure' for male Greek migrants where the prevalence is some 60 per cent higher than for those born in Australia; however, smoking rates in female Greek migrants are 60 per cent lower.[12] When it came to physical activity, both male and female migrants were over three times more likely than the national norm to report no leisure-time physical exertion (of any intensity) in the past two weeks.[13] Systolic blood pressure (i.e. at each heart beat) was slightly lower in the migrants compared to national norms, though this was not true for diastolic pressure (i.e. between heart beats). When it came to weight, studies have shown that Greek

Table 9.2 Evidence from the Australian Risk Factor Prevalence Studies in 1980, 1983 and 1989 (pooled) on risk factors in migrants from Greece compared to native-born Australians, ages 25–64

	Males	*Females*
Adverse exposures – expressed as age- and study design-adjusted ratios to the Australian born		
Current cigarette smoking	1.65	0.41
No leisure time physical activity in the last 14 days	3.35	3.45
Intermediate outcomes usually associated with increased risk – expressed as age- and study design-adjusted differences to the values for the Australian born		
Body mass index (kg/m^2)	1.5	2.7
Systolic blood pressure (mmHg)	−3.6	−1.9
Blood cholesterol (mmol/l)	0.03	0.07

Source: S.A. Bennett, 'Inequalities in Risk Factors and Cardiovascular Mortality among Australia's Immigrants', *Australian Journal of Public Health*, 1993, 17, pp. 251–61

migrants have a higher incidence of obesity and their blood cholesterol concentrations were certainly not below those of the Australian born. In short, the evidence, especially in the case of males, is against the Greek migrants having any advantage due to lower levels of the major established risk factors for chronic diseases.

Could it be that Greek migrants enjoy favourable influences in early life, the effects of which endure beyond the age of migration? One influence claimed to be of this kind – growth-favouring nutrition – is unlikely to be operating as Greek migrants are short.[14] High social interaction is characteristic of Greek culture and it has been shown in some, but not all, studies to be independently associated with lower mortality risk; available evidence suggests that Greek migrants maintain very strong social networks.[15] However, few epidemiologists would consider this evidence sufficient to explain a substantial mortality advantage across a whole population. On the other hand, the very low mortality from suicide (both in Greece and in the migrants) does point to some specific 'cultural protection'.

What, finally, of higher exposure to potentially favourable influences on health – most obviously to protective constituents of the diet, such as fish and antioxidant vitamins? Food consumption data is available for the pooled group of 'southern European' migrants from the 1983 Risk Factor Study. It is combined in Table 9.3 with apparently comparable data from Britain.

Seafood consumption does not appear to be especially high amongst southern European migrants, although there is other evidence that it might be higher if Greeks alone were considered.[16] On the other hand, there is a much higher intake of other putatively protective foods in the southern European migrants – salad foods (tomatoes and leafy greens) and, showing the biggest differences, fruits typically consumed in winter such as oranges, apples and pears. Thus, a dietary pattern typified by such intakes must currently stand as the most plausible, though still speculative, explanation of their low mortality. It still remains though, to explain why mortality should be so much lower in migrants to Australia than in the source population where intakes of protective foods are perhaps even higher *in season*. To stretch untested speculation still further, it could be that a consistent intake of protective foods is important and that their off-season availability is much better in Australia.[17]

Table 9.3 Estimated mean daily consumption, in grams, of selected foods, by Australians born in southern Europe, Australia and the UK (1983) – with data of uncertain comparability from Great Britain (1986–7)

	Australia (by birthplace)[a]			
	South. Europe	*Australia*	*United Kingdom*	*Britain*[b]
Seafood	20.0	18.5	23.5	26.5
Tomato and tomato products[c]	36.5	27.0	22.5	
Tomatoes – raw + fresh[c]				17.9
Leafy greens[d]	39.5	14.5	13.5	16.0
Citrus fruit (excluding juice)	82.0	51.5	51.5	10.0
Apples, pears (excluding juice)	82.0	71.0	68.5	28.0
Fruit juice (excluding diluted types)	39.5	59.0	52.0	38.0
Additional information				
Total energy (MJ)[e]	8.4	9.4	9.4	8.6
Mean age (approx.)	46.0	44.0	45.0	39.0

Notes:
a Data shown are simple means of 24-hour recalls for each sex.
b Data shown are simple means of 7-day weighed intakes for each sex divided by 7.
c The exact comparability of these categories is not clear from the sources.
d The exact comparability of this category in the two sources is not clear.
e This is mainly useful as a guide to whether total food intake is likely to have been over- or underestimated by the methods used.

Sources: K. Cashel, R. English, S. Bennett, J. Berzins, G. Brown and P. Magnus, *National Dietary Survey of Adults*, 1983: No. 1 Foods Consumed, Canberra, 1986. J. Gregory, K. Foster, H. Tyler and M. Wiseman, *The Dietary and Nutritional Survey of British Adults*, London, 1990

DISABILITY, CHRONIC ILLNESS AND MEDICAL BEHAVIOUR

The very favourable position of the Greek migrants in relation to fatal conditions does not extend to self-reported disability. In a 1988 survey of disability:

> Greek-born persons reported the highest level of disability [from among the eight country and regional groups that were compared]. The level among the men exceeded the level for the Australian [total] male population by 22 per cent while the corresponding excess for the women born in Greece was 34 per cent.[18]

Severe handicap was deemed to be present when personal help or supervision was reported to be needed, or when it was reported that the person had problems with self-care, mobility, verbal communication, schooling or employment. For severe handicap the Greek excess was greater still – over 114 per cent above the national rate for men and around 87 per cent above it for women. These high rates of self-reported disability and handicap in Greek migrants are currently unexplained. They are not generally consistent with the proportions reporting chronic illness in the 1989–90 national health survey – especially in the case of males as shown in Table 9.4 – or with the differences in disease prevalence that would be expected to parallel the differences in mortality rates.

The most plausible hypothesis, though one which in the absence of detailed studies must remain speculative, is that a culturally determined 'response bias' is operating. Other evidence suggests that Greeks have a strong sense of bodily integrity so that when they perceive this to be violated, they consider themselves unable to carry out ordinary daily activities. The medical behaviour of the Greek migrants may be relevant here and has been summarised, relative to the total Australian population, as follows:

Awareness of women's health issues:	Poor, but better at younger ages
Use of hospitals:	Very low (men), moderate (women)
Use of doctors:	Very high (both)
Use of medication:	Sleeping tablets and tranquillisers, both very high Pain relievers moderate (men) and high (women)[19]

These characteristics are easier to reconcile with a hypothesis that the Greeks cope well with stress than with a hypothesis that they experience less stress.

While the evidence reviewed above is suggestive in many ways, several questions still need to be answered to explain fully the 'migrant advantage' of Greeks in Australia. Why has their mortality pattern not converged with that of Australian manual workers? What enables Greek migrants, having no seeming advantage with the conventional risk factors for cardiovascular disease, to still enjoy low mortality? How do we explain the paradox of low reported rates of chronic illness with high reported rates of disability? Why do migrants use self-medication and ambulatory professional care, but not hospital services? Some of these issues, especially the balance of

Table 9.4 Prevalence of self-reported chronic illnesses, by illness category, among persons aged 15–74 and born in Australia or in Greece, expressed as an age-standardised ratio to prevalence in total population (value set to 100), National Health Survey, 1989–90

Illness category	*Males*		*Females*	
	Birthplace			
	Aust.	*Greece*	*Aust.*	*Greece*
Diseases of the nervous system	101	73	101	76
Diseases of the circulatory system	105	67	102	108
Diseases of the respiratory system	104	68	107	65
Diseases of the digestive system	102	78	102	105
Diseases of the musculoskeletal system	102	78	101	106

Source: C. Young and A. Coles, 'Women's Health, Use of Medical Services, Medication, Lifestyle and Chronic Illness: Some Findings from the 1989–90 National Health Survey', in J. Donovan, E.M. d'Espaignet, C. Merton and M. van Ommergen, eds, *Immigrants in Australia: A Health Profile*, Canberra, 1992, pp. 122–91

retained and acquired advantages, were explored in more detail in a case study, carried out in 1983–4, of the experience of migrants from one small area of Greece – the island of Levkada.

THE LEVKADIAN MIGRANT HEALTH STUDY

The island of Levkada is located in the Ionian sea, south of Corfu. The subjects for this study came from approximately forty villages in the rural areas of the island (i.e. excluding the provincial town) constituting a base population of approximately 12,300. The economy of these areas was based on subsistence agriculture; olive oil, olives for eating, and wine are the main products, supplemented by pulses, nuts and other garden produce. Fishing makes a small contribution in the coastal villages, but most large fish are exported. Tourism and money sent by family members working outside the island provide additional income. There is very little rain in summer and the rocky terrain presents limited opportunities for modernised agriculture. Impressions suggest that the island would be below the rural Greek average for 'affluence' and 'modernisation'. It provided, therefore, an especially sharp contrast in levels of wealth and lifestyle to conditions in Melbourne, the main destination of Greek migrants to Australia.[20]

This study looked at 628 subjects – siblings, their spouses and their offspring aged more than 11 years – seen in Levkada in the northern summer of 1983, and 846 subjects seen in Melbourne in the southern summer of 1983/84. At the time of fieldwork, most migrant siblings had been in Australia for between 15 and 30 years.

The first question to be clarified was, 'who emigrated and who stayed behind?', because the selective migration of fitter persons might explain a large part of Greek migrant advantage. As might be expected, emigration was more likely in larger families with more brothers. Within our selected set of sibships, 40 per cent of surviving siblings were still living on Levkada, 16 per cent were elsewhere in Greece and 39 per cent were in Melbourne. There was a slight tendency for younger rather than older brothers to emigrate to Melbourne, though among sisters this tendency was marked. Of those who stayed behind, 57 per cent were the eldest or second eldest in their families compared with only 26 per cent of the migrants. Migrating sisters were 1.9 cm taller, on average, and were much less likely to be illiterate: 1 per cent signed their consent form with a cross compared to 30 per cent of those who stayed. Migration was thus socially selective, especially for females, but the variables on which differences were observed were not associated with the main risk factors for chronic disease, so these differences offer little or no insight into explaining differences in mortality risk.

In Levkada, 75 per cent of the brothers were working as farmers or fishermen and the sisters were mostly doing household work. In Melbourne, while some brothers were working as fishermen and some as drivers and building workers, the most common occupations, for both sexes, were in manufacturing. In each location, 75 per cent fully owned their homes; the sense of financial adequacy was similar and the most common suggested uses of an extra $100 per month were saving, debt repayment and house purchase in each location. Household facilities were at a much lower level in Levkada: 55 per cent of houses had no bathrooms, 67 per cent no phone and 80 per cent no car. The net implications for health of this low level of domestic capital are far from clear. It is conventional to consider a limited command of material resources as unfavourable to health, but there may also be advantages. For example, villages were typically on hillsides with fields on the valley floor – an arrangement which, with limited access to cars, should confer benefits to health from the higher levels of habitual muscular activity required in everyday life.

Diet was also investigated. All subjects were asked about the frequency with which they consumed a limited range of foods and a photographic record was made of food and drink consumed over two days in samples of sixty subjects in Levkada and seventy subjects in Melbourne.[21] Quantities of foods consumed have been estimated from the photographs. Olive oil consumption was high in both locations – but not easy to measure except by overall usage (as distinct from ingestion). In Levkada, households used 125 grams per person per day and in Melbourne 50 grams per person per day. Much of the latter oil was actually a blend of olive and other vegetable oils. On Levkada, fruit and vegetables accounted for over 60 per cent of the weight of food consumed (excluding alcoholic drinks) during the summer observation period. In Melbourne this fell to 43 per cent in males and 49 per cent in females. Consumption of red meat and poultry rose to high levels in Australia,[22] though the meat tended to be grilled and the trimmed fat left on the plate. The movement to a cash economy in Melbourne had drastic effects on alcohol consumption. Without home-produced wine, the migrants tended to reduce their intakes or to purchase beer. Mean alcohol consumption in male migrants was estimated at only 16 grams per day compared to 54 grams per day in non-migrants; the corresponding difference for females was 2 grams per day compared to 16 grams per day.[23] Because moderate intakes of alcohol protect against circulatory disease, the *net* effects of alcohol on mortality (deaths caused minus deaths prevented) are not easy to estimate. The optimal intake is not zero but probably in the range of 10 to 20 grams per day.[24] Intakes may thus have been more favourable for males in Melbourne and for females in Levkada. Much of the harm attributable to alcohol is that associated with peak drinking and intoxication, but such drinking patterns are uncommon in the Mediterranean.

The evidence collected on cardiovascular risk factors presented a complex picture. The levels of cholesterol in the blood of the non-migrants and migrants were not notably different from each other, nor from the values for southern Europeans found in the Australian National Risk Factor Survey. Blood pressure levels were, however, inexplicably low on the island – despite high alcohol and salt intakes and a tendency to overweight. In Melbourne, blood pressures in the migrants were half way between those of non-migrants and those of the host population.[25]

Migrants appeared to have less social interaction than their counterparts remaining in Levkada. Marriage rates were high except for non-migrant sisters, 12 per cent of whom were unmarried. Non-migrants were likely to have more contact with close relatives, though 50 per cent of them reported little contact with their grown up children – an unsurprising consequence of rural depopulation. There was a minority of non-migrant women who reported relative isolation on the island, with little contact even with close friends. The direction of differences in reported 'life satisfaction', measured on the bipolar Bradburn scale, might have been predicted from a knowledge of the sexual division of labour in Greek villages and in Melbourne. Men were more likely to report happiness on the island; women were less likely to report unhappiness in Melbourne. The replies of nearly half the women on the island placed them at the top of a five-point 'unhappiness scale'; in Melbourne, this proportion was one third. Perceptions of the relative attractiveness of life in Melbourne and life on the island were striking. At the time of the survey the net flow of migrants was back to Greece, and migrants were asked what they had enjoyed most in Australia, the commonest (open ended) responses were those coded to 'nothing, can't think of anything' (22 per cent), next came 'more economic opportunity' (21 per cent) and 'family life' (16 per cent). There were relatively few mentions of characteristics of the wider host society unrelated to economic opportunity for themselves or schooling for their children. Only 21 per cent of migrants thought the way of life in Australia was better for health; 62 per cent thought Levkada healthier. When the migrants were asked why the rate of flow from Levkada was falling, nearly 60 per cent commented on economic and other improvements on the island. Nearly 40 per cent of the migrant respondents said they intended returning permanently to Levkada. Figure 9.2 shows that when asked to consider their preferences 'if they could have had their life all over again', a majority of both migrants and non-migrants would have preferred to stay on the island.

Positive comments about migrating to Australia were lowest with non-migrant brothers and highest with migrant sisters – a pattern consistent with the life-satisfaction scores.

Greek migrants from Levkada found Australia economically convenient, but viewed its social institutions and lifestyle unfavourably. This is somewhat ironic given the often patronising attitudes towards Greeks of many 'old Australians' interested in 'migrant welfare'.[26] Evidence from within the study and elsewhere points to the strength and tenacity of the Greek sense of 'ethnos'. Bottomley, who studied Greeks in Sydney during the 1970s, noted that 'although the homeland is the focus of Hellenism, Greek ethnicity is not geographically defined'.[27] Australia has never had a strongly integrationist ('melting

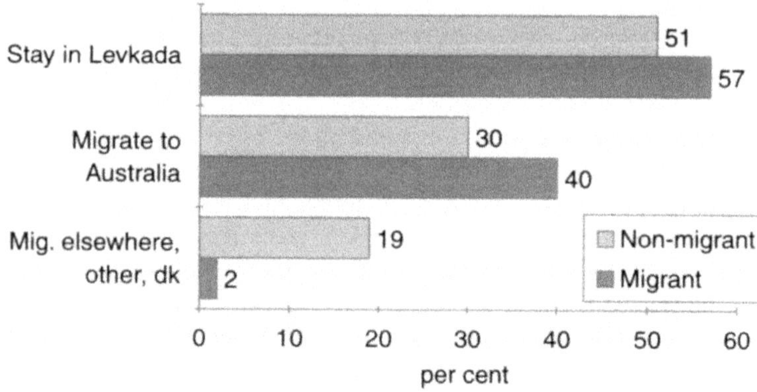

Figure 9.2 Distribution of responses to the question: 'If you could have your life all over again, would you choose to stay in Levkada, migrate to Australia, migrate elsewhere in Greece, etc. . . .?'

Source: Levkadian Migrant Health Study (Powles. unpublished)

pot') policy and today the formal policy is one of 'multiculturalism'. In this setting, Bottomley reports, 'Greeks have taken the opportunity to develop those traditions that have already demonstrated their hardiness over centuries of the Diaspora. To many Greeks, the value of these traditions is unquestioned; they form the basis of ethnic honour'.[28] At the start of our study I had naively assumed that economic success in Australia would be associated with 'Australianisation'. We found the situation to be less simple. Our findings that dietary acculturation showed little apparent association with affluence was in accord with Bottomley's earlier failure to find any correlation between economic status and the retention of Greek cultural traits; indeed, 'Greeks who become wealthy in Australia distribute a large part of their wealth to the homeland'.[29] Since 1980 the proportion of second-generation ethnic Greeks marrying other ethnic Greeks has been rising.[30]

The Levkadian study has filled in some of the details surrounding migration from rural Greece to Australia. It has uncovered a further unexplained health advantage – the low blood pressures in this part of rural Greece. It has stimulated and helped to refine hypotheses for further testing. But it has not, of itself, found an answer to the remarkable mortality advantage of this group of migrants. I turn now to the wider issue of the influence of migration on the fortunes of the host society.

MIGRATION, MULTICULTURALISM AND THE PROTECTION OF HEALTH IN MATURE INDUSTRIAL SOCIETIES

The Greek migrants have not merged into a presumptively homogeneous Australian society, rather they have constituted one dynamic element of an increasing ethnic diversity. It is of interest to consider whether the creation and acceptance of cultural diversity in lifestyles, especially diet, has facilitated change to healthier lifestyles in the wider Australian society. From the 1930s, mortality from chronic diseases, especially heart attack, rcse in Australia and through the 1960s the life expectancy for males actually fell. The much toted healthy outdoor lifestyle of Australia was not the whole story. One widely canvassed answer to high death rates from heart disease and other chronic afflictions was to renounce dietary 'affluence'. But where to turn? The effects of taking the fat and sugar out of a northern European diet were reminiscent of wartime food rationing in Britain – such a bland diet was out of tune with the 1960s. Another alternative was to look to other European diets, most obviously those of the Mediterranean where heart disease and other chronic disease were less common.

Before the 1960s there were no environmental reasons why Australia could not have produced large quantities of Mediterranean foods; however, the food culture and agricultural production still followed the British 'meat and two veg'. Fruit and salad vegetables were enjoyed in season, but tended not to be bought from shops. Since then, and only partly under the influence of health considerations, dietary preferences and food production in Australia have changed: the supply of fruit and vegetables was taken over by Italians and Greeks, and a dense green bank of salad vegetables became a year-round feature at greengrocers. A growing and substantial proportion of fishermen and fish-shop owners were Greek. Italian cafes and pizza bars began to spread from the inner city ethnic enclaves.

At the Bicentennial Food Conference in 1988, after a series of presentations, some of which documented a radical change in dietary practices in the post-war decades, I found myself sitting at lunch, next to the Australian general manager of a major Italian olive oil marketing company. He told me his sales were doubling every twelve months and he did not know why. Mediterranean diets were seemingly becoming the fashion.

While it is easy to speculate about dietary change, it is much less easy to document it quantitatively. Some, unfortunately not strictly comparable, estimated intakes of selected foods were given in Table 9.3. The higher reported intakes of tomatoes, leafy greens and fruit amongst those Australians born in southern Europe is clear. Equally significant, perhaps, are the stepwise increases, most notable for fruits consumed in winter, from the levels in Britain to those of British- and Australian-born Australians and then to the higher levels still of southern-European-born Australians. It seems that the 'migrant advantage' is infectious, if not directly then perhaps indirectly from the increased range of foodstuffs it encourages, and from the different types of diet that can be tried.

My argument here is not that the switch to a lighter diet with more fruit and vegetables has been confined to Australia, nor that it has been entirely attributable to immigration from the Mediterranean. Rather it is that the change in Australia – and in the United States – has been more marked than in western and north-western Europe. It may not be coincidental that Australia and the United States, which has experienced similar multicultural stimuli to dietary change, have experienced some of the highest falls in mortality from diseases of the circulatory system.[31] The abruptness of the Australian change is shown in Figure 9.3.

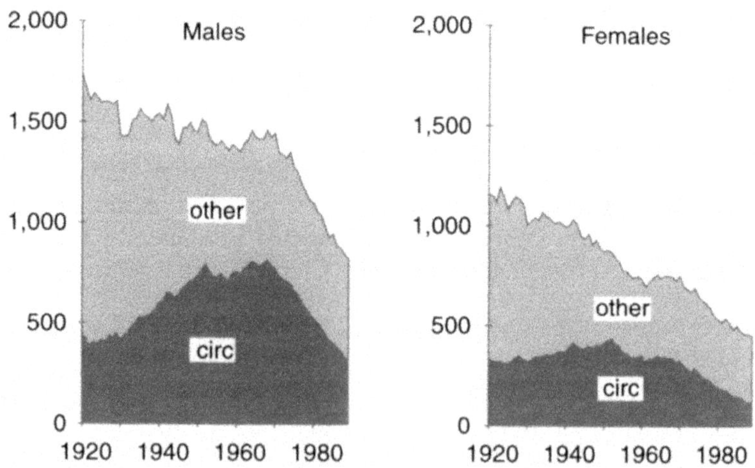

Figure 9.3 Mortality from diseases of the circulatory system and from all other causes, age-standardised rates for Australians aged 45–64, 1920–90

Source of data: Australian Institute of Health

CONCLUSION

It has been conventional to blame adverse exposures associated with dietary affluence for the modern epidemics of cardiovascular and other chronic diseases. But affluence may also bring freedom to experiment: under the stimuli of cultural diversity and rising health awareness, it may also provide a remedy – a post-modernist hygiene with a variety of lifestyles, both healthy and attractive, available 'off the shelf'. The point can be emphasised by comparison with those societies where dietary affluence has not been accompanied by stimuli to qualitative dietary change. In Eastern Europe, the purchasing power for a limited range of mostly traditional foods was enormously enhanced in the decades following the Second World War, but while consumption of meat and butter rose to record peaks, there was little move towards lighter diets with more fruit and vegetables. In increasing contrast to Western Europe, fresh fruit and vegetables were in very short supply – especially in winter. Dietary preferences and practices were unchanged and unable to change. Since the 1970s Eastern Europe has remained a disaster zone for chronic disease mortality. Adult male mortality in Hungary (the worst affected country outside the former USSR) rose to Third World levels.[32] Whilst it would be idle to pretend that the causes of the public health catastrophe in Eastern Europe are fully understood, few experts in chronic disease epidemiology would doubt that diet has played the leading role.

It is therefore plausible to suggest that migrants from cultures that carry dietary protection against chronic disease – most notably the Mediterranean and East Asia – have helped their host societies construct attractive escape routes from the fatal propensities of early, misconsumed affluence.

NOTES

1 R.W. Gardner, *Life Tables by Ethnic Group for Hawaii, 1980*, Honolulu, 1984.

2 D.M. Reed, J.P. Strong, J. Resch and T. Hayashi, 'Serum Lipids and Lipoproteins as Predictors of Atherosclerosis: An Autopsy Study', *Arteriosclerosis*, 1989, 9, pp. 560–4.

3 A. Keys, *Seven Countries: A Multivariate Analysis of Death and Coronary Heart Disease*, Cambridge, Mass., 1980.

4 Australian Bureau of Statistics, *Overseas Born Australians 1988. A Statistical Profile*, Canberra, 1989; C. Young, 'Mortality, the Ultimate Indicator of Survival: The Differential Experience between Birthplace

Groups', in J. Donovan, E.M. d'Espaignet, C. Merton and M. van Ommergen, *Immigrants in Australia: A Health Profile*, Canberra, 1992, pp. 34–70.

5 G. Bottomley, *After the Odyssey: A Study of Greek Australians*, St Lucia, 1979, p. 12.

6 'Women here work more hard because we have to work in production. In the village in Greece, when you want to stay for two hours to lie down a bit you can. But not in the factory. And after, you have to catch transport, come home to prepare the meal, the house, look after the children. You feel more tired than in the village. When the man comes home from work, after he takes his shower, sometimes he goes to visit friends, sometimes to the coffee bar. The woman works four or five hours at home. Women work much more than men. I believe that.' CURA, *'But I wouldn't want my wife to work here': A Study of Migrant Women in Melbourne Industry*, Fitzroy, Victoria, 1976.

7 W. Lowenstein and M. Loh, *The Immigrants*, Melbourne, 1977, p. 139.

8 Young, 'Mortality', pp. 34–70.

9 Keys, *Seven Countries.*

10 Young, 'Mortality'. Rate for diabetes classified as 'high' in source, but the numerical value was not given.

11 The term is used here in its epidemiological sense, i.e. as shorthand for 'environmental exposures' – which are taken to include everything except genes. Thus diet, exercise, stress, etc. are all potential health-determining 'exposures'.

12 S.A. Bennett, 'Inequalities in Risk Factors and Cardiovascular Mortality Among Australia's Immigrants', *Australian Journal of Public Health*, 1993, 17, p. 256.

13 S.N. Blair, H.W. Kohl, R.S. Paffenbarger and D.G. Clark, 'Physical Fitness and All-Cause Mortality. A Prospective Study of Healthy Men and Women', *Journal of the American Medical Association*, 1989, 262, pp. 2395–401.

14 D.J.P. Barker, 'The Fetal and Infant Origins of Adult Disease', *British Medical Journal*, 1990, 301, p. 1111; J. Powles and D. Ruth, 'Diet-Mortality Associations: An Overview', in M.L. Wahlqvist and J.S. Vobecky, *Medical Practice of Preventive Nutrition*, London, 1994.

15 Compare the studies of: K. Orth-Gomer and J.V. Johnson, 'Social Network Interaction and Mortality: A Six Year Follow-up Study of a Random Sample of the Swedish Population', *Journal of Chronic Disease*, 1987, 40, pp. 949–57 and B. Hanson, S. Isacsson, L. Janzon, et al., 'Social Network and Social Support Influence Mortality in Elderly Men', *American Journal of Epidemiology*, 1989, 130, p. 100, with M. Davis, J. Neuhaus, D. Moritz, et al., 'Living Arrangements and Survival of Older US Adults [abstract]', *American Journal of Epidemiology*, 1990, 132, p. 789. Also see: Bottomley, *After the Odyssey*, pp. 107–32.

16 J. Powles, B. Hage and M.-A. Cosgrove, 'Health Related Expenditure Patterns in Selected Migrant Groups: Data from the Australian Household Expenditure Survey, 1984', *Community Health Studies*, 1990, 14, pp. 1–7.

17 A hypothesis that a year-round intake of protective foods was especially important would also help explain the very high mortality in Eastern

Europe where 'off season' intakes of protective foods have been dramatically lower than in the West.

18 E.M. d'Espaignet and M. van Ommeren, 'Differences in Levels and Types of Disabilities', in Donovon et al., *Immigrants in Australia*, p. 221.

19 C. Young and A. Coles, 'Women's Health, Use of Medical Services, Medication, Lifestyle and Chronic Illness: Some Findings from the 1989–90 National Health Survey', in Donovan et al., *Immigrants in Australia*, p. 147.

20 Data from 1986 Australian census.

21 J. Powles, D. Ktenas, C. Sutherland and B. Hage, 'Food Habits in Southern-European Migrants: A Case Study of Migrants from the Greek Island of Levkada', in A.S. Truswell and M.L. Wahlqvist, eds, *Food Habits in Australia*, Melbourne, 1988, pp. 201–23.

22 This pattern for our subjects was consistent with that observed in the national household expenditure data for Greek-headed households. Powles et al., 'Health Related Expenditure Patterns'.

23 J. Powles, G. Macaskill, J. Hopper and D. Ktenas, 'The Effects on Alcohol Consumption of Migration from a Greek Island to Melbourne, Australia: A Study of Sibships', *Journal of Studies on Alcohol*, 1990, 52, pp. 224–31.

24 R. Doll, R. Peto, E. Hall, K. Wheatley and R. Gray, 'Mortality in Relation to Consumption of Alcohol: 13 years' Observations on Male British Doctors', *British Medical Journal*, 1994, 309, pp. 911–19.

25 J. Powles, J. Hopper, G. Macaskill and D. Ktenas, 'Blood Pressure in Subjects from Rural Greece: Comparing Individuals Migrating to Melbourne, Australia with Non-Migrant Relatives', *Journal of Human Hypertension*, 1993, 6, pp. 419–29.

26 D. Cox, 'Medico-Social Problems in the Greek Population in Melbourne: Social and Cultural Background', *Medical Journal of Australia*, 1972, 2, pp. 879–81 – which ends 'I find the Greek to be a fascinating person, a loveable person, but one whom it is essential to understand.'

27 Bottomley, *After the Odyssey*, p. 175.

28 Ibid., p. 180.

29 Ibid., p. 103.

30 Dr C. Price, Australian National University, as cited in *The Age* (Melbourne), 10 April 1989, p. 11.

31 J. Powles and D. Ruth, 'Diet-Mortality Associations'. K. A. Steinmetz and J. D. Potter, 'Vegetables, Fruits and Cancer: I Epidemiology; II Mechanisms', *Cancer, Causes and Control*, 1991, 2, pp. 325–57, 427–42.

32 Compare, for example, Hungary and Sri Lanka in the *World Health Statistics Annual* (WHO, Geneva).

10

SOUTHERN ITALIAN IMMIGRATION TO THE UNITED STATES AT THE TURN OF THE CENTURY AND THE PERENNIAL PROBLEM OF MEDICALISED PREJUDICE[1]

Alan M. Kraut

In July 1994, La Quinta High School in Orange County, California, experienced the worst epidemic of drug-resistant tuberculosis ever reported in a secondary school in the United States. More troubling still, it could all be traced to a 16-year-old Vietnamese girl, an immigrant, who contracted the disease in her homeland. At a time when California's governor, Republican Pete Wilson, was railing against the burden immigrants placed upon his state's health care system and other politicians were lending their voices to a growing nativist chorus, Jody Meador, the local tuberculosis control officer, refused to join in. He told the press that the youngster bore no blame for what had happened:

> The point that should be made is that regardless of the ethnicity of the source case, the problem originated largely as a result of a delay in diagnosis of treatment and not as a result of this source case being an immigrant. TB does not discriminate. It is everybody's problem.[2]

With these words the public health officer deviated from the perennial pattern of equating the affliction with the afflicted, especially in the case of the foreign born.

Throughout American history, nativists have portrayed immigrants as public health menaces. The current resurgence of tuberculosis coming, as it does, in the midst of a large wave of immigration, has stirred public apprehension and echoes events of a century ago. Once again, newcomers and native born wrestle over differences in defining wellness, disease, hygiene, health care and therapeutics. Understanding past negotiation of these definitions illuminates current debates over public health issues, the inevitable by-product in a pluralist society of international migration and what happens when peoples meet.

Conflict over health issues between the host society and southern Italian immigrants at the turn of the last century is a model worth consulting. Between 1880 and the 1920s almost 24 million newcomers arrived on America's shores, most of them from southern and eastern Europe, though many others came from Asian countries, Mexico and Canada. Southern Italians were the largest group among the newcomers at the turn of the century. Approximately 4.5 million Italians entered the United States (US) between 1880 and 1921, after which restrictive legislation curbed the flow. Over 80 per cent were from Il Mezzogiorno, the southern provinces of Italy. Many, men in particular, journeyed back and forth between their villages in southern Italy and the seasonal labour markets of the US, often to particular cities, like New York, where more than 80 per cent of the newcomers worked at some time. American immigration officers dubbed these labour migrants 'birds of passage'.

The negotiations between natives and Italian newcomers over definitions of health and hygiene were complex. The groups were separated by a wide gulf in their understanding of disease, prevention and therapy. From the perspective of some native-born Americans, the Italians were the source of their own distress. In New York City and elsewhere, native-born critics of immigration denigrated southern Italian immigrants as dangerous because their overcrowded and insanitary living conditions produced endemic and sometimes epidemic disease. In 1890, Richmond Mayo-Smith, a Columbia University professor of political economy described Italian immigrants in New York's tenements: 'Huddled together in miserable apartments in filth and rags, without the slightest regard to decency or health, they present a picture of squalid existence degrading to any civilisation and a menace to the health of the whole community.' Italians, heirs to one of the world's oldest civilisations, seemed to Mayo-Smith to be 'ignorant, criminal and vicious, eating food that we would give to dogs'. Their 'very stolidity and patience under such conditions show that they lack the faintest appreciation of what civilisation means', he added.[3]

In 1914, an equally uncharitable E. A. Ross wrote:

> Steerage passengers from a Naples boat show a distressing frequency of low foreheads, open mouths, weak chins, poor features, skew faces, small or knobby crania, and backless heads. Such people lack the power to take rational care of themselves; hence their death-rate in New York is twice the general death-rate and thrice that of the Germans.[4]

Ross, a sociologist, was far better at polemics than statistics. A careful analysis of mortality data by Louis Dublin, the renowned statistician of the Metropolitan Life Insurance Company, used sex and age data from the 1910 Census for New York State and Pennsylvania to confirm that in New York the Italian death rate was generally lower not higher than that for the native born of the same age and gender and considerably lower than that for the comparable age and sex category of the German group.[5] (See Table 10.1.)

Whatever the statistics might suggest, nativists such as Mayo-Smith and Ross were persuaded that the health and vitality of the American population required restrictive legislation to exclude health menaces borne by travellers from Italy's southern provinces. Medical inspections at New York's Ellis Island and other immigration depots conducted by the US Marine Hospital Service (after 1913, the US Public Health Service) simply did not appear to be adequately excluding the unhealthy, according to restrictionists of Mayo-Smith's and Ross's ilk.[6]

Not all those preoccupied by what seemed the unhealthy and unhygienic ways of Italian newcomers plumped for restriction. Some hoped that preaching the American gospel of good health and hygiene to newcomers would persuade Italian immigrants to adopt American ways. The Daughters of the American Revolution (DAR) in Connecti-

Table 10.1 Mortality rates (per 1,000 population) for native born of native parents, Italian immigrants and German immigrants, all ages in New York State, 1910[7]

	Native born	*Italian*	*German*
Male	15.9	9.2	27.5
Female	13.9	9.7	22.6

cut commissioned John Foster Carr to write a *Guide for the Immigrant Italian in the US of America* in 1911.[8] The DAR was quite explicit about their desire to make Italians 'become Americans', not the least to mitigate the danger they posed to American public health. Although Carr pitched the healthfulness of 'country life' as compared to city life to migrants whose families had been on the land for generations, he recognised that most Italians would gravitate to cities because of the higher wages. His *Guide* preached 'public hygiene' as the means to prevent disease in an urban environment and linked the hygienic with the aesthetic, as in his observation that 'Spitting is not only a disgusting habit; it is the cause of tuberculosis and other diseases'.[9] The lengthiest section of the *Guide* was on 'The Importance of Caring for the Health', as Carr stated, 'A working man's capital is a strong, well body'. After many paragraphs urging bathing, care in the purchase of food, sweeping and dusting, and many other good habits, readers were encouraged to co-operate with government officials and to trust them. Immigrants must not hesitate to report unhygienic or dangerous conditions to the Board of Health, because, 'That is the American way. And in America you should do as Americans do'.[10] He carefully explained that boards of health in American cities had the power to coerce those who disobeyed standards of hygiene and endangered public welfare. Perhaps sensing the hesitation of southern Italians to spend large sums on health care, Carr was careful to emphasise that many aspects of health care in America were paid for by taxes. To encourage cleanliness, fresh air and exercise, he made a point of mentioning 'large public baths', 'playgrounds for children' and 'open air gymnasiums for men and boys'. New Yorkers were advised to avail themselves of 'recreation piers built out onto the river, where mothers can take their small children during the hot weather, and where it is pleasant to promenade in the evening'.

While Carr sketched a general profile of good health and hygiene American-style, he was specific when it came to consumption. By the end of the nineteenth century, physicians and public health professionals in America had come to accept that consumption was caused by rod-shaped tubercle bacilli. These were capable of affecting any part of the body, and more than one part simultaneously, though the pulmonary form of the disease was the most common. The latter was spread primarily through the sputum of those infected, who would spray the air with bacilli when coughing or contaminate food shared by others. The word tuberculosis, meaning the formation of tubercles, first appeared in the early nineteenth century, but did not become the preferred name for this disease until the early twentieth century.[11] Pulmonary tuberculosis was also known as phthisis, from the Greek *phote*, a body shrivelling up under intense heat, while the term consumption derived from the Latin *consumere*, describing the wasting of flesh.[12] Interestingly, as public awareness of the disease was increasing, tuberculosis mortality rates were declining. Well before Robert Koch's 1882 identification of the tubercle bacillus, mortality from tuberculosis began to diminish among all sections of the population, beginning in around 1837 in England and 1870 in the US. The exact reasons for the virtual elimination of tuberculosis are a matter of some historical controversy, but a persuasive case has been made that efforts to reduce the contact between those infected with pulmonary tuberculosis and those still uninfected dramatically shrank the opportunity for victims to spread their infection.[13]

Carr's *Guide*'s advice on consumption started with the reassurance that the disease was not fatal, especially if detected and treated early. The prognosis for a confirmed case had been bleak, but from the 1890s the sanatorium or open-air treatment seemed to offer a cure and a model of the kind of hygienic lifestyle that would protect against infection. Echoing the popular wisdom of the day, Carr described 'pure air and sunshine, outdoor life, and nourishing food' as the 'only cures'. Those who suspected themselves infected were urged to head for Clinica Morgagni in New York, 'an Italian institution that takes special care of the tuberculosis poor, and provides in case of need for sending them to sanatoria'.[14] Carr concluded, however, with the stern warning that 'One sick with contagious disease is liable to be punished if he *exposes himself or another similarly sick* in any public place'.[15] After all, the public health of host and immigrant alike was at stake and tuberculosis was a disease not to be taken lightly by anyone. At the turn of the century, tuberculosis was also controlled to some extent by excluding or removing individuals from the general population. But while some native-born Americans attributed the prevalence of tuberculosis specifically to the presence and habits of immigrants, other Americans conceived of disease prevention as part of the larger struggle to make industrial life viable. Industrial reformers defined many diseases, including tuberculosis, as by-products of tenement residence and the industrial workplace. And in the case of 'homework', in which Italian immigrants were particularly involved, the two were the same.

Italian women homeworkers and their daughters dominated the artificial flower trade. In 1913, Mary Van Kleeck, Secretary of the

Committee on Women's Work of the Russell Sage Foundation, published a study of artificial flower makers.[16] Van Kleeck conducted her survey in lower Manhattan in a section of blocks bounded by Christopher Street running diagonally along the north-west, Canal Street on the south, the Hudson River on the west, and a broken line along Sixth Avenue, West Fourth Street and West Broadway on the east, a district that adjoined one in which most of the flower factories were located. Location was important because, as Van Kleeck observed, homeworkers constantly carried large boxes of finished flowers from their kitchen tables to the factories, and their meagre earnings made carfare a prohibitive expense.[17] Van Kleeck studied 110 families, of whom 371 family members worked on flowers. Most were Italian, a fact the investigator attributed to 'the attitude of Italians toward women and their prejudice against their employment outside the home', especially for married women.[18]

Van Kleeck regarded home manufacture as 'a most threatening aspect of the sweating system' because 'the labour of young children is utilised, and advantage is taken of the urgent need of their mothers to earn money without leaving their homes and children', a need that discouraged labour militancy, leaving the workforce 'cheap and docile'.[19] However, Van Kleeck emphasised, the harm was not to the workers alone, because 'goods manufactured in these crowded tenement homes may carry disease not recognised as a result of the home-work system'.[20] Some homeworkers held outside jobs and did homework at night. However, most spent their days surrounded by family, some of whom also helped in 'dark, dirty bedrooms used as workplaces'. Here Van Kleeck saw flower makers already suffering from tuberculosis or 'bad cases of skin disease', who handled the flowers 'with no thought of the possibility of infection'.[21]

Certainly the working day was gruelling and the financial rewards meagre. One Italian family of ten (parents and eight children) that Van Kleeck found living in Greenwich village was typical of those supplementing a family income of $16.50 per week.[22] The father earned $7.00 a week selling lunches in a saloon, while the eldest daughter made $6.50 in a box factory and the 16-year-old son contributed $3.00 earned as a wagon boy. Four children were in school and two babies at home. All but the babies helped make flowers. The mother worked irregularly during the day, joined by her children after school, and the older daughter and son in the evenings. The family made 7 cents gross per three-petaled violet, earning a weekly wage of $3.00. Their three room apartment where they lived and worked cost

$12.50 per month.[23] The congestion and long hours took their toll. Italian homeworkers had a mortality rate from tuberculosis fourteen times that of some upper-income neighbourhoods of the same city.[24] Forging epidemiological links between homework *per se* and tuberculosis is problematic because it is so difficult to isolate the work experience from the larger milieu of poverty in immigrant neighbourhoods. However, in the minds of many contemporaries, such as Mary Van Kleeck, the connection was irrefutable and the preventive undeniable – industrial reform.

While native-born Americans might argue over why Italian immigrants were vulnerable to disease, especially tuberculosis, and what needed to be done to protect the American population from such scourges, all accepted germ theory as an explanatory model of disease. Tuberculosis was a germ disease to be sure, but one that could be limited in its effect and contagiousness through specific public health precautions and treatment and more importantly, by individual hygienic precautions and measures that 'hardened' the body against infection. Such a construction of disease and adequate preventives and therapies was often met with resistance among the newcomers. Health care workers quickly learned that the millions of Italian workers who disembarked in New York and other American ports had not left their own traditional views of health and disease, prevention and therapy at the dock when they departed.

SICKNESS AND WELLNESS AS UNDERSTOOD IN IL MEZZOGIORNO

As they had been for centuries, illness and remedies were bound closely to a blend of religion and pagan beliefs that varied from place to place in Italy's southern provinces.[25] In the 1930s an American anthropologist, Phyllis Williams, explored the cultural roots that nourished Italian immigrants, tracing them back across time and space to the southern provinces. There Christianity had come to cities long before the countryside and pagan deities continued to hold the attention of peasants.[26] From Rome northward, Italian Roman Catholicism resembled that practised in the rest of northern Europe, but south of Rome it was blended with traditions and customs of pagan origin. Reliance upon superstition and magic remained especially strong and although there were regional differences, certain patterns were generally common in the south.[27]

The preservation of health was closely tied to worship of individual saints. Williams observed that, 'Saint Rocco protected devotees against illness, Saint Lucy guarded their eyesight, and Saint Anna helped during the pangs and dangers of childbirth'.[28] Such saints appear in neither the Bible nor the writings of the early Christian fathers, but were folk substitutes for old Greek and Roman gods and spirits of the forests, rivers and mountains. Along with these protective saints, every Italian child was watched over by a guardian angel. There were house spirits and, of course, village saints who generally kept watch over all within the village borders. The polytheism of the old Roman departmental deities survived in local saint veneration, which accounts for the numerous Madonnas who were objects of prayer and supplication. While they were often represented iconographically as the Virgin Mary, each was an embodiment of some saint or historical figure whose past was associated with a particular village or town, such as the Madonna delle Virgine, the patron saint of Scafati. When peasants prayed to this Madonna for good health or the cure for a particular affliction, they were maintaining a practice that pre-dated Christianity but had been assimilated into Catholicism.[29] The annual celebration of a town's patron saint required worshippers to carry the saint's image from the church in a procession through the streets, and offerings, especially money and jewellery, were cast at the statue's feet. On such festive occasions, the personal clothing of a sick person might be brought and placed before the statue. Believers contended that when the garments were worn again, the goodness of the saint imbued the body of the worshipper and restored health.

Southern Italians often attributed illness to the influence of one who had the *jettatura* or *mal'occhio* (evil eye), a belief that had no basis in Roman Catholic theology and which the Church never succeeded in supplanting.[30] Williams regarded the belief in the 'evil eye' as a typically pre-modern one, where misfortune could not be explained merely 'as something precipitated by natural causation, as due to lack of foresight, error, or the entrance into the situation of forces over which they had no control'. Instead, misfortunes such as illnesses were attributed to the influence of 'an ever-present menace, the power of envy'.[31] Those men or women who possessed the 'evil eye' could, with a glance, cause physical injury, sickness or even death. The *mal'occhio* could be warded off by the wearing of amulets, with those representing animals' horns, claws or teeth, fashioned from actual horns and claws, or coral, silver, gold, bone, ivory and lava being popular. Fish, scissors, knives and a male – but not a female hunchback – were common symbols for amulets. They could be placed over a door post, on a bedroom wall, on a chain around the neck, in pockets or in the lining of clothing. When someone suspected of having the 'evil eye' approached, the amulet was to be grasped and pointed unobtrusively in the offending individual's direction. In the absence of an amulet, one might protect health and well-being by extending the first and pinky fingers from an extended fist to represent a set of horns.[32]

Wizards and witches also survived into the twentieth-century minds of southern Italian villagers, though not all were embodiments of evil. *Maghi* and *maghe* (male and female, respectively) often worked as herb doctors practising folk medicine, curing diseases and healing broken hearts with their potions. Individuals who wished to safeguard their homes from evil witches put salt or garlic in keyholes, on window sills or on the door step. A broom placed behind a door was also regarded as a preventive. In 1910, an American physician, unfamiliar with local beliefs and fears, was puzzled by his failure to persuade his neighbours of the benefits of the common anti-tubercular practice of sleeping with an open window at night. One of their reasons for ignoring medical advice was their conviction that evil spirits travelled through the night air.[33]

Southern Italians coped with illness by applying folk remedies derived from a reservoir of folk traditions and customs and by consulting specialists such as witches, barbers, midwives and herbalists. Qualified doctors were few and far between. Small towns usually had one who was paid by the state out of community coffers and the doctor's salary was fixed, though he often received free use of a house in exchange for treating the most impoverished gratis. Wealthier patients paid for special attention, which allowed the physician to supplement his income. Town physicians were not highly respected, in part because people were suspicious of modern medicine. But equally important, folk wisdom taught them 'when it don't cost anything you might know it is no good'.[34] Folk medicine cost little because it was largely practised by experienced housewives or neighbours. Should a herbalist be called, he or she could make diagnoses and concoct required medicine from materials readily available in nearby fields and forests. The diagnoses of folk healers were grounded in adages associating physiological characteristics with particular patterns of personality or disease, such as 'The face without colour is false' or 'He who has long ears will live long'.[35] People with long necks were thought to be susceptible to tuberculosis.[36] However, fear and loathing of the physician as intruder, common in rural southern towns, was not the case in larger cities such as Naples and Palermo, where a more cosmopolitan view of medicine and its practitioners prevailed.

THE ITALIAN PHYSICIAN IN AMERICA: HEALER, REFORMER AND CULTURAL INTERMEDIARY

Millions of native-born Americans, both rural and urban, maintained popular beliefs about health and illness that organised medicine regarded as mere superstitions or outmoded ideas. Indeed, the gap between the notion that people with long necks were more prone to tuberculosis and medical ideas about ill-formed chests and tubercular constitutions was small. None the less, reports of southern Italian beliefs and customs confirmed general ideas of the backwardness of southern European immigrants, and reinforced the suggestions of Mayo-Smith and Ross that the newcomers were physically inferior to America's pioneering Anglo Saxon and Teutonic stock. However, such views did not go uncontested. Southern Italian immigrants in the US had their own medical spokesman, Dr Antonio Stella, who mediated between them and the larger American community. He compiled data, constructed arguments and published articles defending southern Italian immigrants against those who saw the newcomers as inferior and dangerous.

Antonio Stella's roots were not as humble as the majority of those he treated, nor was his life an epic in overcoming obstacles.[37] He was born in Muro, Lucania, a southern Italian province in 1868, but his father was a lawyer and a noted numismatist. Stella was educated at Naples, where he attended the Royal Lyceum, before going on to receive his MD from the Royal University in 1893. After graduation, he emigrated to the US and was naturalised in 1909. Stella specialised in internal medicine and developed an international reputation for his work on tuberculosis. In New York, he became a prominent figure in the medical community, treating important figures such as opera star Enrico Caruso. He was a consulting physician to Manhattan Hospital and the Italian Hospital, served as a visiting physician at the Columbus Hospital, and was also appointed an examiner in lunacy for the State of New York. The year Stella was naturalised, but prior to his oath, he served as a delegate of the Italian government to the Sixth International Tuberculosis Congress held in Washington, DC. He was the author of many medical monographs and articles on immigration, a fellow of the New York Academy of Medicine, a member of the advisory council of the New York Board of Health and active in many national and local professional societies.

Stella authored a volume entitled *Some Aspects of Italian Immigration to the US*, which aimed to shed the most favourable light upon the Italian contribution to the US. The volume's sub-title, *Statistical Data and General Considerations Based Chiefly Upon the US Census and Other Official Publications*, was clearly an effort to support his positive view of Italian immigration by grounding it in statistical and vital data generated by Americans themselves. Stella boldly asserted that whatever health problems Italians in the US might suffer, especially tuberculosis, they had acquired in America rather than brought with them from Italy. Speaking of the Italian people in their homeland, Stella described them as 'one of the healthiest in the world on account of its proverbial sobriety and frugality, also perhaps as a result of the fact, that natural selection has had there freer play than elsewhere'.[38] His point was that Italian health problems were a result of poor environmental conditions and poverty, not due to innate biological inferiority. He was also quick to absolve American Italians of any charges of slovenliness or weak moral fibre. Stella reminded his readers that:

> The Italians, together with the Slav, more than any other foreign group, engage in dangerous and hazardous occupations, in mines, steel mills, blasting, excavations, besides all sorts of dusty and unhealthy trades – thus many times they pay with their health and life, while adding to the prosperity of the US.[39]

Stella had a special interest in tuberculosis among the Italians, especially as data from the Census of 1900 had shown that Italians in the US had the second lowest rate of mortality from tuberculosis of any ethnic group. Their mortality rate of 113.6 per 100,000 was bettered only by native-born Americans, whose mortality rate from TB was 112.8 per 100,000. Stella attributed part of this ethnic advantage to Italians not remaining in America long enough for their deaths to be counted.

> Any medical man who has been brought into close contact with them, will bear witness to the fact, that only a few of the Italian [sic] tuberculous die in the district in which they have contracted the disease. Their fear of consumption is much greater than among any other nationality, and the belief in climate as the only cure for pulmonary disease is so firmly rooted, that the first

> suggestion of anything abnormal with their lungs leads them to make immediate preparation for a trip to the home country.[40]

Where possible, Stella used statistics to back his assertions. For example, he drew on data for 1903–4 showing only two cases of tuberculosis among Italians coming to America that were treated in ships' hospitals, 'a rate of 0.006 per cent'. Yet, among homeward bound Italians, during the same two years, there were 457 cases treated in ships' hospitals and seventeen deaths at sea. Such figures did not include those who travelled as first and second cabin passengers and thus escaped enumeration.[41]

In 1904, Stella published an article on the prevalence of tuberculosis among Italian immigrants in *Charities*, the publication of the Charity Organization Society of New York. He told readers that 'exact information' was often missing because of Italians' mobility and advised that:

> One must follow the Italian population as it moves in the tenement districts; study them closely in their daily struggle for air and space; see them in the daytime crowded in sweat-shops and factories; at night heaped together in dark windowless rooms; then visit the hospitals' dispensaries; and finally watch the outgoing steamships, and count the wan emaciated forms, with glistening eyes and racking cough that return to their native land with a hope of recuperating health, but often times only to find a quicker death.[42]

Data on Manhattan for 1906, published by William Guilfoy of the New York City Department of Health, gave the number of Italians who died from pulmonary tuberculosis as 290 with a death rate of 276.3 per 100,000. That rate, while hardly as low as the 172.4 per 100,000 for Russians and Poles, who were mostly Jewish, was nevertheless favourable when compared to the pulmonary tuberculosis death rate of 476.7 for the Irish and 339.8 for the Austro-Hungarians.[43]

However, Stella's first-hand experience of the Italian neighbourhood on New York's Lower East Side suggested that the reality was worse than the statistics implied because of chronic under-reporting. In tenements on Elizabeth and Mulberry Streets, there were barely 'twelve and fifteen cases of consumption reported to the Board of Health since 1894', but from his 'personal experiences with some of the houses in that particular neighbourhood', Stella observed that 'the average has been not less than thirty or forty cases of infection for each tenement yearly, the element of house-infection being so great'. Frustrated, the physician rhetorically asked, 'And how could it be otherwise?'[44] Like Mary Van Kleeck, Stella blamed the congested housing and dark, unventilated sweatshops for weakening the bodies of robust Italian agrarians, making them fertile ground for the tubercle bacilli. The knowledgeable doctor told his readers in 1904 that the process of physical degeneration was critical in the acquisition of tuberculosis.

> We know nowadays that the penetration of a pathogenic germ into our system is not sufficient to cause a disease. It must find our body in a state of temporary paralysis of all its natural defences, to be able to give rise to certain morbid processes, the evolution of which constitutes a disease.[45]

Dirty linen and impure air did not cause disease, but Stella warned his readers that:

> Six months of life in the tenements are sufficient to turn the sturdy youth from Calabria, the brawny fisherman of Sicily, the robust woman from Abruzzi and Basilicata, into the pale, flabby, undersized creatures we see, dragging along the streets of New York and Chicago, such a painful contrast to the native population! Six months more of this gradual deterioration, and the soil for the bacillus tuberculosis is amply prepared.[46]

Stella's observations were more than amply confirmed by Italian immigration officials who watched as their 'birds of passage' flocked home wilted and sick. Ship physicians reported that the rate of illness was higher among those returning to Italy than among the westward bound, and that tuberculosis was the most frequently diagnosed ailment. In 1904, a list of the most common diseases treated on ocean voyages back to Italy showed that the 278 cases of tuberculosis detected were greater than all the others combined; malaria was a distant second place with 49 cases, contracted by Italians engaged in rural migrant labour.[47] As bad as it was, the American immigrant experience was still not the worst. In his memoir, Italian Council of Emigration member Luigi Rossi recorded what he had heard about returnees in the port of Genoa. There he heard that returnees from different countries could be distinguished by the condition of their bodies and their wallets; because 'those returning from the US come with sufficient health and money, those from Argentina return with their health but no money, and those from Brazil bring neither health nor money'.[48]

Even if it did not occur as rapidly as Dr Antonio Stella wished, Italian immigrants' definitions of disease and therapy did change. Part of this was due directly to their relocation. Remedies used in traditional cures had to be modified because of the 'inability to procure materials, such as wolf bones, from which to compound accustomed remedies'. However, immigrants found an array of substitutes for the 'medicine cupboard', including 'a bewildering array of mushrooms and other foods as well as . . . plants, berries, and barks'.[49] Plants that did not grow wild, such as basil and rue, were cultivated in gardens or in little window boxes that sat on the sills of tenement apartments high above city sidewalks. First-generation immigrants often continued to define illness as an enemy's curse, or the work of human jealousy, or spite administered through the gesture of the 'evil eye'. Restored health was also considered a divine blessing, perhaps even a sign of the Madonna's indirect intervention.

With the exception of public figures such as Stella, physicians remained unpopular objects of suspicion and distrust amongst immigrants and were often consulted only to mollify authorities. At times, Italian immigrants called upon the assistance of witches, *maghi*, or *iannare* to the Neapolitans, to cure tuberculosis. When a physician was summoned at all, he had to be an Italian. One Italian physician from New York described his group's preferences:

> Italians almost always call an Italian doctor because of the mutual sympathy and common language. The Italians are very fond of their families and will spend every cent to care for a member if ill. They are not satisfied with the American doctors because they make a short visit, prescribe and leave. This leaves the family in much doubt and accounts somewhat for their calling in another doctor if there isn't a marked improvement in a few hours. The Italian doctors tell the family what the malady is, and explain to them all about it, and this is what they expect. . . . They always pay cash and as a consequence they are inclined to call various doctors at different illnesses, just as they patronise different stores.[50]

This behaviour echoes old world healing patterns as well as the contemporary beliefs and practices of equally poor working-class Americans.

Still torn between two worlds, Italian immigrants clung to tradition with a tenacity that made the task of physicians complicated. Individuals who trusted a barber with bloodletting vehemently opposed blood tests. The logic was that blood drawn off by the barber was unhealthy, while that taken for a blood test was healthy blood unnecessarily removed from a healthy arm. Many immigrants echoed the traditional argument so well known among southern Italians that, because diseases often run their course and go away, it is preferable to wait for testing and treatment until it is apparent that the virtue of *pazienza*, patience, will not do. This approach to health is consistent with the broader fatalism that southern Italians brought with them, a view that assumes that one should not expect a great deal from life and disappointment will thereby be minimised.

The relationship of Italian immigrants and their children to modern medicine did not remain stagnant. Customs, traditions and beliefs altered with each succeeding generation raised in the US. A study of southern Italian women in the North End of Boston in the late 1960s suggested what might be described as a one and a half generational retention of traditional beliefs after immigration. Women of the immigrant generation, largely from the regions of Abruzzi-Molise, Campania and Sicily, and their older American-born daughters raised before the Second World War tended to cling more strongly to traditional perceptions of illness and therapy because 'the older women . . . had been recipients or observers of the traditional folk cures in childhood or early adulthood more often than the younger second generation women'.[51] By contrast, those younger second-generation women who had begun to rear their children in the 1940s, 'at a time when effective therapy in the form of vitamins, immunisation and antimicrobial drugs had become generally available', largely avoided the religious aspects of *festas*.[52] Unlike the elderly, they did not 'view the roles of the saints and the physician as complementary', nor did they perceive recovery from illness as 'a miracle wrought by the timely intervention of both the saint and the doctor'.[53] Younger second-generation women tended to attach more importance than their mothers or older sisters to 'the skills and technology of modern medicine', although they, too, sometimes resorted to 'prayer and petition' in an extreme health crisis.[54] At times, traditional beliefs associated with the 'evil eye' as the cause of illness still found expression among all generations, but such beliefs were not pervasive and their prevalence was linked to an individual's class position and personality.

Such generational change was encouraging to modernising Italian physicians, although it often seemed too slow to those bitter over the sickness and suffering they could not spare their patients. In 1904, Dr Rocco Brindisi observed with some sympathy that 'Italians, like all peoples with ancient habits and traditions, cling to many prejudices and superstitions, which often hamper those who work with them'. Brindisi was confident that his countrymen were on the road to 'regeneration' and that he himself was an instrument of change through the healing and education he brought to fellow Italians. Brindisi stated that 'there was not the slightest doubt in my mind that the rising generation of our Italians will be, in regard to sanitary conditions, on the same level with the American people'.[55] While Brindisi's predictions were more or less correct, the path to conformity with the norms and practices of mainstream American medicine was uneven and sometimes took more than a generation or two. Strong cultural ties bound Italians to their unique definitions of health and the aetiology of disease that were integrated in a belief system that was a synthesis of Christian and pagan traditions. Italian immigrants' resistance to alien ways and their distrust of those who were unrelated to them by blood or birthplace proved a powerful obstacle to even well-meaning public health officers and reformers crusading against tuberculosis.

Given that full immigrant compliance with American standards of health and hygiene took so long to develop, it can be asked why compulsion was never employed, especially as immigrants were seen as a threat to the health of the majority? The advice offered in Carr's *Guide* could have been made mandatory and followed up by surveillance and other means of enforcement. In practice, Federal public health officers had no jurisdiction over immigrants once they had passed quarantine and the inspection on Ellis Island or some other immigration depot. State and municipal health officials, though they had the authority to take necessary actions in the interest of the public's health, were hampered by limited resources, public resistance and fears of infringing civil liberties. Only the fear of epidemic disease stirred these officials to intervene in the lives of individual citizens, and even then officials rarely imposed restrictions beyond quarantines and raised standards of public cleanliness. Public health officials did not follow individuals into their domiciles and make them adapt to particular standards of health or hygiene. The imposition of particular therapies was a violation of individual liberty and in those rare cases where the state sought to impose a therapy on an individual against their will, the courts refused to uphold the order.[56] While neither the American public nor the courts had many qualms about excluding individuals as health menaces at the point of immigration, those admitted were accorded the same privacy and civil liberties as American citizens. Tuberculosis was eventually curbed among the Italians as it was among other immigrant groups by changes in life-style and by systematic testing and drug therapies that had little to do with acculturation. The lesson of the Italian experience is that diseases such as tuberculosis, while bacteriological realities, are also constructed differently by different groups in society. These diverse social constructions shape how communities treat the victims of diseases and which therapies and preventives are regarded as legitimate.

POSTSCRIPT

The re-emergence of tuberculosis in the 1990s has seen once again the linkage of immigrants with this dread disease. It appears to epidemiologists that the foreign born are contributing disproportionately to high tuberculosis rates. A 1990 report from the Center for Disease Control and Prevention (CDC) noted that 'Foreign-born persons (as a group) residing in the US have higher rates of tuberculosis than persons born in the US.' In 1989, the overall US tuberculosis rate was 9.5 per 100,000 population; for foreign-born persons arriving in the US, the estimated case rate was 124 per 100,000. In the period 1986–9, 22 per cent (20,316) of all reported cases of tuberculosis occurred in the foreign-born population. A majority of foreign-born persons who develop tuberculosis do so within the first five years after they enter the US.[57] Particular counties and cities with high concentrations of recently arrived immigrants echo at local levels what the CDC gleans from its national data. In 1991, New York City reported a 38 per cent rise in the number of TB cases (3,520 cases up from 2,545 in 1989). Highest rates were in the African American community, which accounted for 58 per cent of the cases, with a rate of 129 per 100,000. However, 'the rate for Hispanic residents was 71.5; for Asians 62.1, and for whites 14.8'.[58] Similarly, Montgomery County, bordering the District of Columbia, had the highest rate of tuberculosis in the state of Maryland in 1992, a figure that county health officials attribute in part to the concentration of Asian and Hispanic resident immigrants. Lynn Frank, chief of communicable diseases and epidemiology for the Montgomery County Health Department, tied the spike in tuberculosis largely to 'the number of immigrants who are from countries where the incidence of the disease is much higher'.[59] Yvonne Richards, nurse manager for the county's refugee and migrant health programme, observed that, 'Poor nutrition, poor access to health care, and inappropriate medical treatment in their countries may have made many people more susceptible to TB'.[60]

In 1992, commenting on Haitian encounters with tuberculosis, Dr Jacques Mathieu of the Mount Sinai School of Medicine and the New York City Department of Health described a cultural negotiation not dissimilar from that involving Italian immigrants ninety years ago. He argues that a reliance on folk medicine and prayer to heal may explain the climbing morbidity rate. Hesitation to seek medical attention promptly in the absence of health insurance cannot be ignored. Some simply stop all medication when they feel well. Others are troubled by the appearance of the pills they are given. When the generic medication stocked by local clinics change, so do the colour of the pills, a change that causes some Haitians to become wary and stop their therapy.[61] Physicians fear that stopping a course of therapy before completion could result in mutations of the bacilli and the development of drug-resistant strains. Now, as in the past, public health officials are chary about using state power to impose therapy. In the interest of public health, active disease remains an excludable condition for immigrants, but in only twenty-four states and the District of Columbia can public health officers even detain those with active tuberculosis and impose treatment. The proper balance of patient rights and public health considerations is heatedly disputed among public officials. In reviewing anti-tuberculosis legislation, Lawrence O. Gostin, Professor of Health Law, Harvard, discovered that many states lacked guarantees to ensure that individuals who were forcibly confined while taking medication would have access to an attorney and a court hearing. Only twelve states, plus the District of Columbia, even protect the confidentiality of patients.[62] Some municipalities have made provision to detain tuberculosis patients who do not complete their treatment. However, resources are in short supply and this measure could require confinement of patients for more than a year. At one such facility in New York City, a riot among detainees called attention to the difficulties of incarcerating individuals who are not convicted criminals, even in the interest of the public's health.[63]

Sick, newly arrived immigrants are seen to contribute to a public health problem by their very presence in the community. Yet, by contrast with immigrants of an earlier era, newcomers from Latin America and Asia have not been widely castigated as health menaces. Health officials have been sympathetic to the victims of illness and sensitive to the potential for a nativist backlash triggered by alarm over public health. Undoubtedly physicians' ability to treat TB successfully has also prevented undue public hysteria. In 1992, the New York Task Force on Immigrant Health sponsored a round-table forum on tuberculosis. Participants agreed that 'it is important to not blame immigrants for the current TB epidemic in New York City'.[64] If fear of the foreign born and fear of illness are locked in a timeless embrace, public awareness of this pernicious partnership suggests the possibility of breaking that bond. The even more recent response to the plight of a 16-year-old Vietnamese girl at California's La Quinta High School suggests that some American health care professionals, albeit not all, are determined that the past should not repeat itself.

NOTES

1 This article is based in part on themes developed in A.M. Kraut, *Silent Travelers: Germs, Genes, and the ' Immigrant Menace'*, New York, 1994. Some of the material was also presented in a paper entitled, 'The *Mal'occhio* Versus Modern Medicine: The Challenge of Italian Health Traditions to Public Health in New York City a Century Ago', at the New York Academy of Medicine, 7 April 1994.
2 *New York Times*, 18 July 1994.
3 R. Mayo-Smith, *Emigration and Immigration: A Study in Social Science*, New York, 1890, p. 133.
4 E.A. Ross, *The Old World in the New: The Significance of Past and Present Immigration to the American People*, New York, 1914, p. 113.
5 L.I. Dublin and G.W. Baker, 'The Mortality of Race Stocks in Pennsylvania and New York,' reprinted from the *Quarterly Publication of the American Statistical Association*, March 1920, located in Papers and Speeches file of the Louis Dublin Papers at the Metropolitan Life Insurance Company Archives. Because Italian labourers with tuberculosis and other potentially fatal diseases frequently went home to Italy to die among friends and family, Dublin and Baker's data may be somewhat distorted. However, such distortion was probably insufficient to alter the larger pattern of lower mortality rates among the Italians than among the native born.
6 For a thorough description of this inspection process, see Kraut, *Silent Travelers*, pp. 50–77.
7 All data in the table was excerpted from Dublin and Baker, 'Mortality of Race'.
8 J.F. Carr, *Guide for the Immigrant Italian in the United States of America*, New York, 1911, rep. 1975.
9 Ibid., p. 38.
10 Ibid., p. 48.

11 Valuable historical studies of tuberculosis are: R. and J. Dubos, *The White Plague: Tuberculosis, Man, and Society*, 1952; rep., 1987; J.A. Myers, *Captain of All These Men of Death: Tuberculosis Historical Highlights*, St Louis, 1977; G.P. Youmans, *Tuberculosis*, Philadelphia, 1979. A useful study of the public health campaign against tuberculosis is M.E. Teller, *The Tuberculosis Movement: A Public Health Campaign in the Progressive Era*, Westport, Conn., 1988. An intriguing dissertation on the transformation of the tubercular patient's image from the romantic perception of the eighteenth and nineteenth centuries to the impoverished, wasted figure of the late nineteenth- and twentieth-century victim is N.M. McMurry, '"And I? I Am in a Consumption": The Tuberculosis Patient, 1780–1930', Ph.D. diss. Duke University, 1985. Even more recent is S. Rothman, *Living in the Shadow of Death, Tuberculosis and the Social Experience of Illness in American History*, New York, 1994.

12 The precise origins of the term 'white plague' are unclear. J. Arthur Myers claims that Oliver Wendell Holmes coined the term in 1891. See Myers, *Captain of All*, p. xi.

13 The eminent demographer of disease, Thomas McKeown, in his influential volume, *The Modern Rise of Population*, London, 1976, concluded that non-medical factors, particularly improvements in nutrition and other general aspects of the standard of living, contributed to the decline of infectious diseases, including tuberculosis. However, more recently, historian of medicine Leonard G. Wilson has argued that McKeown was mistaken and that the decline in TB mortality was a direct result of removing pulmonary tuberculosis patients from their families and co-workers to the confines of institutions, increasingly in the US to TB sanatoria. See L.G. Wilson, 'The Historical Decline of Tuberculosis in Europe and America: Its Causes and Significance', *Journal of the History of Medicine and Allied Sciences*, 1990, 45, pp. 366–96; and idem 'The Rise and Fall of Tuberculosis in Minnesota: The Role of Infection', *Bulletin of the History of Medicine*, 1992, 66, pp. 16–52.

14 Carr, *Guide for the Immigrant Italian*, p. 50.

15 Ibid., p. 51.

16 M. Van Kleeck, *Artificial Flower Makers*, New York, 1913.

17 Ibid., p. 92.

18 Ibid., p. 116.

19 Ibid., p. 93.

20 Ibid.

21 Ibid., p. 99.

22 This Italian family's combined annual income of $858 was typical of New York's working-class families. A Russell Sage Foundation sponsored study found 318 of 391 working families reporting incomes between $600 and $1,100 per year, with 57 per cent of the Italian families included in the study in this range. See R.C. Chapin, *The Standard of Living Among Workingmen's Families in New York City*, New York, 1909, p. 38.

23 Van Kleeck, *Artificial Flower Makers*, pp. 98–9.

24 H. White, 'Perils of the Home Factory', *Harper's Weekly*, 11 February 1911, p. 10.

25 Much of the material to follow is from P.H. Williams, *South Italian*

Folkways in Europe and America: A Handbook for Social Workers, Visiting Nurses, School Teachers, and Physicians, New Haven, Conn., 1938. This volume is one in a series published by the Institute of Human Relations at Yale University. The volume, designed to have practical application for those who would serve the Italian immigrant community, is a valuable study conducted in the best social scientific tradition of its era. In her preface, Williams explains how profoundly she has drawn upon work done in Italy compiling cultural traditions, including Dr Giuseppe Pitre's 25-volume study of popular Sicilian traditions, *Biblioteca delle Tradizioni Populari Siciliane*, Torino-Palermo, 1871–1913. Williams is also careful to note that the people whose folkways and mores she describes do not represent a cross-section of the Italians either in Italy or in the United States, but chiefly 'peasants and fishing folk' from the six southern states, including Sicily.

26 Williams, *South Italian Folkways*, p. 135. Williams observes that 'the word pagan is derived from *paganus*, meaning peasant or country dweller'.

27 A.T. Ragucci, 'Generational Continuity and Change in Concepts of Health, Practices, and Ritual Expressions of the Women of An Italian-American Enclave', Ph.D. diss., Boston University, 1971, pp. 9–10.

28 Williams, *South Italian Folkways*, p. 135.

29 Ibid., pp. 136–7.

30 G. Pitre, 'The Jettatura and the Evil Eye', trans. from *Biblioteca delle tradizioni Popolari Siciliane*, Vol. 17, *Usi e Custumi, Credenze e Pregiudizi del Popolo Siciliano*, 4, Palermo, 1889, pp. 235–49, in A. Dundes, ed., *The Evil Eye*, Madison, Wisc., 1992, pp. 130–42.

31 Williams, *South Italian Folkways*, p. 142.

32 Ibid., pp. 143–4.

33 J. Collins, *My Italian Year*, New York, 1910, p. 10. Also in Williams, *South Italian Folkways*, p. 145.

34 Williams, *South Italian Folkways*, p. 160.

35 Ibid., p. 162.

36 Ibid.

37 Most of the biographical data on Antonio Stella is drawn from *The National Cyclopaedia of American Biography*, New York, 1929, pp. 20, 80–1.

38 A. Stella, *Some Aspects of Italian Immigration to the United States: Statistical Data and General Considerations Based Chiefly Upon the United States Censuses and Other Official Publications*, New York, 1924, rep. 1975, p. 66.

39 Ibid., pp. 66–7.

40 Ibid., p. 68. The tendency that Stella describes may also have somewhat distorted the mortality data collected by statisticians such as Louis Dublin of the Metropolitan Life Insurance Company. However, it is unlikely that this tendency was as important as the youth and health of most Italian arrivals in accounting for ethnic differentials in mortality data. See note 5 above.

41 Ibid., p. 68.

42 A. Stella, 'Tuberculosis and the Italians in the United States', *Charities* 1904, 121, pp. 486–9. Also reprinted in L.F. Tomasi, *The Italian in*

America: The Progressive View, 1891–1914, New York, 1978, pp. 169–73.

43 W.H. Guilfoy, 'The Death Rate of the City of New York as Affected by the Cosmopolitan Character of Its Population', *Medical Record*, 1908, 74, p. 133.

44 Stella, 'Tuberculosis and the Italians,' p. 170.

45 Ibid., pp. 170–1.

46 Ibid., p. 171.

47 Commissariato dell' Emigrazione, *Bolletino dell' emigrazione*, no. 20, 1905, p. 28, also quoted by B.B. Caroli, *Italian Repatriation from the United States, 1900–1914*, New York, 1973, pp. 66–8.

48 Luigi Rossi as quoted in Caroli, *Italian Repatriation*, p. 68.

49 Williams, *South Italian Folkways*, p. 175.

50 M.M. Davis, Jr, *Immigrant Health and Community*, Montclair, NJ, 1971; orig. 1921, pp. 138–9.

51 Ragucci, 'Generational Continuity and Change', p. 268.

52 Ibid.

53 Ibid., p. 272.

54 Ibid.

55 R. Brindisi, 'The Italian and Public Health', *Charities*, 1904, 121, p. 486.

56 During the bubonic plague scare in San Francisco at the turn of the century, there was sufficient confusion in the language and circumstances to raise doubts over whether Chinese spokesmen and their legal counsel willingly and without coercion agreed to allow mandatory inoculation of Chinese with Haffkine's vaccine as federal officials maintained. However, federal Judge William Morrow ruled against the government's right to inoculate all Chinese as a violation of the equal protection clause of the Fourteenth Amendment. Kraut, *Silent Travelers*, pp. 91–2.

57 Centers for Disease Control, 'Tuberculosis Among Foreign-Born Persons Entering the United States, Recommendations of the Advisory Committee for Elimination of Tuberculosis', *Morbidity and Mortality Weekly Report*, 28 December 1990, 39, p. 1.

58 *New York Times*, 2 March 1991.

59 *Montgomery Journal*, 14–15 October 1992. I am most grateful to Lynn Frank for the information she shared with me in a telephone conversation about tuberculosis data in October 1992.

60 Ibid. I am also indebted to Yvonne Richards for her willingness to share available Montgomery County data with me.

61 Minutes of New York Task Force on Immigrant Health's Roundtable Forum, 'Tuberculosis in the Foreign-Born and in Puerto Ricans', 24 March 1992, p. 5.

62 L.O. Gostin, 'Controlling the Resurgent Tuberculosis Epidemic: A 50-State Survey of TB Statutes and Proposals for Reform', *Journal of the American Medical Association*, 1992, 269, pp. 255–61. Also, *Washington Post*, 13 January 1993.

63 M. Navarro, 'Four Patients At TB Center Are Arrested In Attack', *New York Times*, 27 January 1994, p. 8.

64 New York Task Force, 'Tuberculosis in the Foreign-born,' p. 6.

11

THE POWER OF THE EXPERTS

The plurality of beliefs and practices concerning health and illness among Bangladeshis in contemporary Tower Hamlets, London

John Eade

INTRODUCTION

This chapter describes the public debates about the health requirements of Bangladeshis principally, but not exclusively, in the borough of Tower Hamlets in London. I will argue that these debates have largely defined and treated Bangladeshi health needs in terms of formal health resources, quantitative data and biomedical models of disease, so while concerned with serious disabilities and health problems, remedies are sought only from within the professional structure of health provision. The beliefs and practices of 'ordinary people', such as Bangladeshi residents, are not sought and do not inform the debate. Such a failure to learn about Bangladeshi beliefs and practices continues a long-established and complex pattern. As Cornwell and Donovan have shown in their studies of health and illness among East London's residents, the distance between health professionals and patients is created by a system of knowledge and power where differences between people are reinforced by class and gender as well as ethnicity and race.[1] Similarly, repeated calls for improved health education, however well intentioned, fail to show an awareness of the crucial role played by non-medical discourses and practices among those whom health professionals wish to help. Without a real engagement with local people's beliefs and coping strategies, the delivery of more resources and schemes developed by health professionals also tend to proffer a one-sided solution.

In this chapter I explore the plurality of discourses and practices concerning health and illness caused by the co-existence of medical and non-medical beliefs and practices. My approach is to analyse the views advanced by other experts (religious and secular community leaders) who claim to speak for Bangladeshi residents in the UK, as well as the limited ethnographic material on the beliefs and practices of ordinary Bangladeshis. As I show, such sources reveal a picture of a diverse and sometimes conflicting world where health and illness are constructed in terms of the relationship between the human and spirit world, and where different experts propose their specific, ostensibly competing, remedies. In exploring this world it is clear that ethnic cultural traditions play an important role in the discourses and practices of health and illness. These cultural traditions can be defined as 'ethnic' because they refer to a country of origin (Bangladesh), language (standard Bengali and Sylheti dialect) and religion (Islam), but they are neither static nor uncontested by 'insiders' and 'outsiders'. Bangladeshis in Britain are engaged in social, economic, cultural and political changes which entail a conscious assessment of the uses to which 'traditions' brought from their country of origin can be put within a new context. Different practices concerning health and illness are caught up in this creative process of cultural reconstruction.

THE SETTLEMENT OF BANGLADESHIS IN BRITAIN

Like other settlers from the New Commonwealth, Bangladeshis came to this country in large numbers during the post-Second World War period.[2] The first generation arrived during the 1960s and early 1970s, their wives and dependants joining them afterwards – a process that gathered pace during the 1980s and which is still incomplete. While these immigrants joined other black and ethnic minority settlers in Britain's urban centres, they were much more heavily concentrated than the other minority groups in metropolitan London.[3] According to a Commission for Racial Equality survey in 1986, by the early 1980s, 44.7 per cent of the Bangladeshi population was located within the Greater London area and the only other areas of significant concentrations were in the West Midlands (14.2 per cent) and the north-west (11.4 per cent). The largest centre of Bangladeshi settlement was within Tower Hamlets in Greater London, where Bangladeshis comprised 9.2 per cent of the borough's inhabitants (12,596 persons). The next largest Bangladeshi settlement in Greater London was in Camden where they constituted 1 per cent of the total population.[4] Other urban areas showed similar concentrations – the Bangladeshis clustering in inner Birmingham within the West Midlands, and in Oldham in the north-west. The survey probably underestimated the numbers of Bangladeshis in Britain, as was suggested by the results of the 1991 Census. In Tower Hamlets, for example, the Census recorded 36,955 Bangladeshis (22.94 per cent) nearly three times the earlier estimate. However, part of the discrepancy was due to continuing settlement by wives and dependants as well as an increase in births. By the early 1990s, the Bangladeshi population in Tower Hamlets and across the country was a predominantly young population. Although Bangladeshis constituted nearly a quarter of the Tower Hamlets population, over half the borough's school population was Bangladeshi. In certain wards, the proportion of Bangladeshi residents had risen to 35 per cent and above (Spitalfields 61 per cent, St Mary's 42 per cent, St Dunstan's 38 per cent, Shadwell 36 per cent, St Katharine's 35 per cent) while the Bangladeshi proportion of the school population was undoubtedly higher.[5]

Most of these immigrants have arrived through a process of chain migration which has largely ensured that these settlers have come from a particular district of Bangladesh – Sylhet – and from certain constellations of villages within Sylhet. Migration to Britain as well as to the Middle East has been a long-established strategy for Bangladeshi families to improve their rural socio-economic status.[6]

The Bangladeshi population now comprises three generations. The first is relatively minute and its members are predominantly men who were *lascars* on ocean-going ships and who found work in manual

Table 11.1 Main concentrations of Bangladeshis in England and Wales c.1980

Inner London	71,016
West Midlands	18,074
Outer London	14,722
Greater Manchester	11,445
West Yorkshire	5,978
Bedfordshire	5,882
Tyne and Wear	2,772
South Glamorgan	1,671
Total	131,560
Total Bangladeshis in England and Wales	161,701

Source: Commission for Racial Equality, 1986

Table 11.2 Population of Bangladeshis in Tower Hamlets 1991 by ward

Ward	*Total population*	*Bangladeshis*	*Percentage*
Spitalfields	8,861	5,379	60.7
St Katharine's	13,807	4,824	34.9
St Dunstan's	10,015	3,757	37.5
Shadwell	10,038	3,565	35.5
St Peter's	10,360	2,383	23.0
St Mary's	5,659	2,351	41.5
Holy Trinity	9,410	2,269	24.1
Limehouse	8,476	1,683	19.8
Bromley	9,632	1,572	16.3
Redcoat	6,571	1,559	23.7
Millwall	13,771	1,082	7.8
Blackwall	4,780	875	1.8
Lansbury	8,383	753	8.9
St James'	5,940	721	12.1
East India	6,881	541	7.8
Bow	8,203	396	4.8
Grove	5,182	297	5.7
Park	5,302	201	4.0
Total	151,271*	34,208*	22.6

Source: 1991 Census
* These totals differ from another Census table I have relied on which gives 161,064 residents and 36,955 Bangladeshis.

occupations within industry, hotels, hospitals, shops and restaurants during the 1950s and 1960s. They have now largely retired or are unemployed. The second generation has also entered similar jobs in the local garment trade and service sector, but a small number have become white collar workers in the public sector. In local voluntary organisations this group is mounting a challenge to the claims of the first generation to represent the Bangladeshi community to outsiders.[7] Most of the second generation came to Britain during the 1970s as young children, but the third generation has largely been 'born and bred' in the East End and constitutes the most 'Westernised' section of the Bangladeshi population.

Social and economic changes in Sylhet in recent decades, and the consequences of migration itself, have resulted in ideological changes and reinterpretations of religious beliefs and practices in both Sylhet and migrant settlements across the world.[8] This can be most clearly seen within the wider context of Islamisation – a process that has been closely linked to political as well as social, cultural, ideological and economic changes. What emerges as a common theme is the essentialisation and reification of Islam, as powerful experts or high-status people define what are 'pure' or 'authentic' Islamic beliefs and practices.[9] In so doing they distance themselves from non-Islamic beliefs and practices espoused by their poorer neighbours. Despite such socio-economic differences in the reformulation or reinvention of Islam, this process has ramifications for all Bangladeshis since Islam is understood as a complete way of life that ideally transcends the divisions of wealth, status, gender, age and nationality. This process of Islamisation is, therefore, important in considering the ways in which the Bangladeshis approach health and illness in London and elsewhere. Later in this chapter I describe beliefs and practices around health and illness which can, in my view, be understood partly in terms of current debates about what it means to be a 'correct' or 'real' Muslim.

HEALTH AND ILLNESS BELIEFS AND PRACTICES

In considering health and illness, it is important to distinguish between three arenas in which beliefs and practices are formulated and sustained: medical, Islamic and folk. Following Kleinman, these spheres can be understood as containing and helping to construct 'distinct forms of social reality', i.e. they 'organise particular subsystems of socially legitimated beliefs, expectations, roles, relationships, transaction settings and the like'.[10] Too much emphasis should not be placed upon the boundaries between these arenas, nor upon their internal cohesion. Indeed, they are continually being contested and redefined in an ideological struggle over what are 'correct' beliefs and practices. Similarly, despite the formulations of experts, which is the focus here, individuals are not confined to a particular arena since they may make use of different beliefs and practices according to the situation in which they find themselves. Strategic choices between different social realities and arenas can be made by Bangladeshis and others within structures where inequalities are shaped by class, gender, 'race' and ethnicity. In this respect the Bangladeshis are not some exotic 'other' – they are similar to local non-Bangladeshi residents in their engagement with different arenas and models of social reality.[11] Within this commonality, people express their engagement in somewhat different ways according to the situation and through reference to particular cultural constructions and practices.[12]

With these reservations in mind the three categories can be defined broadly in the following way. First, the medical model emphasises the analysis and treatment of *disease* and treats the body as a physical entity whose functioning can be objectively and rationally investigated without, for example, recourse to non-medical criteria shaped by religious belief systems. This paradigm has dominated the training of health professionals who are taught to interpret *illness* and the symptoms presented by patients accordingly. However, this model is not uncontested as is revealed by recent debates among various levels of the health professional sector over 'alternative' practices and perspectives, and in recent attempts to reform the medical curriculum. Much of this struggle can be located within the hierarchical structure of health provision where medical orthodoxy is 'usually associated with the medical schools and with acute hospital medicine rather than with general practice, chronic care, or preventive medicine'.[13]

Second, Islamic models of health and illness are similarly contested, with religious experts offering interpretations of 'correct' Islamic belief and practice. These teachings are grounded in understandings of the *Quran* and *Hadith* (traditional sayings of the Prophet Muhammad) and subsequent authoritative texts. *Unani* medicine is the official body of Islamic medical knowledge rooted in the writings of Hakim Ibn Sina (Avicenna) and located within a humoural model of the body.[14] However, what local religious leaders describe as Islamic practice refers less to this highly specialised, historic body of knowledge and more to what they define as Islamic in the context of current ideological debates that elaborate 'a "new traditionalism", an increasing Puritanism which seeks to reject the old, localised [syncretic] ways'.[15]

Third, there are the folk beliefs and practices of Bangladeshis that have developed in the context of these local, syncretic customs. In the Sylhet countryside the customs have to do with beliefs in spirits (*bhut*, *petni*), sorcery and witchcraft which cut across religious boundaries, especially those between Muslims and Hindus. Cults focusing on the shrines of holy men (*pir*) celebrate the miraculous and the ecstatic.[16] Other folk remedies are available to villagers through the services of midwives (*datri*), magicians (*ojja*), herbalists (*kabiraj*), itinerant holy men (*fakir*) and religious teachers (*mullah*).[17] Their expertise is sought especially in the areas of physical and social danger, i.e. pregnancy, birth, early childhood and death. These folk beliefs and practices are particularly sought by poorer families and, to some extent, by women regardless of class. While Muslim religious leaders describe these beliefs and customs as unIslamic, in both Syhlet and

London these syncretic folk beliefs and practices have been given an 'Islamic' reinterpretation. Thus *pir*ism and other cultic practices are reconstructed by the powerful and wealthy in terms of what they define as religious correctness.[18] Such reinterpretations are largely developed by high-status males and directed towards the traditional users of folk remedies – women in general as well as poor, low-status people.

I have presented the three types of belief system as though they were distinct. The differences between them are frequently emphasised by the various experts – at least in the context of medical and Islamic models. None the less, as Gardner warns in her discussion of Islamic reformism and the mystical *pir* cults in the Sylhet countryside, 'rather than being discrete and bounded, there are numerous cross-over points between the different modes of faith'.[19] We are dealing here with various elements that can be presented as belonging to different models for analytical purposes while in people's understandings they may not be so clearly separated.

During the 1980s the emergence of a vigorous group of second-generation Bangladeshi community activists was encouraged by the expansion of public sector support for black and ethnic minority needs in various areas, for example housing, education, youth provision as well as health and welfare. The Greater London Council (GLC) and the Inner London Education Authority (ILEA) was in the vanguard of this movement, but such support also came, albeit unintentionally, from central government through the Department of the Environment and the Department of Health and Social Security in particular. A complex political struggle involved local community groups, the borough council, GLC, ILEA and central government as different political factions began to court the support of competing Bangladeshi groups and leaders.[20] In this context, during the 1980s a number of conferences and workshops were held and reports produced detailing Bangladeshi needs and demands. As I have already argued, these needs were largely defined in terms of health provision and resources. In accordance with this, solutions are viewed as being achievable largely through ascertaining the particular health needs of the Bangladeshi community, which in turn would enable a proper delivery of health services for this group to be developed.

A classic example of this approach can be found in the Tower Hamlets Health Inquiry Report of 1987. It was produced by a collection of senior medical practitioners, community health specialists, a medical sociologist (Jocelyn Cornwell) and distinguished representatives of various interest groups including Kumar Murshed from the Bangladeshi community.[21] After discussing the demography of the borough and introducing two categories of people, the elderly and children, where deprivation was particularly serious, the Report discussed health in relation to employment, unemployment and social class, and lastly focused on ethnicity, racism and health. Referring to a recent training handbook for health professionals, the Report described the way in which health professionals' ignorance concerning 'the needs of minority ethnic groups' can 'increase the danger of under diagnosis and misdiagnosis' for such groups.[22] This point was illustrated by reference to 'religious or cultural customs' and to the difficulties 'Muslim women' face with a male doctor. Drawing on Donovan's research in Newham, the authors emphasise the importance of avoiding 'victim-blaming' with rickets and criticise the DHSS suggestion that Asians should 'spend more time outside and westernise their food'.[23] Similarly they argue that the high incidence of underweight babies may be due not necessarily to mothers' inadequate antenatal measures, but to 'a lack of knowledge about antenatal facilities, unfamiliarity with transport and language barriers', and stress that it was 'up to the health service to provide appropriate facilities'.[24] The section of the Report that deals specifically with the Bangladeshis relies heavily on a study by the House of Commons Home Affairs Committee that attributed the high levels of deprivation experienced by Bangladeshis in terms of 'their recent arrival from a rural peasant society to an urban industrial society, their poor command of English and discrimination'.[25] Other socio-economic factors are addressed in the Report (e.g. homelessness, unemployment, overcrowding) and the issue of mental health was eventually raised with isolation and racial attack, language difficulties, and the lack of 'Bengali speaking' health professionals.[26] The bulk of the document deals with the relationship between socio-economic factors and the structure of the health service in the borough, viz. housing, environment, primary health care services, priority services and care in the community, hospital services and the race awareness programme. The last chapter made general recommendations that concentrated on improving the level of resources and their delivery.

A similar approach was adopted in a more recent report produced by the Camden and Islington Health Authority. Whereas the Tower Hamlets Health Inquiry did not explicitly address the crucial issue of 'needs', the 1993 report virtually began with a definition that significantly concentrated on health provision:

> Needs commonly implies the ability to benefit from an intervention or service provided. Measurement of need requires knowledge of the size of the health problem in a local population, the burden both social and economic on that population and the impact that a service or intervention is likely to have. Needs assessment examining the health and health care needs of black and minority ethnic people is necessary because of the unique problems faced by this population in terms of health, lifestyles and access to health care.[27]

In the following section, on the sources used in needs assessment, the importance of 'listening to local voices' is mentioned, but in the subsequent six chapters of the report these local voices appear to be principally those belonging to community groups and representatives.[28]

While I am not denying the importance of the issues raised by community representatives, clearly this report was a typical example of the way in which questions and answers are framed within terms set by health professionals and by their relationship with other professionals. These assume an unproblematic relationship between needs as defined by health professionals and by those outside the health service. Furthermore, it illustrated the presumption that needs can be defined and quantified objectively. Other modes of discourse concerning need and the complex, differentiated character of people's lifestyles did not impinge on this agenda. Providers of health services were encouraged to learn about black and ethnic minority lifestyles, but the rare references to 'religious and cultural customs' of ethnic minority citizens did not convey the variety of discourses and practices concerning health and illness as described in the preceding section.

The scant attention paid to religious and cultural traditions is, in one sense, not surprising given the lack of careful research so far undertaken in Britain on black and ethnic minority beliefs and practices concerning health and illness. This contrasts with the large number of studies published by medical sociologists and anthropologists on health and illness issues in South Asia. Epidemiological studies and discussions of racism[29] in the UK have not been matched by ethnographic explorations of non-medical discourses and practices. While researchers have discussed some aspects of South Asian beliefs and practices, few of them have provided searching examinations of non-medical systems that dispense with standard clinical questionnaires and interpreters and rely on qualitative data collected through participant observation with 'ordinary' people.[30] Such a stress on the importance of hearing the views of 'ordinary' people and not dismissing them as 'ignorant' or 'superstitious', while clear in the ethnographic literature on non-medical health beliefs and practices in South Asia and Britain, have not been given official sanction. This has meant that their voices have often been ignored and challenges to the power of expert knowledge have rarely been permitted.

MUSLIM BELIEFS AND PRACTICES AROUND HEALTH AND ILLNESS: ISLAMISATION AND THE VIEWS OF THE EXPERTS

During the 1980s the rapid formation and elaboration of a Bangladeshi community infrastructure encouraged the emergence of a public debate concerning the 'needs' of Bangladeshis as Muslims. The debate was spurred by local and more global developments, i.e. the growth of Muslim community organisations, mosques and prayer halls supported by national and international Islamic organisations as well as changing local political alliances especially after the defeat of the Labour Party in the borough elections of 1986. In the local political arena much of this debate took the form of disputes over prayer hall facilities and the functions of mosques,[31] as well as appeals for greater sensitivity to the needs of Bangladeshi Muslim students in the educational sector.[32] Such local conflicts were related to wider controversies over Salman Rushdie's book *The Satanic Verses*, political and ideological developments in the 'heartland' of the Muslim world (the Middle East) and in South Asia, as well as military confrontations in the Gulf War and in Bosnia. In addition, there was the process of Islamisation, a reformist movement that has a global character connecting local communities across national boundaries through the flow of both peoples and information. Within Tower Hamlets the elaboration of Islamic institutions and discourses was demonstrated by the establishment of mosques, *madrassahs* and prayer halls, the growth of Muslim youth groups and missionary activists, the increasing pressure for 'Muslim schools' and a trend towards female 'covering up' through the wearing of scarves, cardigans, overcoats and even *burqa*.

Certain religious leaders also provided for the health needs of Bangladeshis through the provision of folk remedies. These were practices, however, that few secular community leaders knew about or were prepared to acknowledge to white outsiders. Such reticence is not shared by everyone, however, and a conference held in May 1992 indicated that some were prepared to discuss formally the issue of non-medical (Islamic and folk) beliefs and practices among Bangladeshi residents.[33] The conference was organised by the Community Mental Health Team, and professionals and community workers representing local black and ethnic minority groups were invited to discuss 'cultural practices and professional issues concerning service delivery'. Since most of the participants were Bangladeshis or were professionally involved in the delivery of health services to Bangladeshis, discussions inevitably ranged over issues that concerned them in particular. One of the themes that emerged was the relevance of Islam to discussions about service needs and the role of religious experts in providing for those requirements.

Part of the debate was provoked by a paper from a local *imam* that contrasted the low level of Islamic knowledge and the 'superstitious' customs held by most local Bangladeshis with what he believed to be correct Islamic beliefs and practices concerning health and illness:

> The majority are not well acquainted with Islamic knowledge. What information they have usually comes from local *Imams* (ministers of religion), *pirs* (saintly people), and traditions passed through the generations. Superstitions also play a great role in the life of these settlers.

He then proceeded to describe some of these superstitious beliefs and practices:

> (a) *Wind* Some Bangladeshis believe that if someone [has] bad wind it will affect him or her both physically and mentally. At first the person will experience pains in certain parts of the body, and gradually it engulfs the whole body, resulting in mental restlessness.
> (b) *Bad spirits* (*Bhut*) It is a widely held belief among Bangladeshis that *Bhut* (ghosts) or bad spirits affect certain people and cause immense mental disorder, which in turn affects the body as well.
> (c) *Jinn (supernatural bodies composed of vapour or flame) [Encyclopaedia of Islam] Jinn* possesses certain people, who either become speechless, or talk in a foul way. Such people will act in an unusual manner.

(d) *Black magic, etc.* The curse of an enemy, bad dreams and the shade of some unseen beings are also widely believed by Bangladeshis to have adverse mental effects, with noticeable physical consequences.

The *imam* then described the experts in this area of non-medical healing:

> When affected by any of the above, people will turn to a *Mulla* (religious teacher) for healing; he will write Qur'anic verses on a piece of paper, and fold it round for the patient to wear on the affected part of the body. This prescription of amulets is called *tawiz*, and prescribed on almost every occasion of mental or physical problems.
>
> There are other types of healers:
>
> *Pir/Fakir (a saintly person)* – who will blow over water after a recital of the Qur'an and the patient will drink the water. Both the *mulla* and the *pir* also seek to cure people by placing a hand on the affected part of the body, whilst reciting verses from the Qur'an. The *mulla* also writes verses on a piece of paper which could be put into a bowl of water and left overnight, to be drunk the following morning.
>
> *Exorcist, sorcerer, magician* – these people have peculiar practices for healing a possessed or otherwise affected person. The exorcist gives the person hot chilli powder, which is poured down the throat; mustard oil is put in the eyes and nose, and the person is beaten with sticks so that the *jinn* or evil spirit will wither away.
>
> *Kabiraj (herbalist)* – an expert in Ayurvedi medicine who prescribes herbs that are expected to heal the patient.

After describing the heterodox traditions of folk medicine the *imam* depicted what he considers to be the 'Islamic view on the causes and practices' concerning illness. According to him a belief in *jinn* and the evil eye is Islamically acceptable. Thus he states:

> As far as the causes of mental illness are concerned, there is no denial of the fact that the existence of *jinn* [and the] effect of bad [evil] eye are mentioned in the Quran and the sayings of the Prophet of Islam [*Hadith*]. Human beings, however mighty and protected they may be, are vulnerable to supernatural power.

On the other hand, the *imam* regarded the belief in *bhut* and the practice of sorcery ('curse by enemy') as definitely unIslamic. While, as he argued, black magic has existed 'from time immemorial' and affected the Prophet Muhammad, to 'make tawiz or blow in water or the practice of exorcism [has] no sanction in Islam'. Moreover, the *imam* claimed that practitioners such as 'pir, ojja, witchcrafter, sorcerer' are unacceptable since they 'are in the business of making their living out of the majority of Bangladeshi people'.

One of the interesting aspects of the *imam*'s comments was his dismissal, *inter alia*, of *pirs*, especially since Gardner has shown in the context of Sylhet that the role of *pirs* is being reinterpreted or reinvented. Distinctions are made by reformist Muslims between 'good' *pirs* and 'those who are *marifot* – or part of an ecstatic, tantric tradition'.[34] One young reformist student, for example, described those who followed the ecstatic tantric tradition in the following terms:

> Bad pirs are those who play music for prayer. For us this is bad; we call them pretender pirs. There's one like that I know of, who smokes ganja, drinks, and plays drums and sings as he prays.[35]

Good *pirs* were understood in terms of a purism that is largely defined 'not so much by what it represents, but more by what it opposes',[36] i.e. 'activities which are closer to Hindu or tantric [ecstatic] practices than those of Sunni orthodoxy'.[37]

Having described these beliefs and practices, the *imam* offered his own suggestions about improving health provision to local Bangladeshis. He advised doctors to be discerning about their patients' beliefs, 'as everything held by the patient is not superstition, the blanket rejection of all ideas . . . will be counter-productive'. Rather the role of the doctor should be to try gradually 'to dispel the superstitions from the mind of the patient by acceding to some of his ideas as facts'. In accordance with this he stresses that patients should be given 'religious counselling and spiritual advice' and that the assistance of religious leaders should be enlisted to counter the activities of unIslamic healers.

Not surprisingly perhaps, given the background of most participants at the conference, the paper led to a vigorous and sometimes impassioned debate. A senior Asian psychiatrist strongly objected to the idea that any religious specialist should intervene between the health practitioner and the patient. However, a number of speakers supported the paper's emphasis on the role that Islamic teachings and

Muslim leaders could play in health provision. During the debate it also became clear that some drew a very firm line between religion and culture. According to some contributors, Muslims should, in effect, purify their religious beliefs and practices from the influence of non-Islamic (implicitly Hindu) cultural traditions inherited from their country of origin.

The establishment of a superordinate Islamic identity over all others has important implications for the delivery of health resources, as Khalida Khan makes clear in *Q News*, which proudly calls itself 'Britain's first Muslim weekly'.[38] In reviewing a study of South Asian women and mental health in Bristol undertaken by Steven Fenton and Azra Sadiq, Khalida Khan applauds the authors for acknowledging religion in their study.[39] None the less, Khan proceeds to claim that, 'By mixing up the women in a multi-religious pot the study ends by dangerously diluting the severity of the problem particularly within the Muslim community.' She argues that while the importance of religion to the women was recognised by Fenton and Sadiq, they 'cop out: "religion" is conveniently substituted by "culture"'. The consequence of this substitution is that the authors 'are hardly explaining to unaware professionals where the crucial differences lie'. If drop-in centres, for example, are provided

> on ethnic/racial lines such as 'Asian' and 'Afro-Caribbean' then as far as Muslims are concerned at least, the study might as well have not been carried out because facilities provided on a racial basis misses out the Muslim community, splitting it on racial lines (other Muslim women from other racial origins also share the experience of South Asian Muslim women but are excluded) and are useless in resolving their practical problems.[40]

The prioritisation of Islam over other social identities is a discursive process that is evident in more academic debates concerning ethnicity and race.[41] The question raised by this process is the extent to which constructions of Islam as devised by experts and others who claim to know what Islam 'really' means are shared by 'ordinary' people. The process of Islamisation involves many contested themes and 'Islam' can mean various things to different kinds of people. So far we lack detailed evidence to assess how far this process has developed among Bangladeshis in Tower Hamlets, although some insight can be gained from local studies as well as reports in other parts of the country.[42] Despite the Islamic reformism of religious leaders, journalists, community workers and others who represent

Bangladeshis and Islam to outsiders, the *imam*'s comments at the conference indicate that there is a continuing market for the kinds of 'superstitious' services that were denounced at earlier meetings of experts. Other evidence is provided by references to consultations with 'a Hakim or Priest' by Craissati and to the belief in 'bad eye' by Dr Dutt, a local GP.[43]

During my research on other issues in Tower Hamlets during the last twelve years I have gained second-hand information about these non-medical beliefs and practices. Bangladeshi and white welfare workers over the years have discussed their experiences of working with Bangladeshi clients and I have talked to two experts in particular – a Bangladeshi GP and the son of a celebrated local Muslim healer/ *mullah*. The account provided by the *mullah*'s son closely conformed to what other people had told me. His father apparently used a wide range of techniques – blowing over water (*phani phura*), blowing directly at painful parts of the body, touching the sources of pain and spreading honey which had been blessed on affected areas, or the drinking of water which contained a piece of paper on which had been written an appropriate extract from Qur'an. Evidently this *mullah*'s understanding of what was correct Islamic practice differed from the religious leader who contributed to the 1992 health conference and the difference may well have been due to divergences of interpretation between *barelvi* and *deobandi* traditions.[44]

Both religious experts, however, were agreed that witchcraft and sorcery were unIslamic as was the belief in *bhut*. Their denunciation of sorcery is particularly interesting because while beliefs in *jinn* and *bhut* refer to supernatural beings who act largely independently of human beings, sorcery locates misfortune in a social world of envy and competition. In the West and other areas of the world, sorcerers are credited with 'the power to manipulate and alter natural and supernatural events with the proper magical knowledge and performance of ritual'.[45] Those initiating sorcery were to be found within the kinship network, and in at least one area of rural Bangladesh the immediate causes were largely economic since envy 'changes into outright jealousy and unconcealed malice when a previously poor family gradually improves its economic position and starts to compete with the rich in money, wealth and power'.[46]

Admittedly our knowledge about alternative healing beliefs and practices among Bangladeshis in Tower Hamlets and other areas of Britain is very sketchy. However, Khanum's pioneering study in 'Ochingram', north England[47] confirms the impression that many of the beliefs and practices that Gardner has described in the context of rural Sylhet have been transferred to this country. The extent to which they are maintained in Britain appears to be shaped by generation, education and social status. Khanum makes much of the status differential between *borolok* (wealthy people) and *chotolok* (low-status, poor people). The same division was pointed out by two Bangladeshi professionals at the 1992 health conference discussed above. In their paper on Bangladeshi women they distinguished between the *chotolok* who was 'literally "the small person" – working class or peasant' and the *borolok* or '"the big person" – middle class or landed gentry'. They argue that 'given that class is so pervasive it is surprising that this is rarely picked up on as an issue by practitioners'.[48] The way in which class differences are related to the process of Islamisation has yet to be explored. My discussions over the years with Bangladeshis who have entered white collar jobs in local government, education and the health and welfare sector suggest that they attach greater significance to professional discourses concerning secular issues than do Bangladeshis outside this particular arena.

The influence of these secular discourses was illustrated in the same paper which discussed class above. The authors considered the involvement of Bangladeshi women in such issues as racist immigration laws, family structure, marital relations, isolation and depression, and links with the outside world. Racism was a persistent theme in this account, the authors concluding their survey with the argument that 'the centrality of race needs to be more explicitly acknowledged in the assessment process and cultural explanations need to be considered in the context of racism'. The relevance of this argument to 'ordinary' people's assessments of needs would have to be assessed in terms of detailed research into what 'ordinary' people are thinking and doing about secular and religious issues.

As the conference paper makes clear, issues confronting Bangladeshis in Tower Hamlets have to be considered in the context of not only racism but also gender. It should have become obvious by now that all the different modes of non-medical healing involve male experts treating a large proportion of women and young children. Gardner has pointed to the ways in which these beliefs and practices contribute to the social control of females and help to sustain the power of male elders.[49] Everyday practices described as *purdah* are also relevant, given their emphasis on 'protecting' the female from an alien outside world. Significantly, evil *jinns* and *bhuts* are most likely to assault women and young children in dangerous places beyond the household. Moreover, loose hair and clothing could attract the amoral and lustful *bhut*. Males, of course, are not excluded from this moral world of close physical and social control in rural Bangladesh at least. Modesty, proper conduct with others, especially women, and strict observance of Islamic beliefs and practices are seen as helping but do not ensure freedom from spirit possession and sorcery for adult males.

CONCLUSION

This chapter has focused on official discourses developed by 'experts' who are involved in the provision of health and welfare services to 'ordinary' people. While we learn only indirectly about the beliefs and practices of those whom they are supposed to serve, there is clearly a wide divergence between official and lay discourses and procedures. 'Experts' sometimes reveal an awareness to this divergence, but they are not led thereby to question the principles on which their judgements about health and illness are made: they prefer to 'educate' lay people into a 'correct' understanding of what to believe and do.

The discourses of the 'experts' do not, of course, form a unitary whole. We have seen a crucial divide between 'secular' providers of health services and the 'religious' leader who advanced his understanding of correct Islamic belief and practice. However, it is also evident that tactical alliances are struck between these different experts where their interests converge, as in the religious leader's proposal to act as a Muslim 'chaplain' – an intermediary between the medical experts and the Muslim patient whose 'superstitious' ideas could be purified during the healing process. To what extent Bangladeshi professionals supported this Islamising process remains unclear, but evidently some did (perhaps partly for their own tactical reasons). The 1992 conference that the religious leader addressed was organised by the Community Mental Health Team and was attended by health professionals who serviced the 'needs' of Bangladeshis and other 'ethnic minorities' in Tower Hamlets.

The definition of lay people's 'needs' could, therefore, be defined by 'experts' in terms of both secular health and welfare provision (principally through the institutional structure of the National Health Service) and Islamic resources based on local mosques, *madrassahs* (schools for Islamic teaching) and prayer halls. Medicalisation and Islamisation are categories that can be used to describe the ways in which 'experts' construct the 'needs' of others in the context of these different institutional structures. These constructions are not necessarily coherent, nor are they uncontested, since 'experts' disagree with each other concerning 'correct' medical or Islamic practice. The line that the religious leader wished to draw between Islamic and unIslamic belief and practice, for example, could be challenged by other Muslim providers of health services who relied on folk remedies and yet claimed to be acting in an appropriately Islamic manner.

These different claims to know what is right and proper are constructed in the context of the power and distribution of institutional resources to local populations. Bangladeshi secular and religious 'experts' occupy less prestigious positions within the hierarchy of secular welfare institutions, while they are seen as powerful gatekeepers to official healing resources by lay Bangladeshis. The position of these 'experts', however, is always open to challenge from other Bangladeshis who draw on 'unIslamic' folk beliefs and practices (the *pir*, *fakir*, exorcist, sorcerer, magician and herbalist). 'Ordinary' Bangladeshis evidently adopt the strategy of other lay people within this country – try different 'experts' and different remedies and do not bother too much with the boundaries that a doctor or a *mullah* try to place around their particular treatments.

The ways in which Bangladeshi settlers in Tower Hamlets and other areas of Britain approach health and illness reveal the dynamic, contested process of cultural construction as traditions are adapted to the conditions of urban life in Western Europe. I have been uncomfortably aware throughout of the danger of presenting folk beliefs and practices as exotica and confirming racist stereotypes about uneducated 'immigrants'. I wish to repeat that the existence of non-medical beliefs and practices are not particular to Bangladeshis and other 'ethnic minorities' in this country. 'White' people also occupy a plural, contested world of diverse beliefs and practices concerning the body. These beliefs and practices are shaped by more than ethnic, cultural processes, and therefore people move within a world where boundaries of class, gender, racisms and nationalisms cut across ethnic frontiers. Different, exclusivist ideological claims to pure belonging may be made, but the people whom they wish to contain within these ideological territories are not so easily captured. In this chapter we have seen the 'experts' engaged in the ideological work of representing to other 'experts' what their 'community' needs. Further research is now needed to show how lay people accept and resist these claims to know what their needs really are.

NOTES

1 J. Cornwell, *Hard Earned Lives*, London, 1984, and J. Donovan, *We Don't Buy Illness, It Just Comes*, Aldershot, 1986.

2 S. Carey and A. Shokur, 'A Profile of the Bangladeshi Community in East London', *New Community*, 1985–6 12/3, pp. 405–29; J. Eade, *The Politics of Community: The Bangladeshi Community in East London*, Aldershot, 1989; Y. Choudhury, *The Roots and Tales of Bangladeshi Settlers*, Birmingham, 1993; K. Gardner and A. Shukur, ' "I'm Bengali, I'm Asian, and I'm Living Here": The Changing Identity of British Bengalis', in R. Ballard, ed., *Desh Pardesh: The South Asian Presence in Britain*, London, 1994.

3 I am using the terms black and ethnic minority to describe those who have settled in Britain and are seen as different by the majority of the population on the basis of 'race' and/or culture. Racism plays a large part in popular definitions of majority/minority boundaries but I will focus here on ethnicity as a dynamic, cultural process.

4 Commission for Racial Equality, *Ethnic Minorities in Britain: Statistical Information on the Pattern of Settlement*, London, 1986, p. 7.

5 Tower Hamlets Education Strategy Group, *Ethnic Background of Pupil Population*, Tower Hamlets, 1993, pp. 2–3.

6 K. Gardner, 'Mullahs, Migrants, Miracles: Travel and Transformation in Sylhet', *Contributions to Indian Sociology*, 1993, 27/2, pp. 213–35, and K. Gardner, *Global Migrants, Local Lives: Travel and Transformation in Rural Bangladesh*, Oxford, 1995.

7 Carey and Shokur, 'Bangladeshi Community'; C. Adams, *Across Seven Seas and Thirteen Rivers*, London, 1987; Eade, *Politics of Community*.

8 Gardner, 'Mullahs, Migrants, Miracles'.

9 M. Abaza and G. Stauth, 'Occidental Reason, Orientalism, Islamic Fundamentalism: A Critique', in M. Albrow and E. King, eds, *Globalization, Knowledge and Society*, London, 1990.

10 A. Kleinman, 'Concepts and a Model for the Comparison of Medical Systems as Cultural Systems', in C. Currer and M. Stacey, eds, *Concepts of Health, Illness and Disease*, New York, 1986, pp. 33–4.

11 J. Eade and M. Albrow, 'Constructing New Identities in a Globalised World', unpublished paper given at the World Congress of Sociology, University of Bielefeld, July 1994.

12 J. Craissati, 'Stress and Coping in a Bangladeshi Community', unpublished Dissertation, B.P.S. Leicester, 1988.

13 Cornwell, *Hard Earned Lives*, p. 121.

14 H. Chishti, *The Traditional Healer*, Wellingborough, 1988, p. 11.

15 Gardner, 'Mullahs, Migrants, Miracles', p. 223.

16 Ibid., pp. 227–8.

17 M. Islam, *Women, Health and Culture*, Dacca, 1985; T. Blanchet, *Meanings and Rituals of Birth in Rural Bangladesh*, Dhaka, 1984.

18 Gardner, 'Mullahs, Migrants, Miracles', p. 229.

19 Ibid., p. 232.

20 Eade, *Politics of Community*, and idem, 'Nationalism and the Quest for Authenticity', *New Community*, 1990, 16/4, pp. 493–503.

21 Kumar Murshed was a long-established community activist from the second generation who has taken a leading role in local campaigns concerning Bangladeshi health and educational issues. He was a non-executive member of the Tower Hamlets Health Authority for six years, during which time he set up and chaired the Equal Opportunities Implementation Committee.

22 Tower Hamlets Health Inquiry, *Report*, Tower Hamlets, 1987, p. 8.

23 Ibid., p. 9.

24 Ibid.

25 Ibid., p. 10.

26 Ibid., pp. 10–11.

27 Camden and Islington Health Authority, *Health Needs Assessment of Black and Minority Ethnic People in Camden and Islington*, Department of Public Health, Camden and Islington Health Authority, 1993.

28 *Health Needs Assessment*, p. 4.

29 R. Cochrane, F. Hashmi and M. Stopes-Roe, 'Measuring Psychological Disturbance in Asian Immigrants to Britain', *Social Science and Medicine*, 11, 1977, pp. 157–64; P. McKeigue et al., 'Diet and Risk Factors for Coronary Disease in Asians in Northwest London', *Lancet*, 1985, pp. 1086–9; P. McKeigue et al., 'Diabetes, Hyperinsulinaemia and Coronary Risk Factors in Bangladeshis in East London', *British Heart Journal*, 1988, 60/5, pp. 390–6; Craissati, 'Stress and Coping'; B. MacCarthy and J. Craissati, 'Ethnic Difference in Response to Adversity: A Community Sample of Bangladeshis and their Indigenous Neighbours', *Social Psychiatry and Psychiatric Epidemiology*, 1989, 24, pp. 196–201; B. Ineichen, 'The Mental Health of Asians in Britain', *British Medical Journal*, 1990, 330, pp. 1669–70; J. Beliappa, *Illness or Distress? Alternative Models of Mental Health*, London, 1991; S. Fernando, *Mental Health, Race and Culture*, London, 1991; P. McKeigue, 'Patterns of Health and Disease in the Elderly from Minority Ethnic Groups' in A. Squires, ed., *Multi-cultural Healthcare and Rehabilitation of Older People*, London, 1991.

30 The few studies that do engage with the accounts of 'ordinary' Southern Asian people include C. Currer, 'Concepts of Mental Well- and Ill-being: The Case of Pathan Mothers in Britain', in C. Currer and M. Stacey, eds, *Concepts of Health, Illness and Disease: A Comparative Perspective*, Oxford, 1986; G. Ahmed and S. Watt, 'Understanding Asian Women in Pregnancy and Confinement', *Midwives Chronicle and Nursing Notes*, 1986, pp. 98–101; S. Dobson, 'Cultural Awareness: Glimpses into a Punjabi Mother's World', *Health Visitor*, 59, 1986, pp. 382–4; I.-B. Krause, 'The Sinking Heart: A Punjabi Communication of Distress', *Social Science and Medicine*, 1989, 29, pp. 563–75; G. Dutt, 'Stresses in the Bangladeshi Community in the U.K.', *Practice News*, 1993, 4, pp. 5–7; S. Khanum, '"We Just Buy Illness in Exchange for Hunger": Experiences of Health Care, Health and Illness among Bangladeshi Women in Britain', Unpublished Ph.D. thesis, University of Keele, 1994.

31 Eade, 'Nationalism', pp. 493–503; idem, 'The Political Articulation of Community and the Islamisation of Space', in R. Barot, ed., *Religion and Ethnicity: Minorities and Social Change in the Metropolis*, Kampen, The Netherlands, 1993.
32 See G. Wemyss, 'The Politics of Multiculturalism and Equal Opportunities in a College of Education', Unpublished M.A. dissertation, University of Sussex, 1992.
33 *Report of Tower Hamlets Community Mental Health Team Conference*, 1992.
34 Gardner, 'Mullahs, Migrants, Miracles', p. 228.
35 Ibid.
36 Ibid., p. 227.
37 Ibid., p. 223.
38 *Q. News*, 1993, 1/44.
39 S. Fenton and A. Sadiq, *Sorrow in My Heart*, London, 1993.
40 *Q News*, 1993, 1/44.
41 See, for example, T. Modood, '"Black", Racial Equality and Asian Identity', *New Community*, 1988, 14/3, pp. 397–404; T. Modood, 'British Asian Muslims and the Rushdie Affair', *Political Quarterly*, 1990, 61/2, pp. 143–60; A. Brah, 'Difference, Diversity and Differentiation', in J. Donald and A. Rattansi, eds, *'Race', Culture and Difference*, London, 1989.
42 Carey and Shokur, 'Bangladeshi Community'; Adams, *Across Seven Seas*; J. Eade, 'Quests for Belonging', in A.X. Cambridge and S. Feuchtwang, with J. Clarke and J. Eade, *Where You Belong: Government and Black Culture*, Aldershot, 1992; Y. Chowdhury, *The Roots and Tales of Bangladeshi Settlers*, Birmingham, 1993; Centre for Bangladeshi Studies, *Routes and Beyond: Voices from Educationally Successful Bangladeshis*, London, 1994; S. Khanum, '"We Just Buy Illness in Exchange for Hunger"'.
43 Craissati, 'Stress and Coping'; G. C. Dutt, 'How Cultural Beliefs Hamper Psychiatric Treatment', *ODA News Review*, 1991, 2/17.
44 While there appears to be considerable debate among my Bangladeshi informants as to whether these traditions are recognised by congregations in local mosques, various scholars have pointed to theological schools of thought originating within North India. See F. Robinson, *Varieties of South Asian Islam*, Research Paper No. 8, Centre for Research in Ethnic Relations, University of Warwick, 1988. Rex describes Deobandis and Barelvis as 'traditionalists', but claims that Deabandis 'are concerned to eliminate Hindu and pagan elements from South Asian Islam' while the Barelvis (the 'largest single group in Britain') 'add to ordinary Islamic teaching the teachings of the Sufis [mystical leaders], placing great emphasis upon a discipline which liberates the spirit from the flesh'. Barelvis, not surprisingly, acknowledges the role of *pirs* within Islamic belief and practice. See J. Rex, 'Religion and Ethnicity in the Metropolis', in Barot, *Religion and Ethnicity*, p. 24.
45 C. Helman, *Culture, Health and Illness*, Bristol, 1986, p. 79.
46 Islam, *Women, Health and Culture*, pp. 113–4.
47 Khanum, 'We Just Buy Illness'.

48 They refer to Adams' book, *Across Seven Seas and Thirteen Rivers*, in support of their argument. They quote Adams' claim that the first generation of male migrants were 'petty bourgeois in the village context' and had left Sylhet to 'look for work elsewhere rather than work as manual labourers in their villages'. For a more detailed and sophisticated analysis of the rural Sylhet context see K. Gardner, 'International Migration and the Rural Context in Sylhet', *New Community*, 1992, 18/4, pp. 579–90.

49 K. Gardner, 'Jumbo Jets and Paddy Fields: Migration and Village Life in Syhlet', unpublished Ph.D. thesis, University of London, 1990. A revised version of this thesis has been published as *Global Migrants, Local Lives: Travel and Transformation in Rural Bangladesh*, Oxford, 1995.

12

WHO'S DEFINITION?

Australian Aborigines, conceptualisations of health and the World Health Organisation

Maggie Brady, Stephen Kunitz and David Nash

The famous preamble to the constitution of the WHO, which contains the definition of health as 'complete physical, mental, and social well being and not simply the absence of disease or infirmity', is often treated as if it were a singular statement at variance with the Western tradition. Certainly some of the men involved in promulgating it in 1948 saw it as something new, and indeed in important respects it was new. But there was much that was not new. The WHO definition of health is part of the very fabric of the Western tradition. It derives from deeply held assumptions about progress and perfectibility, and the role that science can and should play in the direction of human affairs. Whether the idea of progress is a creation of the seventeenth century, as J.B. Bury maintained, or derives from classical antiquity, as Robert Nisbet argues, there is no doubt that it is deeply embedded in Western thought and that, as Bury wrote, it was in the late seventeenth and early eighteenth centuries 'that the idea of intellectual progress was enlarged into the idea of the general Progress of man'.[1] Its history thereafter has been traced by numerous authors and need not detain us. What is important for our argument is the way the WHO definition, embodying as it does deeply held Western assumptions about the nature of progress, is used in contemporary debates about the health of indigenous peoples in liberal democracies.

We should like to show, first, that the men who developed the WHO definition were quite clear about the tradition of Western thought upon which they were drawing. Yet, and this is our second theme, the definition is now often associated with non-Western medical traditions, such as those of the Aboriginal peoples of Australia. One of the supporting pieces of evidence often adduced for the holistic nature of Aboriginal conceptions of health, which distinguishes it from Western reductionist notions, is that Aboriginal languages do not contain a word for health. How much we should read into the fact that there is no word found so far that exactly translates the English word 'health' is our third major theme.

Our argument is that the complexity of both the Western and Aboriginal traditions has been simplified as a result of political struggles. Such simplification is perhaps inevitable. Certainly it is understandable, for it has proved useful in resisting assimilation, in defending Aboriginal self-determination, and in sustaining or recreating Aboriginality in opposition to the culture of the dominant society. But there is also a price to be paid, for the result has been that complex, cultural constructions have been turned into one-dimensional caricatures.

THE WHO DEFINITION OF HEALTH

The history of international collaboration on health-related matters goes back to the nineteenth century, but our story begins just after the Second World War at the United Nations Conference on International Organisation in San Francisco where it was proposed by the delegations of Brazil and China that an international health organisation be formed. A memorandum from the Brazilian delegation quoted Archbishop Spellman to the effect that 'Medicine is one of the pillars of peace.'[2]

The declaration proposed by the Brazilians and Chinese was approved unanimously by the delegates, and soon after a Technical Preparatory Committee was appointed whose membership consisted 'not of States, but of individuals chosen for their expert qualifications.'[3] The chairman was Professor René Sand, of the Ministry of Health of Belgium. Among the other members were Dr Brock Chisholm, Deputy Minister of National Health of Canada; Dr Andrija Stampar, Professor and Rector of the University of Zagreb in what was then Yugoslavia; Dr Thomas Parran, Surgeon-General of the United States Public Health Service; and Dr Karl Evang, Director-General of Public Health of Norway.[4] It was the sixteen members of this committee who drafted the preamble and constitution which was accepted with little change by the International Health Conference that met in New York in 1946.[5] Evidently Dr Stampar was largely responsible for the broad vision of health that was enunciated in the preamble.[6] In his presidential address to the First World Health Assembly in 1948, he said:

> Disease is not brought about only by physical and biological factors. Economic and social factors play an increasingly important part in sanitary matters which must be tackled not only from the technical, but also from the sociological point of view. Although medicine is over 5,000 years old and modern science about 150, it is only during the last 50 years that this idea has gained ground. Health should be a factor in the creation of a better and happier life. Since health for everyone is a fundamental human right, the community should be obliged to afford all its peoples health protection as complete as possible. The preamble to our Constitution represents, therefore, a great victory, embodying as it does this correct conception of public health, and thus throwing a guiding light on the long and difficult path ahead.[7]

And Brock Chisholm, who was also a member of the Technical Preparatory Group and subsequently became the first Director-General of the WHO, wrote:

> There can be no longer any question of purely defensive and limited barricades in the fight against disease. Gone are the days when the activities of the international health officer were limited to quarantine measures and immunisation. His approach today must be a positive one, an aggressive one, which recognises the close relationship between international health problems on the one hand and economic and social conditions on the other hand.
>
> The specific inclusion in the Constitution of responsibility in the fields of mental hygiene, nutrition, medical care, and environmental sanitation, etc., demonstrates a wider conception of public health than has been promulgated heretofore.[8]

The positive definition of health was what most participants, as well as subsequent writers, believed was particularly original, but they also believed that it was the inevitable result of human progress.[9] In his 1936 volume, *Health and Human Progress*, René Sand traced the evolution of what he and others called 'sociological medicine', what has also been called social medicine. He wrote:

> Deaf to the appeal of its prophets, medicine did not approach the social domain spontaneously, but was dragged into it by the development of hygiene, of public assistance, of social insurance, of labour legislation.
>
> Nevertheless, this evolution was logical; medicine had been nourished by physics and chemistry, and afterwards by physiology, bacteriology and parasitology. It remained for medicine to receive the contributions of psychology and sociology.
>
> This evolution was also necessary; to be preventive, medicine must regulate individual and social life; then it comes to understand that social factors command even curative methods, for the working of our organs is the mirror of living conditions. From this moment on, medicine wants to recognise the whole nature of man, as shaped by his home, his surroundings, his work, his recreation, his struggles and aspirations. Thus every part of medicine becomes social.[10]

Several authors have pointed out that the generation of social medicine physicians, which included the men who wrote the WHO Constitution, believed deeply in the idea of progress and in the ability of natural and social scientists to understand and control what had hitherto been social developments beyond the control of human beings. This was reflected in their readings of the history of their field, which of course differed but none the less all assumed the inevitability of progress.[11] Like René Sand, they saw themselves as the inheritors of a complex tradition. For George Rosen it began in the Enlightenment.[12] For Iago Galdston, 'Social medicine is primarily a derivative of the progress of medicine itself. It represents a maturation of medicine, the attainment of a new high point.'[13] For Henry Sigerist it began with the social insurance reforms of Bismarck in the 1880s.[14] From that time through the Russian Revolution, which gave all citizens the constitutional right to all health services, to the creation of the British National Health Service and to the French Constitution in the 1940s, which guaranteed all citizens the protection of health; and culminating with the preamble to the Constitution of the WHO, the history of social medicine according to Sigerist had been one of progressive extension of the right of all peoples to good health.

No matter how they might understand the history of their field, however, they all saw social medicine as battling with the interests of the established medical profession. Andrija Stampar had said, for instance, that, 'In the past the most progressive ideas in public health were often put forward by those who were not physicians themselves, while the physicians stood aloof in hostile attitudes. This should not happen in future,' he concluded.[15] According to Stampar and the other commentators, history was on the side of the progressives and thus the hostility of the majority of the medical profession would simply have to change. The social medicine physicians of the 1930s, 1940s and 1950s understood the definition of health they had created to be the result of the inevitable if slow progress of Western civilisation and the medicine that was its product. If Western civilisation had been pregnant with the new idea of health, they were the midwives who were both to deliver and name it.

ABORIGINAL UTILISATION OF THE WHO DEFINITION

The WHO definition of positive health, as René Dubos has pointed out, describes a potentiality, rather than a state.[16] It is an *ideal*: 'what ought to be rather than what is'.[17] Dubos, himself a keen supporter of the ecological or holistic model of health, nevertheless argued that the notion that humankind can attain perfect health and happiness is an illusion – a *mirage* – which has flourished in many different forms throughout history.[18] Other commentators have ventured to suggest that the definition is all-inclusive and ponderous, that it has no clearly defined edges, uses words that have no self-evident meanings, and is unworkable as a basis for the measurement of health.[19] Lewis observes that in practice an individual doctor has no reliable positive indications of when such an ideal balance has been achieved.[20] Nevertheless, the original definition was reaffirmed at Alma Ata in 1978 and has become something of a slogan for public relations, taken up by governments and, perhaps even more enthusiastically, by indigenous groups.[21]

Australia endorsed 'health for all' as federal policy in 1979, although it was slow to follow up this commitment. It has been in the area of Aboriginal health that primary health care principles have been most energetically acted upon.[22] Nevertheless, a recurring theme in the discourse about health is the tension between definitions of health as an 'absence of disease' as opposed to the broader formulations of 'wellness' and the WHO definition. Rather than seeking to resolve the perennial debate on which is the 'correct' position, recent work by the National Centre for Epidemiology and Population Health (NCEPH) in Canberra has focused on the *significance* of the debate.[23]

The key to understanding why the broad WHO definition of health has found such currency among Aboriginal health activists lies in its co-existence with their model of primary health care. As a NCEPH report on primary health care observes, at the heart of the WHO definition is the relationship between health care and wider social practice – the broader enterprise of social development which recognises the weight of evidence linking improvements in population health to broad social progress.[24] Politically it links primary health care to ideals of equity, participation and sustainability. In Australia these principles have been actively linked by Aboriginal people to their right to self-determination and community control.

While the federal government was given constitutional responsibility in 1967 to legislate for indigenous Australians, and had the opportunity to take over direct servicing of Aboriginal health care, the provision of health services has remained primarily in the hands of state governments who largely rejected the argument that Aboriginal health required special attention or that it had anything to do with community control. Until the 1970s then, Aboriginal health care was grossly inadequate: in urban and rural regions Aboriginal people had to rely on hospital outpatient departments or charitable GPs, while in remote regions, missions and government settlements employed nursing sisters who delivered basic health care.[25] This meant that many Aborigines did not seek help until they were seriously ill, and because health care services were not co-ordinated with the provision of environmental health infrastructure (water, sewerage, adequate housing), the result was appallingly high rates of infant mortality and adult morbidity and mortality.[26]

Eventually, in association with increasing Aboriginal political mobilisation on other issues (land rights, legal aid, poor wages and conditions, segregation), independent, Aboriginal-controlled health services were established which employed their own medical officers, nurses and health workers. These medical services began in 1971, as a result of pressure from Aboriginal activists and sympathetic health professionals, aiming to provide acceptable primary health care. They have been funded largely by the Australian federal government, bypassing the states.

The Aboriginal medical services have been represented by a national umbrella organisation since 1974, and in concert have constantly lobbied for greater federal commitment and more resources for Aboriginal-controlled services, as well as drawn attention to the economic, social and political aspects of Aboriginal health. Their spokespeople have also drawn increasingly on the discourse linking primary health care, self-determination and the special cultural status of indigenous peoples. Janice Reid, a leading medical anthropologist, observed,

> In Australia, the spirit of primary health care is most nearly captured not by government departments but by the Aboriginal Medical Services. [They] see their role not only as providers of health care but as health promoters and facilitators of community development projects outside the customary province of a medical service.[27]

The larger services also function as centres for political activism and lobbying. Frustrated in earlier years by the reluctance of state and federal governments within Australia to endorse the important role of these Aboriginal-controlled services, and constantly threatened by cuts in funding, Aboriginal spokespeople and health activists turned to the international arena. This has entailed exposing the poor health status of Aborigines to the court of world opinion, primarily the United Nations, WHO and the Working Group on Indigenous Peoples, and making good use of the politics of embarrassment.[28]

By embracing the Alma Ata principles of primary health care and the broad definition of health, Aboriginal organisations have been able to lobby for ideals of social justice, equity and access, and fend off suggestions that separate services are a luxury that the government cannot afford. As recently as 1988, for example, the federal Department of Aboriginal Affairs asserted that Aboriginal medical services would ultimately merge with state and national provision.[29]

It has been within the context of this struggle to reinforce the unique role of separate, Aboriginal-run services that the contested definitions of health have come to prominence. In order to justify their presence and highlight the continued need for special services for Aborigines that are respectful of cultural differences, Aboriginal people have asserted that their conceptualisations of health are different from (and superior to) what is frequently designated as the 'Western biomedical model'. They have harnessed the broad WHO definition to assist in this task:

> The Aboriginal approach to both prophylaxis and curing is a holistic one. It recognises the physical, personal and spiritual dimension of life and health. In many ways, the Aboriginal

> perspective on health and illness is closer than that of Western medicine to the WHO's definition of health as 'a state of complete physical, mental and social well-being, not merely the absence of disease'.[30]

An opportunity to test Australian government approaches to Aboriginal health care against WHO principles presented itself in the mid-1970s. In 1974, the Australian federal government had invited two WHO experts to examine health care delivery to Aborigines. Their report concluded that there was insufficient Aboriginal involvement in the delivery of primary health care and criticised the emphasis on hospital-type curative health care. Health services, the report stated, must be soundly based in order to give Aborigines the chance to develop to their full potential and optimal health.[31] Four years later, Congress, the Aboriginal-controlled health service in Alice Springs, made good use of this and other WHO reports in its submission to a federal Standing Committee enquiry into Aboriginal health. Congress asserted that the Northern Territory health department had failed to apply methods recommended by WHO, and that the department considered such methods to be radical and dangerous. Another submission observed that for all the enlightened rhetoric, the biomedical model was still current in the Northern Territory.[32] The 1979 Standing Committee, advised by two sympathetic experts with grass-roots involvement in Aboriginal health, and taking the Congress criticisms seriously, recommended that an independent team should 'evaluate the effectiveness of all Aboriginal health care services and programs in accordance with the WHO's definition of health and the principles of self-determination'.[33] In 1980, however, a confidential review of the effectiveness of Aboriginal health programmes articulated the perceived disadvantages of the broad WHO conceptualisation of health:

> The Committee accepts the WHO's definition but recognises that as soon as attempts are made to measure health, problems arise in relation to lack of information and cultural, social and subjective interpretations. The Committee has based its assessment of physical ill health on available conventional indices and has relied on anecdotal evidence with respect to mental and social well-being.[34]

THE ABORIGINAL ELABORATION OF THE WHO MODEL

Fifteen years later, the debate continues. Aboriginal health activists are still promoting the principles of primary health care, and associating these with community control and participation. They continue to stress that Aboriginal definitions of health are synonymous with that of WHO, and are in stark contrast with the biomedical model. For example, a South Australian report on Aboriginal health status observes, '*Pukulpa* [a Pitjantjatjara word] . . . translates more readily to 'happiness' and implies a state of well-being not dissimilar to that described by the WHO definition of health'.[35] A chapter entitled 'Health. A holistic approach' in a recent textbook on Aboriginal studies contains this quotation:

> Aboriginal conceptions of health are radically different from [the] biomedical perspective . . . It is imperative that medical authorities take cognisance of the Aboriginal perspective with regard to health and well being and accept that in contrast to the more focused clinical and disease oriented approach of non-Aboriginal health professionals, Aboriginal peoples' collective concerns are to regain their land, to ensure that their children have tucker [food] and to be able to undertake social obligations including ceremonial duties.[36]

Aborigines have increasingly enlarged upon the three WHO meanings of 'health': 'physical', 'mental' and 'social'. They have argued that the elaboration is necessary in part because the word 'health' is understood differently by Aboriginal people, and that indigenous languages have no similar word. An example of an elaboration on the three-pronged WHO definition comes from South Australia, where a combined Aboriginal health services forum defined health as 'a state of complete physical, psychological, social, spiritual, emotional and cultural well-being for the individual and his community'.[37] However, the most influential and oft-quoted document in this regard is the report of the working party on the National Aboriginal Health Strategy (1989). In this report, health is defined as physical as well as social, emotional and cultural well-being:

> In Aboriginal society there was no word, term or expression for 'health' as it is understood in Western society . . . The word as it is used in Western society almost defies translation but the nearest translation in an Aboriginal context would probably be

> a term such as 'life' is health is life . . . This is a 'whole of life' view and it also includes the cyclical concept of life death life.[38]

While this assertion is not strictly correct (as we shall show shortly), the exegesis provided by this report has become conventional wisdom and has been reiterated in numerous subsequent documents, including Aboriginal submissions, government reports, the Royal Commission into Aboriginal Deaths in Custody, dissertations and medical journal editorials.[39] It has become the 'mission statement' for the health branch of the Aboriginal and Torres Strait Islander Commission, a major source of funding for Aboriginal health services.[40]

In New Zealand a similar process of elaboration has been underway, and Maoris have provided a number of consciously refined definitions. In 1982, a definition of health was proposed to be the four-way interaction between spiritual, mental, physical factors, and the extended family. Later, a model with eight dimensions was discussed, known as the 'octopus'.[41] The Maori writer Mason Durie observed that this was a reminder to the world that there was more to health than the absence of biological malfunction.[42] Indeed, these definitions are continually positioned as being antithetical to the biomedical, technological, one-dimensional, Cartesian-dualism model of 'Western' medicine.

But is the 'Western' model of health quite so monolithic and unreconstructed? As Lyn Payer warns, the widespread ignorance of the diversity of medicine and medical traditions in highly developed countries has a number of implications.[43] There is, after all, a long history of acceptance in the West of the relationship between affective and physical states, and the influence of the mind on illness. Descartes has long been depicted as the villain who destroyed this holistic tradition, but as Brown points out, this 'mythic image' disintegrates in the light of historical enquiry.[44] He urges a more nuanced and unfolding interpretation. Even Pasteur suggested that the psychologic state could influence resistance to microbes.[45] 'Morale' and the psyche are now thought of more than ever in connection with organic disease.[46] The land itself – its 'spiritual' ambience as well as its medicinal flora, frequently referred to as being peculiar to indigenous discourse – also has a place in Western notions of healing. In parts of Europe – whether a legacy of romanticism or not – the wildness of nature, homoeopathy, long walks, cold baths, fasting, herbal medicine, spas, 'Kneipping' (a combination of hydrotherapy and diet) and

Steiner's notions of 'balance' are all accommodated as healing and healthful strategies. The French notion of the *terrain* (loosely translated as 'constitution') influences diagnoses of illness, results in less aggressive use of drugs in treatment, and allows for regimes such as rest and stays at spas as a means of shoring up the individual's immune system.[47] Western models of health also include Polgar's 'elastic', processural view of accumulated resistance and of the process of balance between the individual and his environment.[48] Engel, as part of his bio-psycho-social model, points out that the dichotomy between 'disease' and 'problems of living' is by no means a sharp one.[49]

There is more than a suggestion of a false dichotomy, then, in the portrayal of 'the West' as the bearer of a hegemonic, egocentric and solely biomedical model of health, as opposed to the other which concerns more 'holistic' peoples who are socio-centric and harmonious and for whom health is so much more.

A CLOSER LOOK AT ABORIGINAL CONCEPTUALISATIONS

In much the same way as selective representations and simplifications of a supposedly monolithic Western health model are at variance with the more nuanced reality, so too are many of the brief summaries that claim to reflect pan-Aboriginal conceptualisations of health. These too invite more detailed scrutiny and subtle interpretation. Apart from the linguistic issue of whether Aboriginal languages contain a 'word for health' (which we examine shortly), it is through the work of fieldworkers (anthropologists, linguists and health professionals) and the Aboriginal people with whom they worked closely that we can begin to delve more deeply. Health and well-being are certainly associated by Aboriginal people in particular regions of Australia with *social* harmony. Hamilton, a social anthropologist, writes of the Yankunytjatjara in north-west South Australia that

> health is the outcome of good feelings, which are signalled by harmonious social relationships, the absence of fear or insecurity . . . and health can only be maintained by a balance between the correct social relationships and correct observation of the required ritual behaviours.[50]

These factors are associated with beliefs about the causes of sudden illness and death associated with sorcery and with sites on the land, beliefs that are prevalent in parts of central and northern Australia. Sorcery involves ill-intent which must be analysed and resolved socially. The land contains dangerous sites that can provoke sickness and death if they are misused, and damage to particular sites can result in physical symptoms being experienced by individuals with special connections to those locations.

A variation on this theme is expressed by Pitjantjatjara speakers who were resettled on land that was not their own at the time of the British atomic testing programme (1952–62) in South Australia: they refer to this 'new' country by a term that has negative connotations: 'grey ground' (*pana tjilpi*), ground that makes people aged and grey-haired prematurely, as opposed to the red sand of the spinifex country from whence they came.

Social and spiritual elements are therefore significant contributors to the health of individuals, and social health is given a higher priority than ensuring physical health. For example, many health maintenance activities (maintaining a clean and uncrowded living area, eating a balanced diet, intervening in the harmful behaviour of others) are compromised by the social compulsions of generosity and non-authoritarian dealings with others. 'The maintenance of good social relationships is more important than the improvement of certain physical aspects of living advocated by the health staff' wrote a doctor working at Oenpelli in the Northern Territory.[51]

Webber, a psychologist, drew attention to the significance of the social world in the definitions of degrees of ill-health or wellness among people living on Groote Eylandt off the Northern Territory coast. He found that people differentiated between the 'strong', 'weak', 'wounded' and 'sick'. While the 'weak' were those who were suffering from common complaints such as headache, infected eyes, ears or skin, or were simply 'below par', the 'sick' on the other hand were those whose mental and spiritual aspects were affected as a result of magic, 'singing' or poisoning by someone.[52] Someone who has been 'sung' becomes fearful and ill, and the search for causes and the appropriate interventions are undertaken by kin. Webber identifies the element of fear as being a key difference between the beliefs of this Aboriginal language group and Europeans:

> It is clear that the Groote Eylandt people have an idea of good health and injury similar to that found in European society. Their differentiation between the sick and the weak is quite different

from our notion, however, as is the relative association of fear in these categories.[53]

Webber (writing in the mid-1970s) goes on to observe that we are only just beginning to appreciate once more the effect that the conduct of one's life has upon one's health, something of which Groote Eylandt people are well aware. F. S. Soong (a doctor) stressed the Oenpelli residents' 'social-medical' theory of health, which he thought differed from the definition suggested by WHO, because of the Aboriginal emphasis on good social relations and participation in rituals.[54]

'Health' has a *number* of definitions and associations that vary across the country and do not always fit with the public and official glosses presented in some of the documents referred to earlier. Examples of this wide variation range from the definition of well-being given by an urban Adelaide Aboriginal man as 'feeling powerful about my Aboriginality'[55] to those common among people living in remote Mornington Island, Queensland. Johnson (a non-Aboriginal health psychologist)[56] notes that in Queensland and in the Utopia region,[57] older people perceive plumpness, even fatness, as an indicator of health.

Peile (a linguist and Pallotine father) criticises those who suggest that health for Aborigines is a 'state of harmony' between all animate and inanimate things, saying that people living at Balgo, Western Australia, hold two basic concepts of health: the body being cold and dry, and the spirit residing in the navel and stomach. He also demonstrates that there is a strong relationship between health and the spirit, and health and a (hunted) meat diet. The spirit or *kurrunpa* is a term used for the invisible principle of life, but also for the physiological manifestations such as the activity of the heart, throat, lungs, diaphragm and pulse. The spirit is equated with the stomach, so that people place their hands on the stomach to indicate mental pain or anguish (this is also the case for Pitjantjatjara-speaking people in South Australia). He offers detailed phrases translated from Kukatja that are indicators of health: having a 'strong', 'hard' head; having a 'good nose' (for sensing); having 'good breathing', having a 'good spirit' which is lodged in the region of the stomach. Peile is adamant that the whole Aboriginal concept of health in the area where he lived and worked rests on the 'foundation of hot–dry, wet–cold. Health is derived from blood, for blood is life and the source of this life is primarily meat'.[58] Peile elicited a long text from an elderly desert man, in which he spoke in Kukatja about how the body functioned. Peile's translation includes the following:

> Meat always keeps my brain cold. Without it my head would get a headache, so I go out, kill an animal and eat it . . . [a young man] feeds himself with meat, he gives himself blood, he gives himself spirit, he eats the meat together with the fat. He feeds himself with fat . . . Without meat the heart and the soul become dry. Blood gives breath to the heart when a person eats meat. Meat gives blood, meat gives breath to the skull, it gives it to the ears, to the hands, everywhere there is blood from meat . . . I will not die if there is nothing wrong with me. I won't live if I do not eat meat, if I don't kill and eat blood . . . We kill animals and eat the blood, otherwise we would die. We breathe that we may exist, breathing and existing come from having meat.[59]

Peile's evidence suggests two points. First, the fact that health is so intimately linked by these desert people with the destruction of hunted animals suggests a more utilitarian interpretation of the idea of 'harmony' with all animate beings than that allowed by more stereotyped and romanticised versions. Second, that *kurrunpa* is the term for both life and physiological functions draws our attention to an important characteristic of Aboriginal languages.

The vocabularies of Australian languages, generally speaking, tend to express abstractions as part of the range of meaning of terms that also have concrete reference. It is common in any language for the meaning of a single word to consist of several related senses, a phenomenon called polysemy (multiple meaning). One recurrent pattern of polysemy in Australia is for one word to refer both to an entity and to express the potential presence of the entity.[60] Thus, it is common for the one word to cover 'fire' and 'firewood', or one term to cover 'game animal' and 'meat'. Similarly, a word can refer to a concrete entity as well as to the abstraction of which that entity is a prime instantiation; thus, the word for 'fire' also means 'heat'.

In understanding how vocabulary can be so structured, we can look at English where, to a lesser extent, the same abstract–concrete polysemy occurs. The noun *light* can refer to an individual source of light ('That light is broken') or to illumination ('There's not much light in here') or to visible radiation ('Light travels in straight lines'). English tolerates the possibility of more than one sense in some contexts: 'There's no light in that room' could mean the lack of a light fitting (in a room lit by sunlight), or low illumination (in a room with a working light fitting). Note that this is commonplace polysemy: it is not mediated for instance by metaphor: the abstract 'light' is not some metaphorical extension of concrete 'light', but rather both are related senses of the one word. A related concrete–abstract polysemy occurs in the Warlpiri language of central Australia, and probably many other languages. For instance, Warlpiri *langa* 'ear' encompasses 'hearing', *lirra* 'mouth, teeth' encompasses 'voice', *milpa* 'eye' encompasses 'sight', and the term for 'body' (*palka*) also means 'presence' (opposite of 'absence').[61]

It is natural for English speakers without a good grasp of the particular Aboriginal language to take the concrete meaning as the sole sense, reinforced by the concrete English translation equivalent, and probably also by the absence of separate abstract terminology in Aboriginal English. It appears that the first non-Aborigines to draw attention to the absence of Aboriginal language terms for 'health' were two doctors working in the Northern Territory in the 1970s. Both were inspired by notions of biculturalism, the WHO model, the potentially crucial role of Aboriginal people as primary health care workers, and a sense of impending change and progress. (For example, in 1973 traditional healers were hired by the health division in the Northern Territory, an experiment in institutionalisation that was soon abandoned.) In this context, the apparent lack of Aboriginal terms reinforced the view of these health professionals that a 'bicultural' approach was necessary (the 'sharing' of traditional and European concepts and practices, with Aboriginal health workers developing a synthesis). So it came about that the published writings and verbal presentations of these two medical officers set a trend. One of them, Dr F. S. Soong wrote in 1981:

> The Gunwinggu people do not have a word for health. The closest equivalents are strong, not sick, happy and feeling good. Those Aborigines who were fluent in English said good health means . . . *Gamak* [sic] or 'happy with my people' and *Gamak Rowk* [sic] or 'feeling good during and after ceremonies'.[62]

Two years later, a report from Congress in Alice Springs reiterated, 'It is interesting to note that Aborigines do not have terms for "health" or "healthy". The closest Aranda equivalent to "healthy" is *mwarre*, which means "good" or "well" in a much wider sense'.[63]

However, a closer look at another central Australian language, Warlpiri, serves to flesh out these somewhat stark attributions. Warlpiri, like a number of Australian languages, has a term (*wankaru*)[64] covering 'alive, healthy'. The elaborated dictionary entry for this word, and for its opposite, *nyurnu* 'sick, dead', show a number of inter-related senses, which cannot be captured with a few short English glosses. Additional typical usages of *wankaru* have been exemplified by a literate Warlpiri person as follows: (1) When a person falls from a vehicle and emerges OK; (2) When they hit or shoot something and it gets up 'awake' and runs and flies away.[65]

The prosaic usages of *wankaru* given above, along with the meanings 'alive', 'healthy', 'health' and 'life' in one term exemplify the concrete–abstract polysemy pattern. This is extremely important, for it means that people may have a concept while lacking a specific word identifying that concept. The extent to which there is no word for health does not preclude an abstract conception of health as a state independent of its context, any more than the fact that Warlpiri has no separate word meaning just 'sight' means that there is no conception of vision apart from the idea of eyes.

CONCLUSION

It has not been our intention to downplay the fact that reductionism is an important, even dominant, theme in Western medical thought. Neither do we disagree with the proposition that in many regions of Australia, the health and well-being of Aboriginal people are associated with social harmony and with the fulfilment of obligations associated with particular tracts of land (and the eating of hunted meat from that land). Rather, we have argued that both traditions, the Western and the Aboriginal, are complex. The former embraces conceptions of health that go well beyond merely the adequate physical functioning of individuals. The latter embraces conceptions of health that are sometimes abstract as well as some that are essentially practical in ways that on occasions belie more romantic conceptualisations. It is in the process of political struggles over health provision and resource distribution that the complexities of both traditions have been reduced to simple opposites. It is understandable why in the heat of controversy this so often happens. It may even be good tactics in the short run. In the longer run, however, it may serve to impoverish our understanding of ourselves and one another.

NOTES

1 J.B. Bury, *The Idea of Progress: An Inquiry into its Growth and Origin*, 1932; New York, 1955, p. 128; R.A. Nisbet, *Social Change and History: Aspects of the Western Theory of Development*, New York, 1969, p. 106.
2 WHO, *The First Ten Years of the WHO*, Geneva, 1958, p. 38.
3 Ibid., p. 39.
4 Ibid., pp. 476–7.
5 Ibid., p. 47.
6 H. van Zile Hyde, 'A Tribute to Andrija Stampar, M.D., 1888–1958', *American Journal of Public Health*, 1958, 48, p. 1580.
7 A. Stampar, 'Presidential Address', First World Health Assembly, Geneva, 25 June 1948. Reprinted in M.D. Grmek, ed., *Serving the Cause of Public Health: Selected Papers of Andrija Stampar*, Zagreb, 1966, p. 200.
8 B. Chisholm, 'The WHO', *British Medical Journal*, 6 May 1950, p. 1021.
9 See, for instance, C.F. Brockington, *World Health*, Boston, 2nd edn, 1968, chapter 1.
10 R. Sand, *Health and Human Progress: An Essay in Sociological Medicine*, New York, 1936, p. 2.
11 See, for instance, D. Porter and R. Porter, 'What was Social Medicine? An Historiographical Essay', *Journal of Historical Sociology*, 1988, 1, pp. 90–106; E. Fee, 'Henry E. Sigerist: His Interpretations of the History of Disease and the Future of Medicine', in C.E. Rosenberg and J. Golden, eds, *Framing Disease: Studies in Cultural History*, 1992, New Brunswick, NJ, pp. 297–317.
12 G. Rosen, 'In the Enlightenment', in I. Galdston, ed., *Social Medicine: Its Derivations and Objectives*, New York, 1949.
13 I. Galdston, *The Meaning of Social Medicine*, Cambridge, 1954, pp. 5–6.
14 H.E. Sigerist, 'From Bismarck to Beveridge', in Galdston, *Social Medicine*.
15 Stampar, 'Presidential Address', p. 201.
16 R. Dubos, 'Human Ecology', *WHO Chronicle*, 1969, 23/11, p. 504; A.E. Davis and J.E. George, *States of Health: Health and Illness in Australia*, Sydney, 1988, p. 29; G. Lewis, 'Concepts of Health and Illness in a Sepik Society', in C. Currer and M. Stacey, eds, *Concepts of Health, Illness and Disease: A Comparative Perspective*, Leamington Spa, 1986.
17 Ibid., p. 127.
18 R. Dubos, *Mirage of Health. Utopias, Progress and Biological Change*, New York, 1959, p. 2.
19 T. Kue Young, *Health Care and Cultural Change: The Indian Experience in the Central Sub Arctic*, Toronto, 1988, p. 135; P.M. Moodie, *Aboriginal Health*, Canberra, 1973, p. 6.
20 Lewis, 'Concepts of Health and Illness'.
21 Moodie, *Aboriginal Health*, p. 6.
22 National Centre for Epidemiology and Population Health, *Improving Australia's Health: The Role of Primary Health Care*, Canberra, 1992.
23 Ibid., p. 33.
24 Ibid., p. 34.

25 S.J. Kunitz, *Disease and Social Diversity*, Melbourne, 1994.
26 M. Kamien, 'Cultural Chasm and Chaos in the Health Care Services to Aborigines in Rural New South Wales', *Medical Journal of Australia*, Spec. Suppl. 1975, 2, pp. 6–11.
27 J.C. Reid, ed., *Body, Land and Spirit: Health and Healing in Aboriginal Society*, St Lucia, Qsd, 1982, pp. xiv–xv.
28 N. Dyck, ed., *Indigenous Peoples and the Nation-State: ' Fourth World' politics in Canada, Australia and Norway*, St Johns, Canada, 1985.
29 J. Baker, *Nunga's Access to Health Care in Adelaide: Metropolitan Health Needs Assessment Study*, Adelaide, 1989.
30 Reid, *Body, Land and Spirit*, p. 91; also S. Saggers and D. Gray, *Aboriginal Health and Society*, Sydney, 1991, p. 42.
31 Commonwealth of Australia, *Hansard Reports* for House of Representatives Standing Committee on Aboriginal Affairs into Aboriginal Health, 26 June 1978, p. 154.
32 Ibid., p. 3021.
33 Commonwealth of Australia, House of Representatives Standing Committee on Aboriginal Affairs, *Aboriginal Health*, 1979, p. xvii.
34 Department of Prime Minister and Cabinet, 'Program Effectiveness Review, Aboriginal Health', Unpublished Departmental Report, Commonwealth of Australia, 1980, p. 8.
35 K. Kirke, C. Divakaran-Brown, K. Priest and D. Roder, *South Australian Health Statistics Chart Book, supplement 4: Aboriginal Health*, Adelaide, 1993, p. 101.
36 J. Burden, 'Health: A Holistic Approach', in C. Bourke, E. Bourke and B. Edwards, eds, *Aboriginal Australia: An Introductory Reader in Aboriginal Studies*, St Lucia, Qsd, 1994, pp. 169, 172.
37 Kirke et. al., *South Australian Health Statistics Chart Book*, p. 7.
38 National Aboriginal Health Strategy Working Party, *A National Aboriginal Health Strategy*, Canberra, 1989, p. ix.
39 N. Beaton, 'Editorial: Aboriginal Health and a New Curriculum for Rural Doctors', *Medical Journal of Australia*, 1994, 160, pp. 185–6; Burden, 'Health: A Holistic Approach'; Human Rights and Equal Opportunity Commission, *The Provision of Health and Medical Services to the Aboriginal Communities of Cooktown, Hopevale and WujalWujal*, Canberra, 1991; Kirke et al., *South Australian Health Statistics Chart Book*; Royal Commission into Aboriginal Deaths in Custody, *National Report*, Vol. 4, Canberra, 1991; R. Spark, R.J. Donovan and P. Howat, 'Promoting Health and Preventing Injury in Remote Aboriginal Communities: A Case Study', *Health Promotion Journal of Australia*, 1991, 1/2, pp. 10–16.
40 Australian and Torres Strait Islander Commission, *Operational Plan 1993–1994*, Canberra, 1994.
41 M. Durie, *Whairo: Maori Health Development*, Auckland, 1994.
42 Ibid., p. 69.
43 L. Payer, *Medicine and Culture: Varieties of Treatment in the United States, England, West Germany and France*, London, 1988.
44 T. Brown, 'Cartesian Dualism and Psychosomatics', *Psychosomatics*, 1989, 30/3, pp. 322–33.
45 Payer, *Medicine and Culture*.

46 C. Herzlich and J. Pierret, 'Illness: From Causes to Meaning', in Currer and Stacey, *Concepts of Health.*
47 Payer, *Medicine and Culture.*
48 Lewis, 'Concepts of Health and Illness'.
49 G. Engel, 'The Need for a New Medical Model: A Challenge for Biomedicine', *Science*, 1977, 196, pp. 129–36.
50 A. Hamilton, 'Child Health and Child Care in a Desert Community, 1970–1971', in Reid, *Body, Land and Spirit*, p. 67.
51 F.S. Soong, 'Cultural Brokers in East Arnhem Land: A Study of the Role of the Aboriginal Health Worker', Unpublished Dip. Anth. thesis, University of Sydney, 1981, p. 103.
52 D.L. Webber, L.E. Reid and N. Lalara, 'Health and the Groote Eylandter', *Medical Journal of Australia*, Spec. Suppl. 1975, 2/4, pp. 17–20.
53 Ibid., p. 19.
54 Soong, 'Cultural Brokers'.
55 Kirke et al., *South Australian Health Statistics Chart Book*, p. 101.
56 P. Johnson, 'Health Beliefs and Behaviours of the Kaiadilt People of the Bentinck Islands, Northern Queensland, Australia', Unpublished thesis, Grad. Dip. Behavioural Studies in Health Care, La Trobe University, Melbourne, 1993.
57 Personal communication with Dr Jeannie Devitt.
58 Wiminydji and A.R. Peile, 'A Desert Aborigine's View of Health and Nutrition', *Journal of Anthropological Research*, 1978, 34/4, p. 504; H. Valiquette, *A Basic Kukatja to English Dictionary*, Balgo, Western Australia, 1993, p. 408.
59 Wiminydji and Peile, 'A Desert Aborigine's View of Health and Nutrition', pp. 500–1.
60 G.N. O'Grady, 'More on Lexicostatistics', *Current Anthropology*, 1961, 1/4, pp. 338–9.
61 M. Laughren, 'Remarks on the Semantics of Body-part Terminology in Warlpiri', *Language in Central Australia*, 1984, Alice Springs, 1, p. 4.
62 Soong, 'Cultural Brokers', p. 111.
63 P. Nathan and D.L. Japanangka, *Health Business*, Victoria, 1983, p. 18.
64 The Warlpiri term is etymologically related to *wanka* 'raw, alive', cf. Kukatja *wanka* 'awake, conscious, healthy'. Õ.H. Valiquette, *A Basic Kukatja to English Dictionary*, Balgo, Western Australia, 1993.
65 WANKARU – 1. *Ngula ka yapa wantimi rarraly-kajingirli manu ngula ka wilypi-pardimi ngurrju-juku.* (When a person falls from a vehicle and emerges OK.) 2. *Ngula kalu nyiyakantikanti pakarni manu luwarni manu ngula ka yakarra-pardinjarla parnkami manu parrpa-pardimi.* (When they hit or shoot something and it gets up 'awake' and runs and flies away.)
NYURNU – 1. *Ngulaju ngulaka yapa ngunami miyalu murrumurru, miirnta manu ngawu ngulakanyanu purdanyanyi.* (When a person has a stomach pain, catarrh or feels rotten.) 2. *Yirdi-mani karnalu kujaju ngulaka jarntu manu nyiyarlangu mayi palimi.* (We call it this when a dog or something dies.) Personal communication, Grace White Napaljarri, August 1994.

INDEX

Page numbers in **bold** denote major section/chapter devoted to subject. f denotes figure. t denotes table

For Product Safety Concerns and Information please contact our EU representative GPSR@taylorandfrancis.com
Taylor & Francis Verlag GmbH, Kaufingerstraße 24, 80331 München, Germany

www.ingramcontent.com/pod-product-compliance
Ingram Content Group UK Ltd.
Pitfield, Milton Keynes, MK11 3LW, UK
UKHW022111190926
475702UK00013B/1378
9781138868182